Spondylolysis, Spondylolisthesis and Degenerative Spondylolisthesis

Spondylolysis, Spondylolisthesis and Degenerative Spondylolisthesis

Editors

Robert Gunzburg, M.D., Ph.D.
Senior Consultant
Department of Orthopaedics
Centenary Clinic
Antwerp, Belgium

Marek Szpalski, M.D.
Chairman
Department of Orthopaedics
Associate Professor
IRIS South Teaching Hospitals
Free University of Brussels
Brussels, Belgium

LIPPINCOTT WILLIAMS & WILKINS
A **Wolters Kluwer** Company
Philadelphia • Baltimore • New York • London
Buenos Aires • Hong Kong • Sydney • Tokyo

Acquisitions Editor: Robert Hurley
Managing Editor: Michelle LaPlante
Production Manager: Bridgett Dougherty
Senior Manufacturing Manager: Benjamin Rivera
Marketing Director: Sharon Zinner
Design Coordination: Holly McLaughlin
Production Services: Nesbitt Graphics, Inc.
Printer: Edwards Brothers

530 Walnut Street
Philadelphia, PA 19106 USA
LWW.com

Printed in the USA

Library of Congress Cataloging-in-Publication Data
Spondylolysis, spondylolisthesis, and degenerative spondylolisthesis /
editors, Robert Gunzburg, Marek Szpalski.
p. ; cm.
Includes bibliographical references and index.
ISBN 0-7817-7633-3
1. Spondylolisthesis. 2. Spine—Abnormalities.
I. Gunzburg, Robert. II. Szpalski, Marek.
[DNLM: 1. Spondylolysis. 2. Orthopedic Procedures—methods.
3. Spondylolisthesis. WE 725 S7635 2006]
RD771.O88S675 2006
616.7'3—dc22

2005024688

10 9 8 7 6 5 4 3 2 1

Contents

Surgical Treatment: Adults Degenerative

Contributing Authors

Thomas Andersen

S. Aunoble *Spine Unit, CHU Bordeaux, France*

Federico Balagué *Adjunct Associated Professor, Department of Orthopedic Surgery, New York University School of Medicine, New York, N.Y.; Médecin-chef adjoint, Department of Rhematology, Hôpital cantonal, 1708 Fribourg Switzerland*

E. Barbaix, M.D. *Lecturer, Departments of Human Anatomy and Embryology, Ghent University and Vrije Universiteit Brussel, Belgium*

Andrea Barbanera *Department of Neurosurgery, Ospedale Bellaria, Bologna, Italy*

P. Barsa *Department of Neurosurgery, Neurocenter Regional Hospital Liberec Czech Republic*

Y. Basso

Tom Bendix, M.D. *Professor, Department of Sports Science and Clinical Biomechanics, University of Southern Denmark, Denmark; The Back Research Center/Human Locomotion Science, Funen Hospital, Denmark*

Michel Benoist *Consultant Rheumatologist of Paris Hospitals, University of Paris VII, Paris, France; Consultant in Rheumatology, Department of Orthapaedic Surgery, Hôpital Beaujon, Clichy, France*

Ashok Biyani, M.D. *Assistant Professor, Department of Orthopaedic Surgery, Medical University of Ohio, Toledo, Ohio*

B. Bley

Adriana Bogorin *Department of Radiology, University Hospital of Strasbourg*

Prof. C. Bolger *Professor and Head, Clinical Neuroscience Department, Royal College of Surgeons, Ireland; Director of Research and Development, National Center for Neurosurgery, Beamont Hospital, Dublin, Ireland*

Maurice A. Bourlion, Dipl. Eng., Ph.D. *Ceritifed Professor*

P. Buchvald *Department of Neurosurgery, Neurocenter Regional Hospital, Liberec, Czech Republic*

Finn Bjarke Christensen, M.D., PhD., DMSc. *Associate Professor, Department of Orthopedics, Aarhus University Hospital, Norrebrogade, Denmark*

Gianluca Cinotti, M.D. *Associate Professor, Department of Orthopaedics, University La Sapienza, Rome, Italy*

J. P. Clarys *Full Professor, Department of Experimental Anatomy, Vrije Universiteit Brussel, Brussels, Belgium*

Robertson Correia Bernardo, M.D. *Neuroradiologist, Department of Radiology, Mater Dei Hospital, Belo Horizonte–M.G., Brazil*

M. de Kleuver *Spine Unit Department of Orthopedics, Sint Maartenskliniek Nijmegen, The Netherlands*

M. De Maeseneer *Departments of Experimental Anatomy, Manual Therapy and Radiology, Vrije Universiteit Brussel, Brussels, Belgium*

Helton Defino *Associate Professor, Chief of Spine Service, Department of Biomechanics Medicine and Rehabilitation of the Locomotor System, Faculty of Medicine of Ribeirão Preto, University of Sao Paulo, Ribeirão Preto-SP, Brazil*

Alberto Di Martino, M.D. *Department of Orthopaedics and Trauma Surgery, Campus Bio-Medico University, Rome-Italy*

Prof. Jean-Louis Dietemann *Professor of Radiology, Department of Radiology, Faculty of Medicine, Strasbourg, France; Chief and Professor, Radiologie 2, University Hospital of Strasbourg, Strasbourg, France*

P. Donkersloot *Neurosurgical Unit, Virga Jesse Ziekenhuis Hasselt, Belgium*

J. Dudler *Ma tre d enseignement et de recherche (MER), Facult de biologie et de mèdecine, Universit de Lausanne, Lausanne, Switzerland; Mèdecine-associ, Service de Rhumatologie, Mèdecine Physique et Rèhabilitation, Centre Hospitalier Universitaire Vaudois, Lausanne, Switzerland*

Nabil A. Ebraheim, M.D. *Professor and Chairman, Department of Orthopaedic Surgery, Medical University of Ohio, Toledo, Ohio*

Anthony P. Fabrizi *Department of Neurosurgery, Ospedale Bellaria, Bologna, Italy*

Prof. Yizhar Floman, M.D. *Professor Emeritus, Department of Orthopedic Surgery, Hebrew University Medical School, Jerusalem, Israel; Chief, Israel Spine Center, Assuta Hospital, Tel Aviv, Israel*

Brian J. C. Freeman, FRCS (Tr & Orth) *Consultant Spinal Surgeon, University Hospital, Queen's Medical Centre, Nottingham, United Kingdom*

Allister Gibson *Senior Lecturer, Department of Orthopaedic Surgery, The University of Edinburgh, The Medical School, Edinburgh, Scotland, United Kingdom; Consultant Spinal Surgeon, Department of Orthopaedic Surgery, The Royal Infirmary of Edinburgh, Edinburgh, Scotland, United Kingdom*

Phillip Gillet, M.D., Ph.D. *Professor, Orthopaedic Department and Anatomy, Universit de Liège (ULg), Liège, Belgium; Head of Department, Department of Orthopaedic Surgery, University Hospital CHU, Liège, Belgium*

Vijay K. Goel, M.D. *Professor and Chairman, Department of Bioengineering, University of Toledo, Toledo, Ohio*

Robert Gunzburg, M.D. *Eeuwfeestkliniek Harmoniestraat, Antwerp, Belgium*

Tommy Hansson, M.D., Ph.D. *Department of Orthopaedics, Institute of Surgical Sciences, Göteborg University, Thenburg, Sweden*

D. Hoste

W. C. H. Jacobs, M.S. *Coordinator Orthopedic Research Unit, Department of Research, Development and Education, Sint Maartenskliniek, Nijmegen, The Netherlands*

Prof. André J. Kaelin, M.D. *Professor, Department of Pediatrics, Medical School, University of Geneva, Genève, Switzerland; Chief, Department of Orthopedics, Children's Hospital HUG, Geneva, Switerland*

Prof. J. C. Le Huec *Department d'Orthopédie, CHU Pellegrin Tripode, Bordeaux Cedex, France*

F. Liquois *Orthopaedic Clinic J Vilar, Bruges, France*

A. Malik, M.D. *Staff Member, Department of Orthopedics and Traumatology, Hospital Vall d'Hebron, Barcelona, Spain*

J. Michielsen, M.D. *Dept. of Orthopaedics and Traumatology, University Hospital of Antwerp, Edegem-Antwerp, Belgium*

Maryline Mousny *Cliniques Universitaires Saint-Luc, Brussels, Belgium*

Everard Munting, M.D., Ph.D. *Consultant, Orthopaedic Department, Cliniques Universitaires Saint Luc, Universit Catholique de Louvain, Brussels, Belgium; Head, Department of Orthopaedics and Traumatology, Clinique St. Pierre, Ottignies Louvain-La-Neuve, Belgium*

Margareta Nordin, Dr. Sci. *Professor, Department of Orthopaedic and Environmental Medicine, New York University, New York, NY; Director, Occupational and Industrial Orthopaedic Center (OIOC), NYU Hospital for Joint Diseases, New York, NY*

Ferran Pellis, M.D. Ph.D. *Spine Unit, Hospital Vall d'Hebron, Barcelona, Spain*

Prof. Gilles Perrin *Hôpital Neurologique P. Wertheimer, Lyon, France*

Malcolm H. Pope, DrMedSc, Ph.D., DSc *University of Aberdeen, Liberty Safework Centre Aberdeen, Scotland, United Kingdom*

C. Pouders *Research Assistant, Departments of Experimental Anatomy and Radiology, Vrije Universiteit Brussel, Brussels, Belgium*

Abraham Rogozinski, M.D. *Orthopedic Surgeon, Rogozinski Orthopaedic Clinic, Jacksonville, Florida*

Chaim Rogozinski, M.D. *Orthopedic Surgeon, Rogozinski Orthopaedic Clinic, Jacksonville, Florida*

Koichi Sairyo, M.D., Ph.D. *Associate Professor, Department of Orthopaedics, University of Tokushima, School of Medicine, Tokushima, Japan*

Jeff S. Silber, M.D. *Assistant Professor, Department of Orthopaedic Surgery, Long Island Jewish Medical Center, New Hyde Park, New York*

Francis W. Smith, M.D. *University of Aberdeen, Liberty Safework Centre Aberdeen, Scotland, United Kingdom*

Rikke Søgaard MPH *Ph.D. Student, Orthopaedic Research Lab, Institute of Clinical Medicine, Aarhus,*

P. Suchomel *Department of Neurosurgery, Neurocenter Regional Hospital, Liberec, Czech Republic*

Michael. F. Sullivan, M.A., M.B., F.R.C.S. *Hon Senior Lecturer, Department of Surgery, Spinal Surgeon, Royal National Orthopaedic, University of London, London, U.K.*

Jan Sys *Orthopaedics, UZA, Edegem, Belgium*

Prof. Marek Szpalski *Department of Orthopaedic, HIS-Molière Longchamp, Brussels, Belgium*

Alexander R. Vaccaro, M.D. *Professor Department of Orthopaedic Surgery, Thomas Jefferson University, The Rothman Institute, Philadelphia, Pennsylvania*

Prof. Peter Van Roy, P.T., Ph.D. *Full Professor, Department of Experimental Anatomy and Manual Therapy, Vrije Universiteit Brussel, Brussels, Belgium*

Raphael Vialle, M.D. *Chief Assistant of Paris Hospitals, Department of Orthopaedic Surgery, Hôpital Beaujon, Clichy, France*

L. Villet

A.W.J. Vreeling, M.D. *Department of Orthopedic Surgery, Sint Maartenskliniek Nijmegen, The Netherlands*

Gordon Waddell *The Spinal Unit, The Royal Infirmary of Edinburgh, Edinburgh Scotland United Kingdom*

D. Wardlaw *University of Aberdeen, Liberty Safework Centre Aberdeen, Scotland, United Kingdom*

Georg Zöllner *Department of Radiology, University Hospital of Strasbourg*

Mino Zucchelli *Department of Neurosurgery, Ospedale Bellaria, Bologna, Italy*

Preface

Spondylolysis, the interruption of the vertebral isthmus, is one of the most ubiquitous spinal conditions. Its etiopathogenesis has long been a topic of debate, but it is now generally accepted to be the result of nonunion after a stress fracture. The anatomy of the condition as well as the biomechanics and etiopathogenesis are described.

Imaging tools used to coin the type of lesion and its evolution in time differ and are presented together with recent advances such as vertical MRI.

In many instances the diagnosis is fortuitous, which raises the question, "Does it hurt?" The origin of low back and nerve root pain are discussed.

Isthmic spondylolysis requires different approaches in children, adults, and high level sports addicts. These are analyzed and algorithms proposed.

The surgical treatment deserves a large part in this book. Depending on the origin of the pain and the quality of the adjoining intervertebral discs, pars reconstruction or intervertebral fusion may be preferred. Techniques vary widely and proposed implants show an inventiveness seldom seen in other pathologies.

Spondylolisthesis occurs when, due to gravitational forces, the upper vertebra slips forward. The debate on the need to deuce the slip when performing fusion surgery has been occupying the spine community for decades and is still raging. Advocates of the different attitudes expose their reasons and techniques, and the repercussion on the adjacent levels is discussed.

In middle age, a slippage can occur as a result of disc degeneration and concurring facet joint osteoarthritis. This is referred to as *degenerative spondylolisthesis*. It is a self-limiting condition, and requires special attention, as it raises specific treatment challenges.

Surgical instrumentation only serves as internal support while bony fusion occurs, and more recently new techniques have been proposed to enhance this mechanism. Synthetic bone, as well as bone formation enhancing proteins, are discussed.

Finally, some economic aspects of spondylolysis and spondylolisthesis are looked at from a more societal point of view.

The editors hope that readers from many different disciplines will find this book useful as it looks at the pathologies from very different points of view. It can be of help in diagnostic and therapeutic questions as well as medicolegal disputes.

Robert Gunzburg, M.D., Ph.D.
Marek Szpalski, M.D.

1

The Anatomy of the Neural Arch of the Lumbar Spine, with References to Spondylolysis, Spondylolisthesis, and Degenerative Spondylolisthesis

P. Van Roy, E. Barbaix, M. De Maeseneer, C. Pouders, and J. P. Clarys

In spondylolysis, a local bony defect at the level of the pars interarticularis tends to create and may finally lead to an uni- or bilateral cleft within the neural arch. In a complete bilateral pars defect, spondylolysis may lead to spondylolisthesis, whereby the vertebral body together with the pedicles, the transverse processes, and the upper articular facets are separated from the laminae, the spinous process, and the inferior articular facets. In children and adolescents, spondylolytic changes result from overloading, probably with stress fractures as a precursor factor (1) and facilitated by a possible hereditary predisposition (2). This contrasts with degenerative spondylolisthesis in middle-aged or elderly patients, whereby degenerative changes of facet joints and intervertebral discs produce instability, which at a certain point may induce ventral slip of the upper vertebra of a vertebral motion segment without pars defect. Consequently, the morphology of the neuroforamen becomes irregular and flattened (3), compromising the normal topography of its content. The nerve root canal normally has an inverted teardrop- or ear-shaped section and is more oval toward its exit zone (3,4). Its widest part is situated in the subpedicular notch of the upper vertebra. The L5 lateral neurovascular canal is particularly long compared to higher lumbar levels (4) (Fig. 1.1 A,B). The morphology of the lateral neurovascular canal depends on the condition of the adjacent apophyseal rings, the endplates and the interposed intervertebral disc anteriorly, the pars interarticularis of the superior vertebra, the superior articular facet of the vertebra below and the ligamentum flavum posteriorly, as well as on the condition of the pedicles of the motion segment under consideration. A bony indentation originating from the pars defect may provide a bilobulated aspect of the neuroforamen with enlarged horizontal diameter. Transforaminal or corporotransverse ligaments may influence the morphology of the lateral neurovascular canal at its exit zone, reducing the superoinferior diameter or forcing the neurovascular content to pass through the available space within the lateral canal, depending on the localization of the ligaments (5). Besides a general classification of the ligaments related to the intervertebral canal, Amonoo-Kuofi and El-Badawi (6) presented a detailed classification and description of the ligaments at the exit zone, making a clear distinction between the topography of the L5 lateral canal and higher lumbar lateral canals. Some of these ligaments may contribute to entrapment when the neuroforamen becomes flattened in spondylolisthesis.

A B
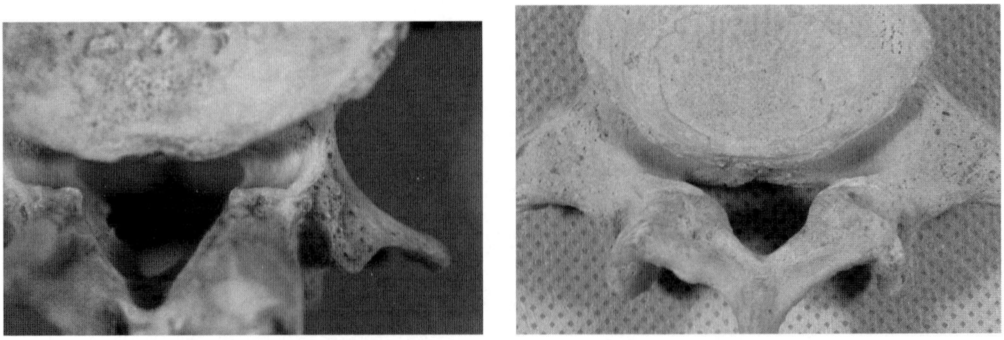

FIG. 1.1. **A:** Typical lateral neurovascular canal at upper lumbar levels. **B:** Typical lateral neurovascular canal at the L5 level.

Spondylolysis, spondylolisthesis, and degenerative spondylolisthesis occur predominantly in the lower lumbar spine (3,7), irrespective of the different underlying mechanisms in isthmic spondylolysis and degenerative spondylolisthesis. This raises the question whether the lower lumbar spine presents a morphology that is more prone to spondylolytic and spondylolisthetic processes and/or is subjected to higher loading than higher lumbar levels. One of the most apparent anatomical differences is the spatial

A B C D
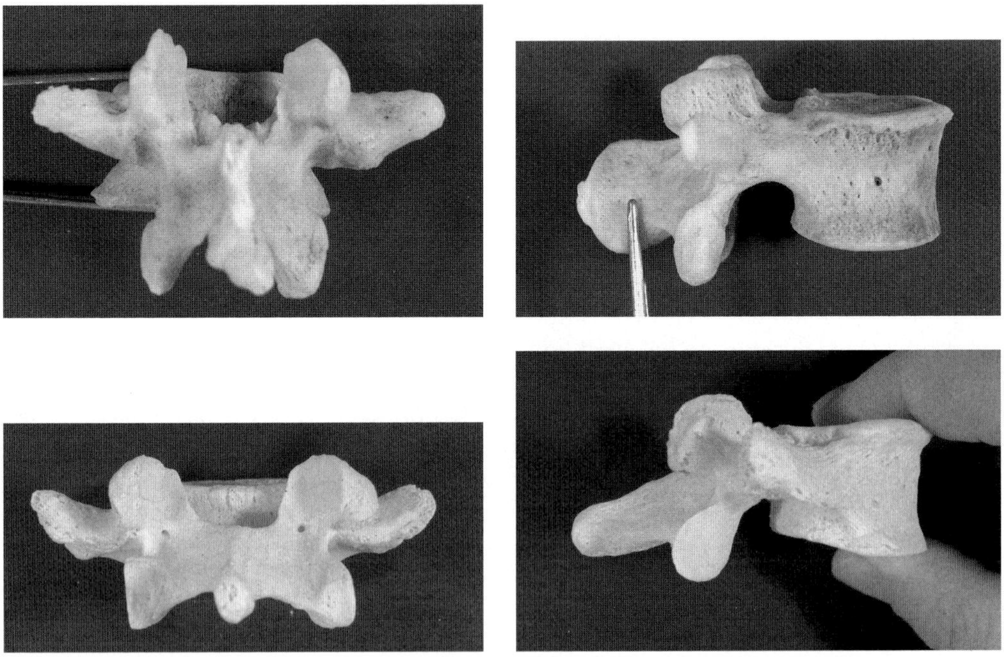

FIG. 1.2. **A:** Typical spatial configuration of the articular facets on the laminae in the upper lumbar spine. **B:** Lateral view of the same vertebra as in (A). Note the horizontal and vertical distance between the right transverse process and the right inferior articular facet. **C:** Typical spatial configuration of the articular facets on the laminae in an L5 vertebra. Note the decreased isthmus height compared to this parameter at higher levels (A). **D:** Lateral view of the same vertebra as in (C). Note the different horizontal and vertical distances between the right transverse process and the right inferior articular facet, compared to the same parameters in (B).

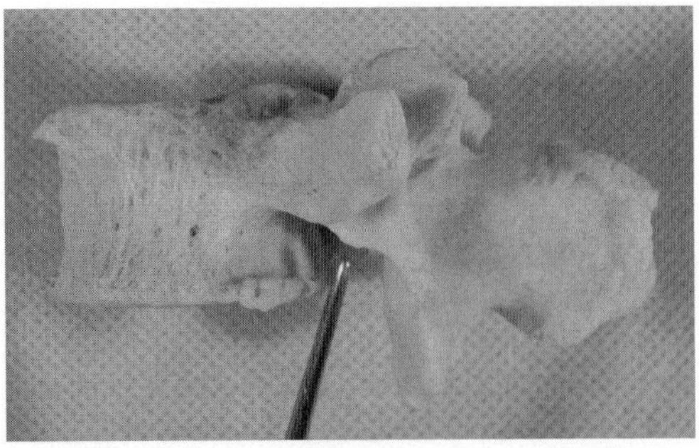
A

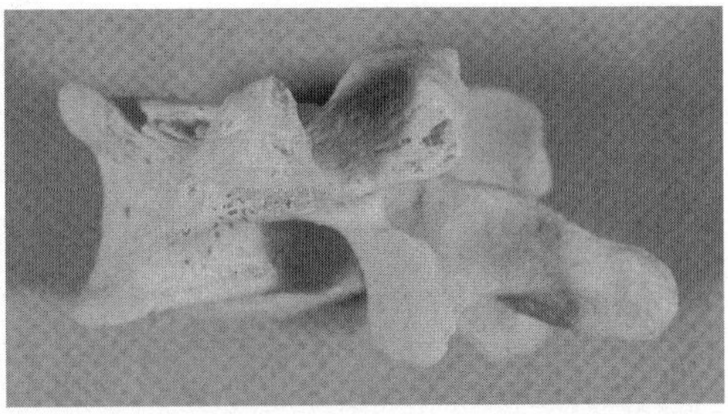
B

FIG. 1.3. A: The stronger lateral buttress* at higher lumbar levels. **B:** The lesser developed lateral buttress* at lower lumbar levels.

distribution of the superior and inferior facets with respect to their laminae. The height of the quadrangle resulting from an outline connecting the lateral margins of the four articular facets of the first lumbar vertebra is much larger than its width, whereas the opposite can be observed at the L5 level (8,9). The four facets of the upper two lumbar vertebrae fit in a trapezium, those of L4 in a square configuration, and those of L5 in a parallelogram whose long sides are horizontally oriented. As a result of a different spatial configuration of the facet joints, depending on their level, the height of the pars interarticularis decreases at lower lumbar levels (10), as does the distance between the transverse processes and the adjacent inferior facets (Fig. 1.2 A–D).

Weiner et al. (11) described "the lateral buttress" of a lumbar vertebra, representing a bony bridge between the superolateral edge of the inferior articular facet and the inferior aspect of the junction between the pedicle and the processus costarius. In the upper lumbar spine, the presence of a larger lateral buttress at the cranial aspect of the lateral foramen provides a stronger bony reinforcement of the pars interarticularis than at lower levels (Fig. 1.3 A,B). Whereas cross-sectional areas of the pars gradually increase from L1 to L4 levels, only a slight increase is observed between L4 and L5 levels (12). However, remarkable local width differences with adjacent levels can be found (13).

DEVELOPMENT OF THE PARS INTERARTICULARIS

The entire lumbar vertebra develops from five ossification centers: one for the vertebral body, two for the apophyseal rings, and two for the neural arch. For a long time it was believed that each half of the neural arch develops from two ossification centers; then Willis (14) illustrated that overlooking the presence of a thin isthmus in these ossification centers caused the misconception. In the upper lumbar segments, the ossification centers appear somewhat earlier than in the lower segments: at 7 to 9 weeks versus 8 to 9 weeks of gestation (15). Endochondral ossification of the pars interarticularis starts at 12 to 13 weeks of gestation. In the upper lumbar segments, the ossification centers of the neural arch originate at the end of the pedicle and result in an isotropic configuration of the trabeculae and cortical bone in the region of the pars interarticularis. In lower lumbar segments, the ossification centers originate in the region of the pars interarticularis and

*see Weiner et al. (11).

lead to an anisotropic configuration of trabecular and cortical bone in this region. Less densely trabeculated pedicles of smaller caliber appear in lower lumbar segments and the superior articular processes reveal a lesser trabecular density compared to the inferior articular processes (15). Cortical layers are thickest in the narrowest region of the pars, with the anterolateral aspect being thicker than the posteromedial one; the thickening is probably related to the amount of stress this part of the neural arch is subjected to during movement (1). Observations of trabecular and cortical bone at the cervicothoracic transition indicated that a layered morphology of the cortical bone of the neural arch and pars articularis deserves attention, especially in case of a poor or heterogeneous trabecular network (16).

Although several congenital clefts of the posterior elements of lumbar vertebrae may occur (retrosomatic cleft, retroisthmic cleft, spina bifida), pars defect reveals a birth incidence of zero (15,17). Changes of the signal intensity of bone marrow on magnetic resonance (MR) images in lumbar pedicles are an ancillary sign of spondylolysis (18) and are often seen in degenerative joint disease (19).

BONY VARIANTS OF LUMBAR VERTEBRAE IN RELATION TO SPONDYLOLYSIS, SPONDYLOLISTHESIS, AND DEGENERATIVE SPONDYLOLISTHESIS

Variants of the Facet Joint Morphology

The shape, inclination, and curvature of lumbar articular facets may reveal important intra- and interindividual differences. The upper articular joint facets often have a C- or J-shaped configuration; others are flat. Corresponding differences exist in the inferior facets, which are usually slightly longer than the superior facets of the underlying vertebra. Curved superior facets can be seen as parts of cylindrical tubes, providing mainly upward and downward gliding of the corresponding inferior facets and thus allowing flexion, extension, and lateral bending but only limited axial rotation. Lateral bending is realized by downward gliding of the ipsilateral inferior facet and upward gliding of the contralateral inferior facet with respect to their articulating counterparts.

At upper lumbar levels, the joint facets are expected to present a preponderantly sagittal orientation; the orientation becomes more frontal at lower levels (8,20,21). However, this statement should not be generalized, because systematic observations of facet type and orientation in collections of dried bones indicated that various configurations and orientations may be present at every lumbar level (8,22). Withstanding to a lesser extent anterior movement, the presence of a sagittal orientation of the articular facets at lower lumbar levels could be a predisposing factor for degenerative spondylolysthesis (23).

Flat-type articular facets and coronal orientation of the articular surfaces are more frequently observed in children and adolescents with pars defect than in those without (24).

Articular Tropism

Several aspects of articular tropism (left–right asymmetry between the articular facets (Fig. 1.4 A–D) may occur, resulting from different shape, curvature, orientation, dimensions, surface area, or implantation of the facets. The background of articular tropism may be either congenital or acquired. Degenerative changes may play an important role.

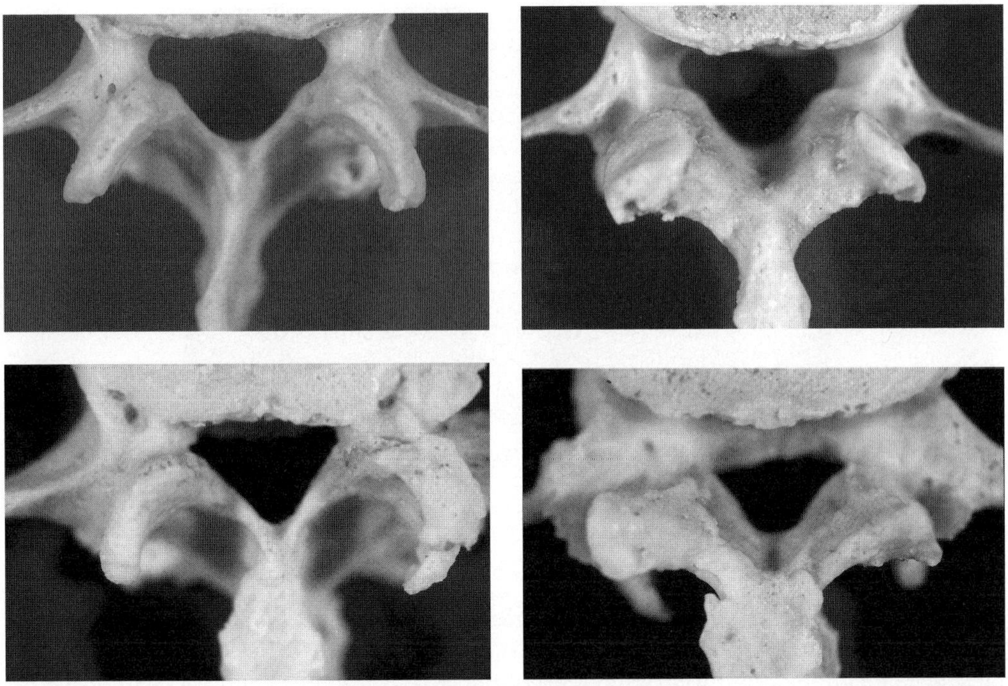

FIG. 1.4. Examples of articular tropism. **A:** Specimen A presenting different shape of the superior articular facets (flat versus J-shaped facet). **B:** Specimen A presenting a slight difference of the curvature of the inferior articular facets. **C:** Specimen B presenting articular tropism of the superior articular facets caused by degenerative enlargement. **D:** Specimen B presenting articular tropism of the inferior articular facets caused by different morphology of the articular processes (mortise joint).

Left–right differences of zygapophyseal joint facets are frequent at the thoracolumbar junction (25). An example of different orientation of superior articular facets at the lumbosacral transition junction is given in Figure 1.5.

Although most articles about articular tropism in the lumbar spine refer to different configurations of the superior articular facets (26–33), it is worthwhile to consider the

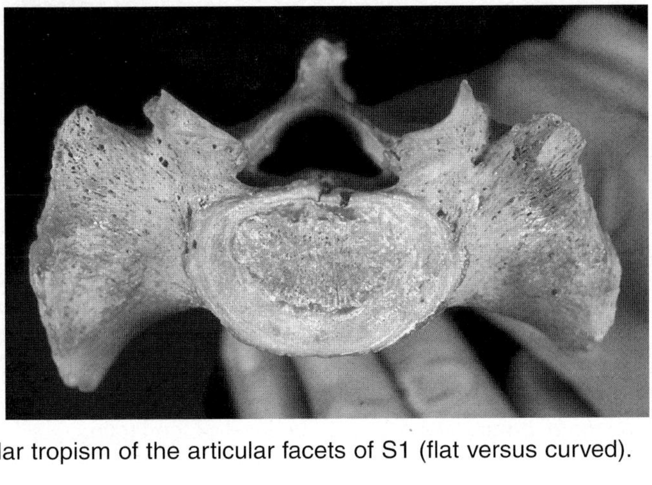

FIG. 1.5. Articular tropism of the articular facets of S1 (flat versus curved).

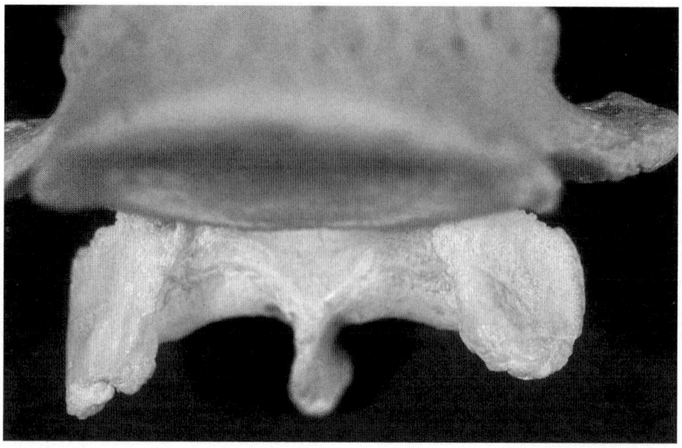

FIG. 1.6. Articular tropism: marked height difference and different orientation of the inferior articular facets.

left–right differences at the level of the inferior articular facets as well (34). One can expect that different height of the left and right inferior facets (Fig. 1.6), as well as the presence of an unilateral fovea at the level of the adjacent lamina (Fig. 1.7) will influence the segmental range of motion, including reciprocal coupled motion between axial rotation and lateral bending.

Spondylolysis is often associated with congenital malformation of the adjacent facets. Enlarged superior articular facets are a characteristic feature of spondylolytic vertebrae; left–right differences in dimensions and surface area of joint facets are often encountered in unilaterally affected vertebrae (35).

Besides congenital malalignment, osteoarthritic facet enlargement and deformation may also contribute largely to articular tropism. Articular tropism is extremely common in degenerative spondylolisthesis (3).

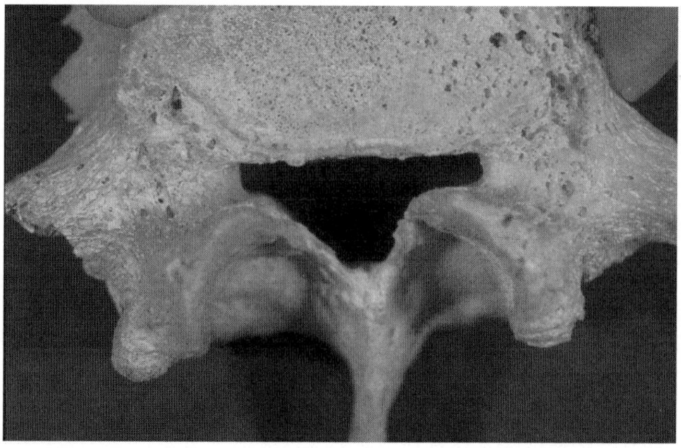

FIG. 1.7. The presence of a unilateral fovea at the level of the lamina.

Other Left–Right Asymmetries of Lumbar Vertebrae

Left–right asymmetries are not restricted to articular tropism but may also result from differences between pedicles or processus costarii, from an oblique spinous process, or from an asymmetric shape of the vertebral body, induced by irregular endplates or by irregular apophyseal rings (36). Marked local width differences of the pars interarticularis were reported by Giles (13). Isthmic spondylolysis may occasionally occur in association with congenital or acquired malformations of the neural arch, causing left–right asymmetry: unilateral shortening, narrowing, elongation (37) or hypertrophy of the pedicles, or pedicular cleft (38). More frequently, isthmic spondylolysis appears in association with spina bifida occulta (39).

TRABECULAR CHANGES AND DISC DEGENERATION

Disc degeneration is considered to be a major factor in producing instability resulting in degenerative spondylolisthesis. It is worthwhile to consider some associated morphologic changes. Loss of trabeculae in the vertebral body and change in vertebral body shape often precede disc degeneration (40). As a consequence, the endplates may become concave, in turn modifying shape and height of the intervertebral disc. The vertebral bodies are often typically wedge shaped in degenerative spondylolisthesis (Fig. 1.8 A–D).

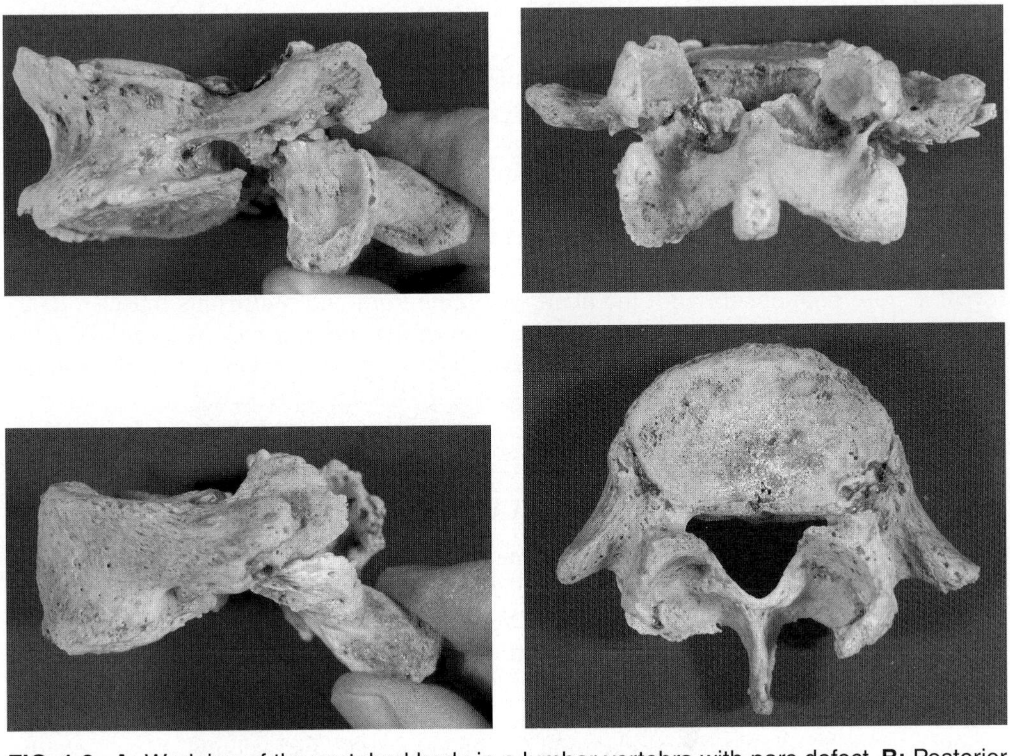

A B C D

FIG. 1.8. A: Wedging of the vertebral body in a lumbar vertebra with pars defect. **B:** Posterior view of the same vertebra as in (A). **C:** Wedging of the vertebral body in a lumbar vertebra in association with degeneration of the articular facets. **D:** Posterior view of the same vertebra as in (C).

SAGITTAL ANATOMY OF THE LUMBOSACRAL REGION

The sagittal balance of the lumbar spine partly depends on sagittal anatomical and positional parameters of the sacrum. The lumbar lordosis and sacral kyphosis largely define the degree of the sacral slope in the erect position. Spondylolisthesis patients often show morphologic parameters that predispose to ventral slip: a more curved sacrum, especially at the level of the first two sacral vertebrae, and a larger incidence angle (41). The incidence angle is the angle between a perpendicular to the middle of the (proximal) sacral endplate and a line connecting the middle of this sacral endplate with the center of the bicoxofemoral axis.

A normal central lumbar canal may be round, triangular, or dome shaped. A trefoiled configuration should be considered a secondary development (42,43); it results from ventral midpoint thickening of the laminae over their full height, which leads to the characteristic indentation of the central canal and narrowing of the anteroposterior dimensions of the lateral recess (4,7). A round central canal provides concave superior and inferior posterior borders of the vertebral body and is usually present at higher lumbar levels. The posterior border of the lumbar vertebral bodies of L4 is rather straight, and that of L5 is often straight and may even be slightly convex. The presence of a straight or concave posterior border of the body of the fifth lumbar vertebra, along with a round or ovoid posterior border of the first sacral vertebra, may mimic anterior corporal displacement (3). Willis (44) reported that slight differences between the anteroposterior diameters of L5 and S1 vertebral bodies are common, as are small pedicle length differences. S1 pedicles may be shorter, equal to, or longer than L5 pedicles. These variants may cause a slightly posterior or anterior projection of the L5 vertebral body with respect to the S1 vertebral body on lateral roentgenograms.

Several types of sacralization or lumbalization may alter the anatomy of the lumbosacral transition. Sacralization mainly occurs between the vertebral bodies of L5 and S1, but unilateral or bilateral additional friction zones or bony bridges may be present between the processus costarius of L5 and the underlying pars lateralis of the sacrum.

Iliolumbar ligaments consist of several bands connecting the processus costarii of L5 tightly with the iliac tuberosity, the iliac crest, and the iliac fossa (45,46). Additional fascicles may provide a connection to the processus costarii of L4. The iliolumbar ligaments reveal a close relationship with the quadratus lumborum and multifidus muscles. They are important structures to withstand ventral slip of the superior part of a pars defect at the L5 level and eventually also at the L4 level. These ligaments also restrict the amount of lateral bending at the lumbosacral transition.

CONCLUSION

L4 and L5 lumbar vertebrae present a number of differences as compared to higher segments: more anterior slope of the endplates resulting from their localization in the inferior half of the lumbar lordosis; a typical spatial localization of their facet joints on the laminae, resulting in a shorter pars interarticularis; a less well developed lateral buttress; less uniform trabeculation of the pedicles and the pars interarticularis, resulting from a slightly different ossification process.

Several aspects of anatomical variation can be associated with spondylolysis, spondylolisthesis, and degenerative spondylolisthesis, and they probably facilitate underlying pathomechanics.

Observation of the following anatomical items is relevant with respect of spondylolysis, spondylolisthesis, and degenerative spondylolisthesis:

- Pars articularis: pars defect, unilateral elongation, thinning, poor trabecular density, hypertrophy
- Pedicles: left–right asymmetry, secondary changes, subpedicular notch, retrosomatic cleft
- Laminae: retroisthmic cleft, spina bifida
- Facet joints: facet type (flat) and orientation (sagittal), articular tropism, secondary changes
- Lateral buttress
- Vertebral body: wedging, poor trabecular density, concave endplates, asymmetry of the apophyseal rings
- Intervertebral disc: shape, degeneration
- Central lumbar canal: shape, size
- Neuroforamen: modification of its shape by surrounding anatomical items (pedicles, apophyseal rings, endplates, intervertebral disc, facet joints, pars interarticularis, ligamentum flavum), especially flattening and superior bony indentation, transforaminal and corporotransverse ligaments
- The lumbosacral transition: articular tropism, sacralization, attachments of iliolumbar ligaments, sacral kyphosis, incidence angle

REFERENCES

1. Krenz J, Troup JD. The structure of the pars interarticularis of lower lumbar vertebrae and its relation to the etiology of spondylolysis. *J Bone Joint Surg* 1993;55-B:735–741.
2. Wiltse LL. The etiology of spondylolisthesis. *J Bone Joint Surg* 1962-A;44:539–560.
3. Rothman SL, Glenn WV, eds. *Multiplanar CT of the spine*. Baltimore: University Park Press; 1985:213–254.
4. Rauschning W. Normal and pathologic anatomy of the lumbar root canals. *Spine* 1987;12:1008–1019.
5. Bakkum BW, Mestan M. The effects of transforaminal ligaments on the sizes of T11 to L5 human intervertebral foramina. *J Manip Physiol Ther* 1994;17:517–522.
6. Amonoo-Kuofi HS, El-Badawi MGY. Ligaments related to the intervertebral canal and foramen. In: Giles LG, Singer KP, eds. *The clinical anatomy and management of back pain series, Vol. 1: Clinical anatomy and management of low back pain*. Oxford: Butterworth-Heinemann; 2001:114–133.
7. Eisenstein S. The trefoil configuration of the lumbar vertebral canal: a study of South African skeletal material. *J Bone Joint Surg* 1980;62-B:73–77.
8. Bogduk N, Twomey L. *Clinical anatomy of the lumbar spine*. Melbourne: Churchill Livingstone; 1991.
9. Fawcett E. A note on the identification of the lumbar vertebrae of man. *J Anat* 1932;66:384–386.
10. Ebraheim NA, Lu J, Hao Y, et al. Anatomic considerations of the lumbar isthmus. *Spine* 1997;22:941–945.
11. Weiner BK, Walker M, Wiley W, et al. The lateral buttress: an anatomic feature of the lumbar pars interarticularis. *Spine* 2002;27:E385–E387.
12. Panjabi MM, Goel V, Oxland T, et al. Human lumbar vertebrae: quantitative three-dimensional anatomy. *Spine* 1992;17:299–306.
13. Giles LG. Miscellaneous pathological and developmental (anomalous) conditions. In: Giles LG, Singer KP, eds. *The clinical anatomy and management of back pain series, Vol. 1: Clinical anatomy and management of low back pain*. Oxford: Butterworth-Heinemann; 2001:196–216.
14. Willis T. The separate neural arch. *J Bone Joint Surg* 1931;13:709–721.
15. Sagi H, Jarvis J, Uhthoff H. Histomorphic analysis of the development of the pars interarticularis and its association with isthmic spondylolyis. *Spine* 1998;23:1635–1639.
16. Verhoef M. Trabecular and cortical morphology at the cervicothoracic transition. MSc thesis in manual therapy (in Dutch), Brussels, Vrije Universiteit Brussel, 2004.
17. Rowe GG, Roche MB. The etiology of a separate neural arch. *J Bone Joint Surg* 1953;35-A:102–110.
18. Ulmer JL, Elster AD, Mathews VP, et al. Lumbar spondylolysis: reactive marrow changes seen in adjacent pedicles on MR images. *AJR Am J Roentgenol* 1995;164:429–433.
19. Morrison JL, Kaplan PA, Dussault RG, et al. Pedicle marrow signal intensity changes in the lumbar spine: a manifestation of facet degenerative joint disease. *Skeletal Radiol* 2000;29:703–707.

20. Adams M, Bogduk N, Burton K, et al. *The biomechanics of back pain*. Edinburgh: Churchill Livingstone; 2002;238 p.
21. Taylor JR, Twomey LT. Age changes in lumbar zygapophyseal joints: observations on structure and function. *Spine* 1986;11:739–745.
22. De Vis JP Articular tropism of the lumbar spine. MSc thesis in manual therapy (in Dutch), Brussels, Vrije Universiteit Brussel, 2000.
23. Grobler LJ, Robertson PA, Novotny JE, et al. Etiology of spondylolisthesis: assessment of the role played by lumbar facet joint morphology. *Spine* 1993;18:80–91.
24. Miyake R, Itaka T, Katoh S. Morphologic analysis of the facet joint in the immature lumbosacral spine with special reference to spondylolysis. *Spine* 1996;21:783–789.
25. Singer KP. Pathoanatomy of the thoracolumbar transitional junction. In: Giles LG, Singer KP, eds. *The clinical anatomy and management of back pain series, Vol. 1: Clinical anatomy and management of low back pain*. Oxford: Butterworth-Heinemann; 2001:183–195.
26. Ahmed AM, Duncan NA, Burke DL. The effect of facet geometry on the axial torque-rotation response of lumbar motion segments. *Spine* 1990;15:391–401.
27. Cassidy JD, Loback D, Yong-Hing K, et al. Lumbar facet joint asymmetry. *Spine* 1992;17:570–574.
28. Gunzburg R, Sandhu A, Fraser RD. The value of computerised tomography in determining lumbar facet orientation. *J Spinal Disord* 1989;2:170–175.
29. Hagg O, Wallner A. Facet joint asymmetry and protrusion of the intervertebral disc. *Spine* 1990;15:356–359.
30. Kénési C, Lesur E. Orientation of the articular processes at L4, L5 and S1: possible role in pathology of the intervertebral disc. *Anat Clin* 1985;7:43–47.
31. Noren R, Trafimow J, Andersson GBJ, et al. The role of facet joint tropism and facet angle in disc degeneration. *Spine* 1991;16:530–532.
32. Tulsi RS, Hermanis GM. A study of the angle of inclination and facet curvature of superior lumbar zygapophyseal facets. *Spine* 1993;18:1311–1317.
33. Vanharanta H, Floyd T, Ohnmeiss DD, et al. The relationship of facet tropism to degenerative disc disease. *Spine* 1993;18:1000–1005.
34. Van Roy P, De Vis JP, Barbaix E, et al. *Articular tropism and asymmetry of incisurae intervertebrales in lumbar vertebrae*. Abstract book of the European forum on Manual Therapy, BVMT-ABTM in conjunction with IFOMT-ECE, Antwerp, Belgium; 2001:35.
35. Eisenstein S. Spondylolysis: a skeletal investigation of two population groups. *J Bone Joint Surg* 1978; 60-B:488–494.
36. Van Roy P, Barbaix E, Clarijs J. Anatomy of the lumbar canal, foramen, and ligaments, with references to recent insights. In: Gunzburg R, Szpalski M, eds. *Lumbar spinal stenosis*. Philadelphia: Lippincott Williams & Wilkins; 2000:7–25.
37. Basu PS, Noordeen MHH, Elsebaie H. Spondylolisthesis in osteogenesis imperfecta due to pedicle elongation. *Spine* 2001;26:E506–E509.
38. Kalideen JM, Satyapal KS, Bayat F. Case report: pedicular cleft associated with bilateral pars interarticularis defects and transverse process hypoplasia of a fifth lumbar vertebra. *Br J Radiol* 1994;67:1136–1138.
39. Kumar R, Niall D, Walsh A, et al. Spina bifida occulta in isthmic spondylolisthesis: a surgical trap. *Eur Spine J* 2002;11:159–161.
40. Twomey L, Taylor JR. Structural and mechanical disc changes with age. *J Man Med* 1990;5:58–61.
41. Marty C, Bisaubert B, Descamps H, et al. The sagittal anatomy of the sacrum among young adults, infants, and spondylolisthesis patients. *Eur Spine J* 2002;11:119–125.
42. Atila B, Yazici M, Kopuz C, et al. The shape of the lumbar vertebral canal in newborns. *Spine* 1997;22:2469–2472.
43. Papp T, Porter RW, Aspden RM. The growth of the lumbar vertebral canal. *Spine* 1994;19:2770–2773.
44. Willis T. Lumbosacral anomalies. *J Bone Joint Surg* 1959;41-A:935–938.
45. Basadonna P-T, Gasparini D, Rucco V. Iliolumbar ligament insertions: in vivo anatomic study. *Spine* 1996;20:2313–2316.
46. Lee D, Vleeming A. *The pelvic girdle: an approach to the examination and treatment of the lumbo-pelvic–hip region*. Edinburgh: Churchill Livingstone, 1999, 17–42.

2

Biomechanics of Spondylolysis and Spondylolisthesis

Malcolm H. Pope and Francis Smith

Spondylolysis is a fracture of the pars interarticularis. If the pars defect is bilateral, it may allow slippage of the vertebra, resulting in spondylolisthesis. Mechanical stresses cause spondylolisthesis, which is most common in the lower lumbar spine at levels L4 and L5. These levels carry more load than higher levels of the spine and have greater shear forces due to the lumbar lordosis. Stresses on the pars interarticularis are accentuated during repetitive hyperextension, which results in increased contact of the caudal edge of the L4 inferior articular facet with the L5 pars. This may result in a stress fracture of the pars.

Many more athletes than nonathletes develop a pars defect. Sports that involve repetitive hyperextension and axial loading of the lumbar spine result in repetitive microtrauma to the pars interarticularis. Such sports include gymnastics, wrestling, hurdling, weight lifting, cricket, rowing, pole vaulting, diving, swimming, American football, baseball, tennis, sailing, and volleyball. Gymnasts are four times as likely as controls to develop spondylolysis, and 50% of American football linebackers have a pars defect. In American football blocking, the average compression force at L5 is 7 times body weight, and the peak shear force is 2.6 times body weight.

The lumbar spine has the functions of support, mobility, housing of neurological structures, and control. The orientation of the facets varies for different spinal levels, and this orientation determines how much flexion, extension, lateral flexion, and rotation the body can achieve at a particular vertebral level. The facets and other posterior elements have a load-bearing function to help support the weight of the upper body and anything that it carries, and they are also acted upon by spinal muscle forces. The posterior elements carry approximately 16% of the total load when a person is standing upright but 30% of the total load in hyperextension. During hyperextension, the vertebrae rotate such that the superior articular processes of one vertebra push against the inferior articular processes of the vertebra directly above it. This contact force causes the inferior articular processes to bend upward and tensile stresses to develop on the underside of the pars. During flexion, the inferior and superior articulating facets of adjacent vertebrae attempt to pull away from each other but are held together by the ligaments that encapsulate the joint, which tends to bend the pars forward.

Fatigue failure occurs due to repetitive loads that are less than the load to cause failure after a single load. The fatigue life is dependent on the amplitude of the cyclic stresses and the method by which they are imposed. Fatigue tests of the lumbar neural arch simulated a man walking quickly in a flexed posture with a 50-kg pack on his back. Over 70% of specimens failed at the pars, and specimens simulating persons aged 14 to 30 years failed much sooner (<50,000 cycles) than those simulating middle-aged people (>500,000 cycles with no fracture).

While there is a complex interplay of muscle forces and ligament tension at intervertebral joints, the facet load is the main force acting on the neural arch. Loading of the inferior articular process and bending in the pars cause high stresses because the pars is the narrowest part of the neural arch and thus has the smallest cross-sectional area with which to resist load. With cyclic flexion and hyperextension, or with repeated high-impact forces on the upper body, the pars is repetitively bent in one direction and then the other, and fatigue life may be reached and a crack will initiate at the point of highest principal stress. The crack will propagate across the pars if loading continues.

In addition to occurring in certain athletic groups who subject their upper bodies to high repetitive forces, spondylolysis seems to develop most often in children, adolescents, and young adults. This could be partly due to the fact that the ossification of their neural arches may not be complete and the bone is therefore less stiff and has a lower fatigue life. Or it could be partly due to the fact that the intervertebral discs of young people are more elastic and therefore allow more shear force to reach the facets, increasing the magnitudes of the forces and stresses on the pars. Another cause could be that most young people engage in more frequent strenuous activity than adults, causing the fatigue life of the pars to be reached sooner.

ETIOLOGY

Spondylolysis is a fracture of the pars interarticularis (pars). If the fracture gap widens, then the fracture is termed spondylolisthesis. Widening of the gap leads to shear forces. If the pars defect is bilateral, it may allow slippage of the vertebra, typically L5 on S1, resulting in spondylolisthesis. Spondylolisthesis can occur at any level of the spine, although it is most common in the lower lumbar spine. Most cases result from minor overuse trauma, particularly repetitive hyperextension of the lumbar spine. Spondylolysis is found in approximately 6% of the overall population (1) but is more common in certain subsets of the population. For example, there is a 2.8% incidence of spondylolysis in black men but up to a 50% incidence in Alaskan natives (2). Those aged 5 to 20 years are much more likely to develop this condition than older persons, and there is a congenital disposition (1). As noted above, a much higher proportion of athletes than nonathletes develop a pars defect. Gymnasts are four times as likely as the general population to develop spondylolysis (3), and up to 50% of American football linebackers have a pars defect (4).

The types of spondylolisthesis are as follows:

Type 1. Dysplastic (congenital) with a defect in the upper sacrum or arch of L5.

Type 2. Isthmic with a pars problem that permits forward slippage of the superior vertebra, usually L5. This type usually occurs in children older than 5 years, usually in those aged 7 to 8 years, and it rarely occurs before walking begins. Slip progression is minimal after skeletal maturity. There are three subcategories:

- Type 2A, or lytic spondylolisthesis, involves a defect in the pars area resulting from recurrent microfractures due to the impact of the articular processes against the pars in extension. This defect usually occurs by age 6 and is sometimes associated with congenital defects such as lumbarization, sacralization, and spina bifida occulta.
- Type 2B is an intact but elongated pars, probably resulting from repetitive microfractures that heal in an elongated position.
- Type 2C, which is rare, results from an acute fracture of the pars from major trauma.

Type 3. Degenerative spondylolisthesis is an acquired condition resulting from chronic disc and facet degeneration, leading to segmental instability and gradual slippage of the vertebra, usually at L4 or L5.

Type 4. Traumatic (at any age) results from fracture of any part of the neural arch or pars that leads to listhesis.
Type 5. Pathologic results from a generalized bone disease, such as Paget disease or osteogenesis imperfecta.
Spondylolisthesis is graded based on the amount of vertebral subluxation in the sagittal plane:

Grade 1. Less than 25% of vertebral diameter.
Grade 2. 25%–50%.
Grade 3. 50%–75%.
Grade 4. 75%–100%.
Spondyloptosis. Greater than 100%.

FUNCTIONAL ANATOMY

The trunk muscles provide stability, control movements, and generate the force necessary to perform many essential activities. The back, glutei, and the hamstring muscles are all active during lifting. The activity is related to the external load moment and is also a function of posture, speed, and asymmetry of the lift. With low back pain (LBP), the muscles lose coordination and speed of response besides losing strength and endurance.

Mechanical stresses play an important role in the process of spondylolisthesis. The erect posture produces a constant downward and forward thrust on the lumbar vertebrae. Stresses on the pars interarticularis are accentuated during repetitive hyperextension, which results in increased contact of the caudal edge of the L4 inferior articular facet with the L5 pars interarticularis. This collective trauma may eventually result in a stress fracture of the pars interarticularis. Spondylolisthesis may occur when bilateral pars defects are present, which allows forward slippage of the vertebra (typically L5 on S1).

Figure 2.1 shows the resolution of forces in the lower lumbar spine that result in a shear force Rs.

SPORT-SPECIFIC BIOMECHANICS

Sports that involve repetitive hyperextension and axial loading of the lumbar spine may lead to repetitive microtrauma to the pars interarticularis, resulting in spondylolysis and sometimes spondylolisthesis. These include gymnastics, wrestling, weight lifting (particularly standing overhead presses), cricket, rowing, pole vaulting, diving, hurdling, swimming (especially the butterfly stroke), American-style football (especially blocking or hitting the blocking sled), baseball (especially pitching), tennis (especially serving), sailing (particularly the hiking maneuver), and volleyball (Figs. 2.2 and 2.3).

The forces in sports can be analyzed by the principles of mechanics. For example in gymnastics and diving, high rates of rotation occur. The principle of the conservation of angular momentum is most simply stated as:

$$\text{Angular momentum} = \text{moment of inertia} \times \text{angular velocity, or } AM = Iw$$

1. Angular momentum can be viewed as the quantity of rotation a body has about some given axis as a result of its speed of rotation and the distribution of mass about the axis.
2. Moment of inertia (I) is a measure of how the mass of body is distributed about the axis of rotation. The farther the mass is from the object, the larger the I and vice

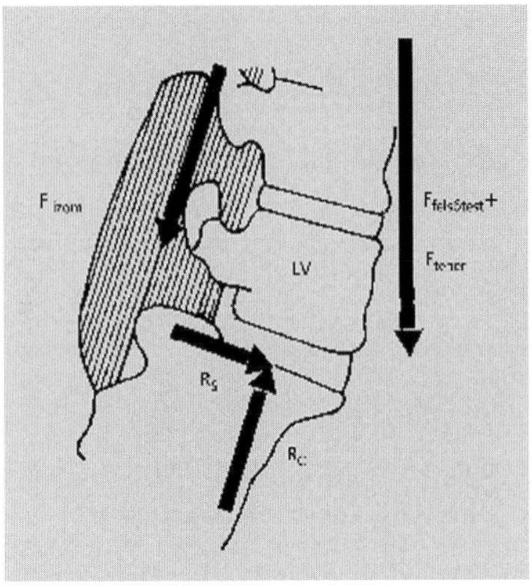

FIG. 2.1. Shear forces on the lumbar spine.

versa. In fact, *I* increases as the square of the distance of the mass and therefore a small increase in distance can result in a relatively large increase in *I*.

3. Angular velocity (*w*) is simply the stated speed of rotation about the axis of rotation.
4. Since *AM* must be conserved (unless an external force or torque is applied) the product of *I* and *w* must stay constant. If a gymnast tucks up in the air, *I* will decrease and thus *AM* will be conserved; *w* will increase accordingly and vice versa.
5. This tuck puts high shear forces on the spine.

Jeff Thomson (Fig. 2.4) was the fastest bowler in the recorded history of cricket. He was not only unique in the execution of his side-on javelin-type action but in having a

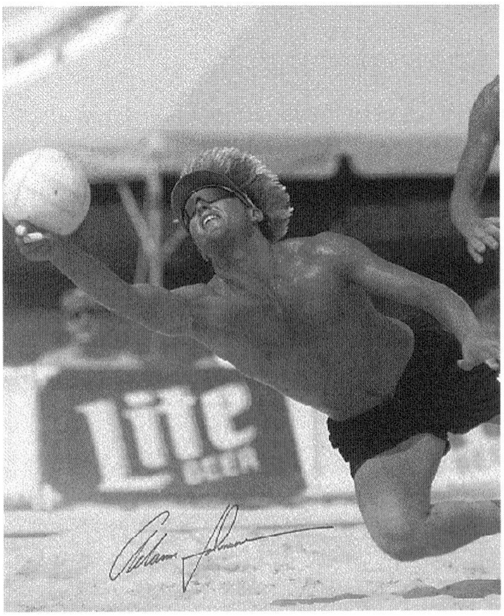

FIG. 2.2. Elite volleyball.

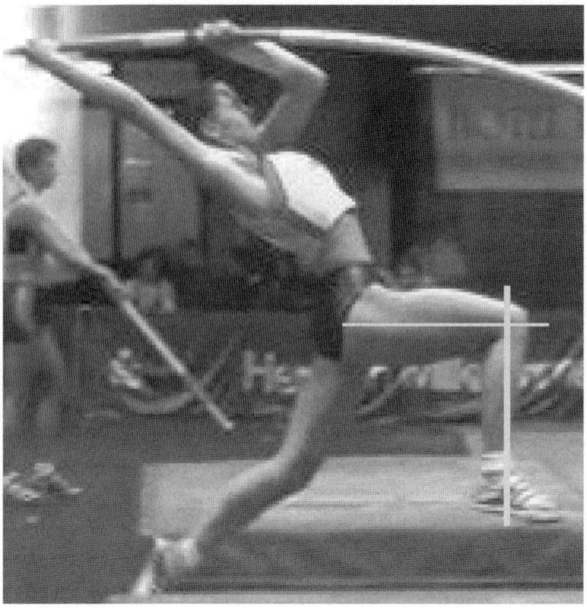

FIG. 2.3. Initial pole vault position.

short, ambling run-up before delivery. What he lacked in run-up speed, he made up in a greater range of trunk flexion and good use of the ground reaction forces.

Gatt et al. (4) analyzed the forces on the lumbar spine during American football blocking. American football linemen subject their spines to highly repetitive impact loads. They also subject the spine to repetitive flexion/compression in going from the three-point crouch stance to upright blocking posture and colliding with another player. Figure 2.5 shows children learning this maneuver. Gatt et al. (4) had players block a practice sled while forces were measured with force transducers and the angles of their trunk were filmed. Static equilibrium was used to find the compressive and shear forces and moment at L5. The average peak compression force at L5 was found to be 8,679 + 1,965 N, or 7 times body weight, and the average peak shear force at L5 was found to be 3,304:t 1,116 N, or 2.6 times body weight. Cyron and Hutton (5) found that a single shear force of 1,200 N to 2,800 N could fracture a vertebra at the pars without cyclic loading. However, the calculated load in Gatt's experiment would also have been resisted by other spinal elements such as the discs and ligaments.

BIOMECHANICS

The lumbar spine is a complex structure, which has the functions of support, mobility, housing of neurological structures, and control. The spine supports the internal organs, the upper and lower extremities, trunk, head, and external load moments. Mobility is required for the physical tasks of daily living, which complicates the spine structure. The basic unit of the spine is the functional spinal unit (FSU), defined as the superior vertebra, the inferior vertebra, the intervertebral disc, and the ligaments. The facet joints have two functions; the first is to guide the motion of the spine. The orientation of the facets varies at different spinal levels, and this orientation determines how much flexion, extension, lateral flexion, and rotation the body can achieve at each vertebral level. Second, the

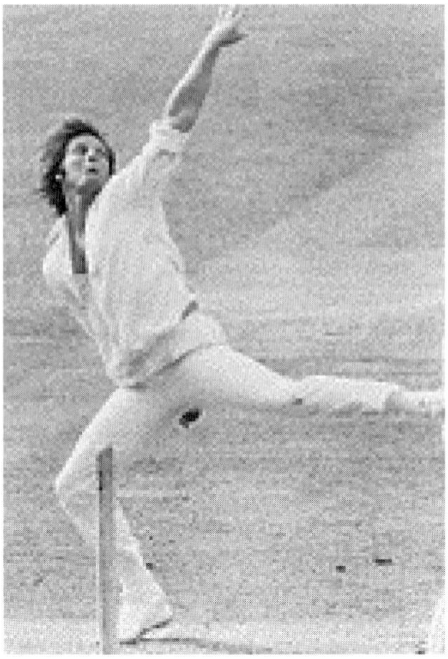

FIG. 2.4. Cricket bowling.

facets and other posterior elements have a load-bearing function to help support the weight of the upper body and anything that it carries, and are also acted upon by spinal muscle forces. The FSU kinematics contributes to the total motion of the lumbar spine and determines the stress distribution. Any component of the FSU can be fatigued by cyclic loading, which can cause failure or an adaptive response. The FSU is viscoelastic, which means that it creeps and has properties that change with the rate of loading. The FSU exhibits coupled motion (a force in one direction may induce motion in another). This phenomenon may be important in the unstable motion segment and possibly in

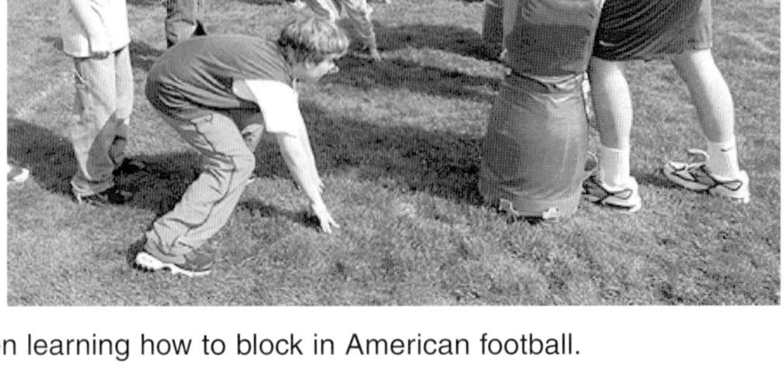

FIG. 2.5. Children learning how to block in American football.

spondylolisthesis. The coupled motion is normally presented in the form of a flexibility or stiffness matrix. The FSU has a balance point at a reproducible location and mechanical response where coupled motion is minimized. It is sensitive to (a) vector magnitude, (b) orientation, and (c) load rate. It is possible that the neuromuscular system applies load(s) and/or torque(s) to each FSU using the minimization of the FSU's 6-degrees-of-freedom motion as its objective function. Large rotations occur in the FSU as it is loaded further from its balance point and paraspinal muscles adjust their activation accordingly. Likewise an injury, degeneration, structural defects, pain, or even fatigue changes muscle recruitment. This could explain some failure patterns and pathologies seen on clinical examination and provides a rationale for rehabilitation.

While a single traumatic impact load can cause a pars fracture, most cases are the result of cumulative microtrauma from cyclic loading, leading to fatigue failure. Fatigue failure is defined as failure due to repetitive loads that are less than the load, which would induce failure after a single application. Fatigue occurs in all the tissues of the body, and it occurs if the rate of repair is less than the rate of injury due to repetitive loading. Cyron and Hutton (5) stated that, in the spine, the fatigue life is dependent on the amplitude of the cyclic stresses and the method by which they are imposed.

If the vertebra is theoretically cut at the point where stresses are to be calculated, the forces can be resolved into a force acting perpendicular to the cut surface, which causes a normal stress; a force acting parallel to the cut surface, which causes a shear stress; and a moment (Fig. 2.6). The moment, in turn, causes normal stresses due to bending. A fatigue crack will be initiated at the point of greatest normal stress, also called the greatest principal stress.

Spondylolysis and spondylolisthesis usually occur in the lumbar spine at L4 and L5. The reason for this is that they carry more loads and are more susceptible to shear forces due to the lumbar lordosis. The vertebral bodies and intervertebral discs share compressive forces, and shear forces are shared by the facets, discs, and spinal ligaments.

Gatt et al. (4) estimated that the posterior elements carry approximately 16% of the total load when a person is standing upright. Figure 2.6 shows a simplified two-dimensional diagram of the forces acting across the pars. Forces on the inferior articulating

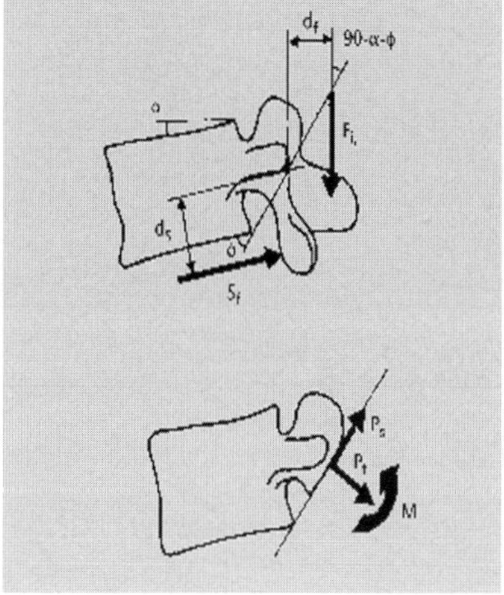

FIG. 2.6. Forces on the motion segment.

facets are resolved into a shear force parallel to the theoretical cut through the pars, a normal force perpendicular to the cut, and a moment. However, Klemenesics and Kiss (6) established that up to 30% of the total load in full hyperextension can be carried by the posterior elements. During hyperextension, the vertebrae rotate so that the superior articular processes of one vertebra push against the inferior articular processes of the vertebra directly above it. This contact force causes the inferior articular processes to bend upward and tensile stresses to develop on the underside of the pars. During flexion, the inferior and superior articulating facets of adjacent vertebrae attempt to pull away from each other but are held together by the ligaments that encapsulate the joint, which tends to bend the pars forward. Higher shear forces develop during flexion due to the increased angle of the vertebra to the horizontal and the increased moment arm over which body weight acts, and the erector spinae muscles, which stabilize the upper body during forward bending, also pull on the posterior elements (2).

Although there is a complex interplay of muscle forces and ligament tension at intervertebral joints (3), the facet load is the main force acting on the neural arch (7). Loading of the inferior articular process and bending in the pars cause high stresses because the pars is the narrowest part of the neural arch and thus has the smallest cross-sectional area with which to resist load (6) (Fig. 2.7). With cyclic flexion and extension/hyperextension, or with repeated high impact forces on the upper body, the pars is repetitively bent in one direction and then the other, and fatigue life may be reached, at which point a crack will initiate at the point of highest principal stress. The crack will propagate across the pars if loading continues.

In addition to certain athletic groups who subject their upper bodies to high repetitive forces, spondylolysis seems to most often develop in children, adolescents, and young adults. Cyron and Hutton (5) suggest that this could be partly due to the fact that the ossification of their neural arches may not be complete and the bone is therefore less stiff and has a lower fatigue life. Or it could be partly due to the fact that the intervertebral discs of young people are more elastic and therefore allow more shear force to reach the facets, increasing the magnitudes of the forces and stresses on the pars. Another cause could be

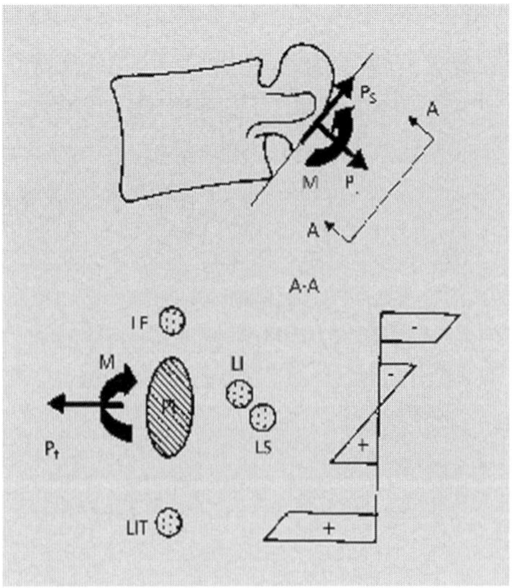

FIG. 2.7. Stresses on the pars.

that most young people engage in more frequent strenuous activity than adults, causing the fatigue life of the pars to be reached sooner.

Cyron and Hutton (5) determined the fatigue life of the lumbar neural arch. They subjected the inferior articular facets of 74 cadaveric human lumbar vertebrae to shear loads cycling between 380 N and 760 N to simulate a man walking quickly in a flexed posture with a 50-kg pack on his back. Over 70% of their specimens failed at the pars, indicating that the neural arch is definitely weakest at the pars, and it was validated that vertebrae from those aged 14 to 30 years failed much sooner (<50,000 cycles) than those from middle-aged people (which still had no fracture even at 500,000 cycles or more). Green et al. (2) suggested that Cyron and Hutton's experiment was perhaps quite unrealistic in dealing with only shear, since in vivo the intervertebral discs and ligaments would limit most of the shear loads going to the facets. Green et al. (2) conducted their own in vitro experiment, in which the ligaments were left intact and gravity and muscle tension were simulated. The greatest deflection and bending indicated the highest stresses. They concluded that when bending and shear were combined, the greatest deflections and stresses, and therefore the greatest risk for pars fracture, would be in hyperextension of the spine.

Inoue et al. (7) evaluated the mechanical effect of the direction of facet load on the isthmus stresses of the lower lumbar neural arch. Stress analyses were performed by using three-dimensional finite element models of isolated L4 and L5 vertebrae. The largest maximal principal stress in the neural arch was quite similar in L4 and L5. The results suggested that the direction of facet load, which may be characterized by the facet orientation, could have mechanical effects on the occurrence and direction of isthmic failure.

CONCLUSION

Biomechanical factors are significant in the development of spondylolysis leading to spondylolisthesis. Gravitational and postural forces cause the greatest stress at the pars interarticularis. Spondylolisthesis can occur at any level of the spine, although it is most common in the lower lumbar spine. Most cases result from minor overuse trauma, particularly repetitive hyperextension of the lumbar spine. Lumbar lordosis as well as rotational and shear forces play a role in the development of lytic pars defects and the fatigue of the pars in the young. An association exists between high levels of activity during childhood and the development of pars defects. A much higher proportion of athletes than nonathletes develop a pars defect. Genetic factors also play a role.

REFERENCES

1. Theiss SM. Isthmic spondylolisthesis and spondylolysis. *J South Orthop Assoc* 2001;10(3):164–172.
2. Green TP, Allvey JC, Adams MA. Bending of the inferior articular processes of lumbar vertebrae during simulated spinal movements. *Spine* 1994;19(23):2683–2691.
3. Motley G, Nyland J, Jacobs J, et al. The pars interarticularis stress reaction, spondylolysis, and spondylolisthesis progression. *J Athl Train* 1998;33(4):351–358.
4. Gatt CJ, Hosea TM, Palumbo RC, et al. Impact loading of the lumbar spine during football blocking. *Am J Sports Med* 1997;25(3):317–321.
5. Cyron BM, Hutton WC. The fatigue strength of the lumbar neural arch in spondylolysis. *J Bone Joint Surg* 1978;60-B(2):234–238.
6. Klemenesics ZL, Kiss RM. The biomechanics of spondylolysis and spondylolysthesis. In: Enderle JD, ed. Proc 22nd Ann Int Conf of IEEE Engineering in Medicine and Biology Society. Piscataway, NJ: IEEE; 2000.
7. Inoue H, Ohmori K, Ishida Y, et al. Finite element analysis of the lower lumbar neural arch under facet loading. *J Spinal Disord* 1998;11(3):241–247.

3

Biomechanics of Spondylolysis with Reference to its Etiology, Diagnosis, Treatment, and Slippage

Koichi Sairyo, Vijay K. Goel, Ashok Biyani, and Nabil Ebraheim

Lumbar spondylolysis is primarily a stress fracture of the pars interarticularis (1–6) and is prevalent in about 6% of the population (7). More than 80% of the cases showing forward slippage, called isthmic spondylolisthesis, accompany this disorder (8). In one fifth of the cases, amount of slippage exceeds 25% of the anterior-posterior (A-P) disc depth. However, the pathomechanism of slippage is still uncertain. For example, there is no consensus about the region in which the slippage occurs: growth plate or the intervertebral disc.

Since spondylolysis and spondylolisthesis are stress-related lumbar disorders, biomechanical studies may help to understand the underlying pathomechanisms. In this chapter, we describe biomechanical investigations for lumbar spondylolysis, mainly from our laboratory, with reference to its etiology, diagnosis, treatment, and slippage.

ETIOLOGY

The etiology of spondylolysis is considered to be a stress fracture at the pars interarticularis. To understand the stress distributions within the spinal elements of a motion segment or functional spinal unit (FSU), we developed a finite element model of the ligamentous L3-S1 segment. The details, including element properties, nonlinear behavior, material properties, and experimental validation, are reported elsewhere (3–5,9–12). Stress distributions in various structures were analyzed in flexion, extension, lateral bending, and axial rotation in response to 400 N axial compression and 10.6 Nm moment. Von Mises stresses at the various structures were computed. The predicted highest stresses were found in the pars interarticularis. Furthermore, the stresses in extension and rotation were higher than in flexion and bending (Fig. 3.1). These results support the clinical observation that pars fracture most often occurs in extension and rotation (13,14).

DIAGNOSIS

For diagnosing spondylolysis, usually plain radiographs, computed tomography (CT) scans, and scintigrams are used. Spondylolysis can be classified into three stages: early, progressive, and terminal (15). The early stage, which follows the stress fracture, shows as a hairline on CT scans. At the progressive stage, the gap at the defect site is clearly visible. The terminal stage is same as pseudoarthrosis, showing sclerosis at the fracture site. Even using CT scan, the early stage is sometimes very difficult to diagnose. The Scottish

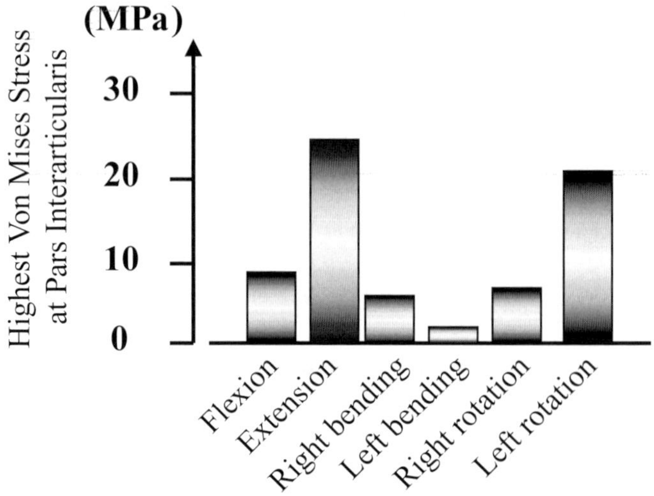

FIG. 3.1. Stresses at pars interarticularis during each lumbar motion.

terrier collar sign on oblique radiographs is the famous and reliable sign. However, the reliability of the sign is questionable in detecting early stages of this disorder.

Magnetic resonance imaging (MRI) is less invasive than computed tomography or plain radiography, and more recently, we have shown that a high signal at the pedicle in an axial slice of T2-weighted MR images can be used effectively for detecting the early stage of the disorder (4). Figure 3.2 demonstrates CT and MRI scans of early stage spondylolysis in two pediatric patients. Both patients show early stage spondylolysis on CT, and the adjoining pedicles show high signal (arrows) on MRI T2-weighted image.

We investigated the pathomechanism of the signal change of pedicle using finite element (FE) analysis. The stresses at the pedicle were second highest, next to the pars interarticularis. Thus, the highest stress at the pars may induce a stress fracture at the site,

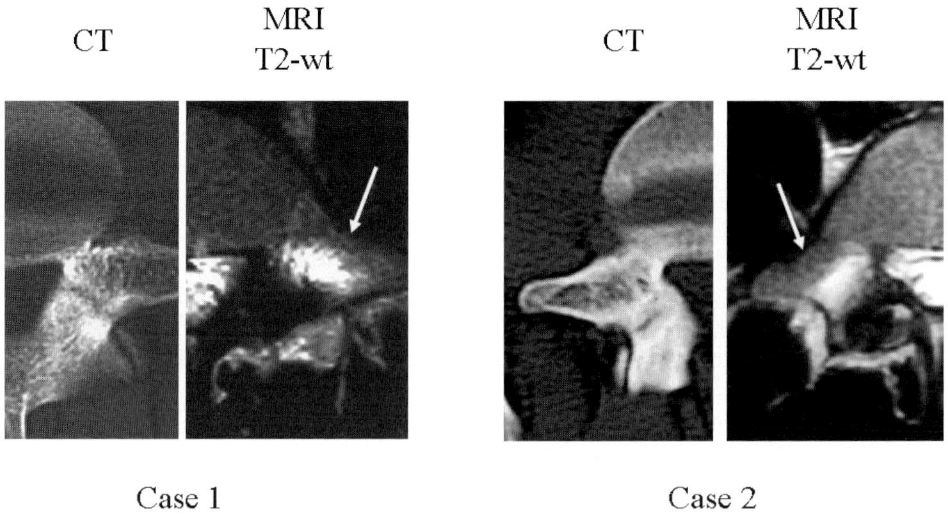

FIG. 3.2. CT and MRI of pediatric patients with the early stage spondylolysis. Arrows on MRI indicate high signal change of the pedicle.

while the second highest stress may cause bone marrow edema due to stress reaction like a condition of bone bruise.

Using MRI, other pediatric lumbar disorders, such as apophyseal bony ring fracture and herniated nucleus pulposus (HNP), can also be diagnosed. Thus, this method can be a valuable tool for screening pediatric patients complaining of low back pain. We propose an axial slice (D) through the pedicle while taking slices around the disc space (A–C) on MRIs (Fig. 3.3). Those slices help diagnosis the apophyseal ring tear and the HNP, while the axial slice facilitates early diagnosis of lumbar spondylolysis. Thus, the addition of the extra MRI slice will assist in correct diagnosis of the three major lumbar disorders in pediatric patients who visit the clinic complaining of low back pain.

TREATMENT

Spondylolysis in its early and progressive stages responds to conservative treatment. Terminal stage defects (pseudoarthrosis) mandate surgical interventions to promote bony union. For conservative treatment, a brace to immobilize the fracture site is usually prescribed along with the cessation of sport activities for at least 3 months (5,15). Finite element analysis was used to determine the relationship between the load type and direction of fracture (Fig. 3.4). This information may help determine the most optimal brace type to prescribe. The stress data indicate that patients can be divided into two categories, extension- or rotation-induced spondylolysis. For patients in whom the fracture indicates a sagittal orientation, the optimal brace would be the one that immobilizes rotary motion. But patients with the fracture angle more coronally oriented need a brace that will effectively immobilize motion in extension. To further prove the hypothesis, clinical prospective trials using a specific brace according to the CT-based fracture angle are essential.

For patients who do not respond to conservative treatment, various surgical options are available in line with the accompanying symptomology. Pars defects repair is indicated in patients with low back pain secondary to pars defect (16). In patients with radiculopathy caused by the impingement of nerve root at the pars defect, decompression of the affected nerve root by removal of loose lamina is essential (17). Intervertebral segmental fusion is routinely indicated to reduce the symptoms due to pars defect and intervertebral discs, such as degeneration and slippage. There is a significant risk of further instability after Gill's laminectomy (18); therefore, concomitant intervertebral fusion has been recommended to prevent further slippage. Most recently, Sairyo et al. (1) have proposed an

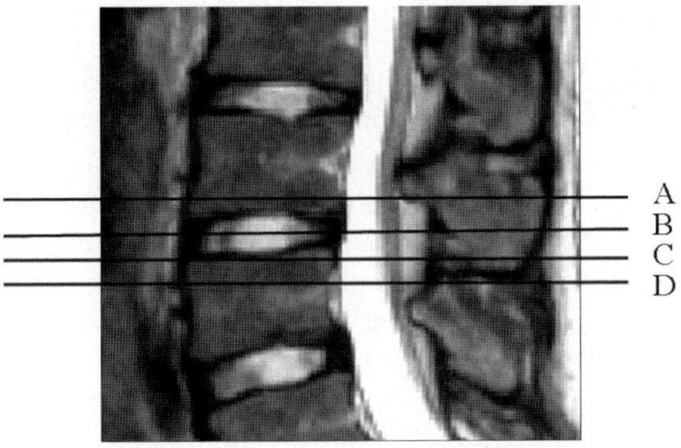

FIG. 3.3. Locations of axial slices on MRI for screening of pediatric patients with low back pain.

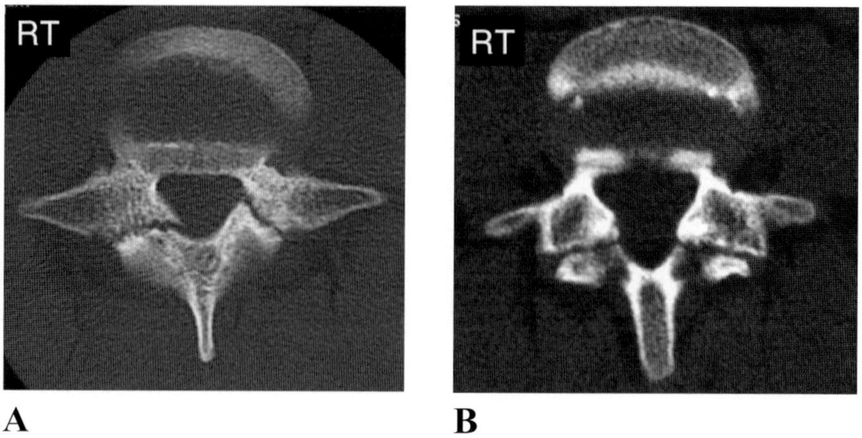

FIG. 3.4. Type of spondylolysis based on the FEM results. **A:** A right defect of (**A**) and both defects on (**B**) are considered to be caused by extension motion. In cotrast, a left defect on (**A**), rotation motion.

endoscopic technique to decompress the impinged nerve root. This procedure leaves the supra- and interspinous ligaments intact; thus, damage to the paravertebral musculature is minimal. Since this technique is minimally invasive, additional arthrodesis may not be necessary. Using FE models, we analyzed the biomechanical changes following laminectomy (as recommended by Gill) and endoscopic decompressive procedure for the spondylolytic spine. Figure 3.5 A–C depicts our models simulating bilateral spondylolysis, Gill's laminectomy, and left-side endoscopic decompression, respectively. In the depictions, the anterior compartment has been removed to highlight the modifications in the posterior structures. The bilateral spondylolysis is simulated at L4 in Figure 3.5A. In Figure 3.5B, the loose lamina at L4 is removed, simulating the Gill's laminectomy. The left side of L4 is decompressed using endoscopic decompression procedure in Figure 3.5C. After the conventional laminectomy (Gill's method), stresses in the disc region increased twofold during flexion, compared to the spondylolysis model (presurgery). The high stresses may facilitate disc degeneration and further slippage. However, endoscopic decompression did not change the stress distribution as compared to the presurgery case (Fig. 3.6). Thus, our analyses support the argument that fusion is not necessary for endoscopic technique although it is an essential accompaniment for Gill's procedure.

SLIPPAGE (ISTHMIC SPONDYLOLISTHSIS)

A consensus is emerging regarding mechanism and site of slippage of the spondylolytic vertebra in children and adolescents. Several biomechanical studies suggest that the most probable site of slippage is the vertebral growth plate; that is, the vertebra slips after the epiphyseal separation, according to these clinical and biomechanical observations (3–5,12,19–24). For example, we conducted a biomechanical study using immature fresh calf spine FSUs with intact growth plates (21,22). After creating the pars defects bilaterally, the FSU was secured into the MTS machine (MTS System, Minneapolis, Minnesota). Anterior shear force was applied to the cranial vertebral body until failure, and the failure site was identified (Fig. 3.7). The superior vertebra slipped forward after the growth plate fracture, indicating that in an immature spine the growth plate is the weakest link against anterior shear force. The calf models are of limited value due to anatomical differences between the calf spine and the human spine; thus, we repeated the

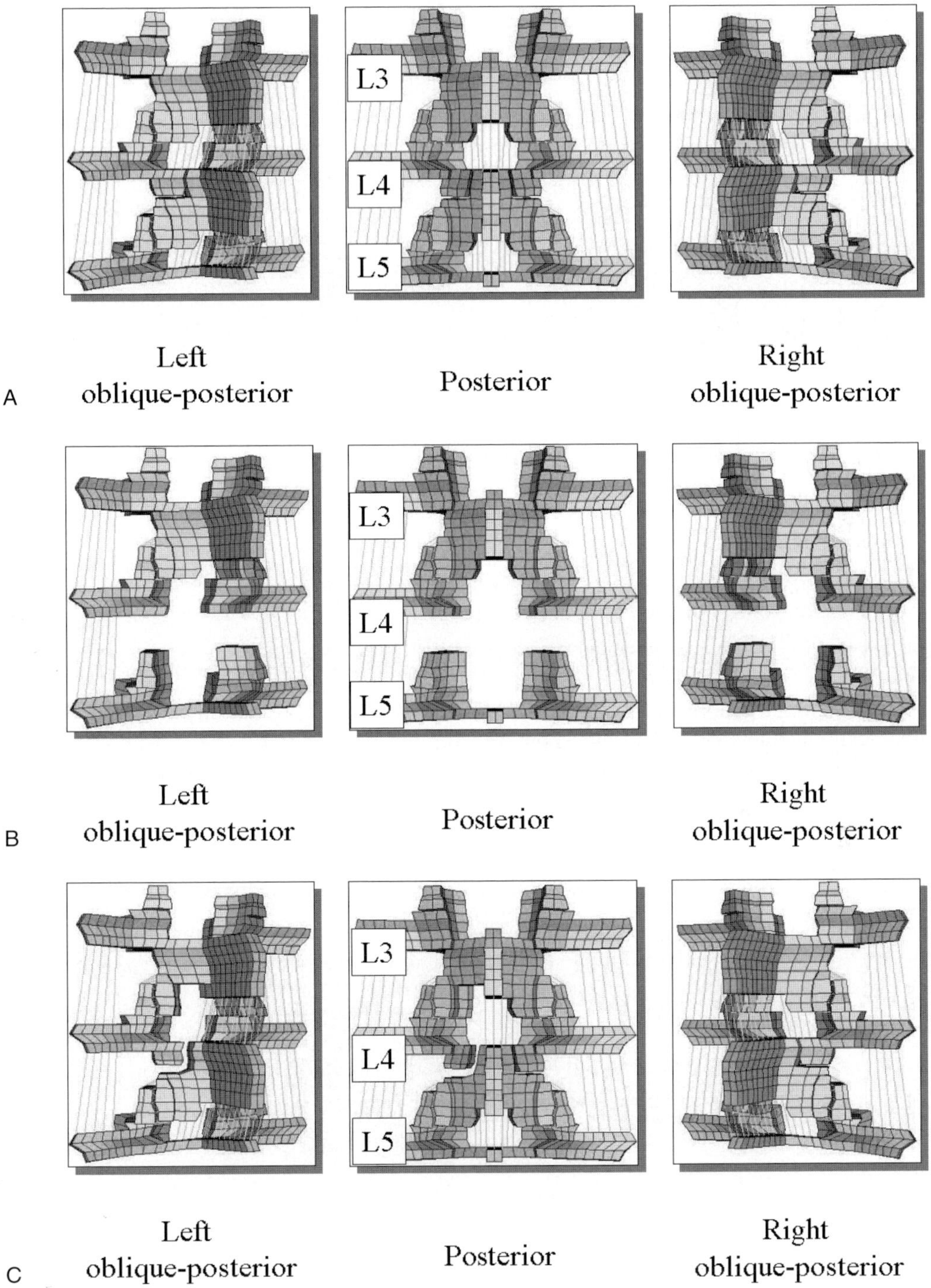

FIG. 3.5. A: Finite element model (L3–L5) of spondylolysis at L4. Bilateral pars defects at L4 are created by creating the gaps. **B:** Finite element model (L3–L5) simulating Gill's laminectomy for L4 spondylolysis. Loose lamina as well as supra- and interspinous ligaments are removed. **C:** Finite element model (L3–L5) after endoscopic decompression at left side for L4 spondylolysis.

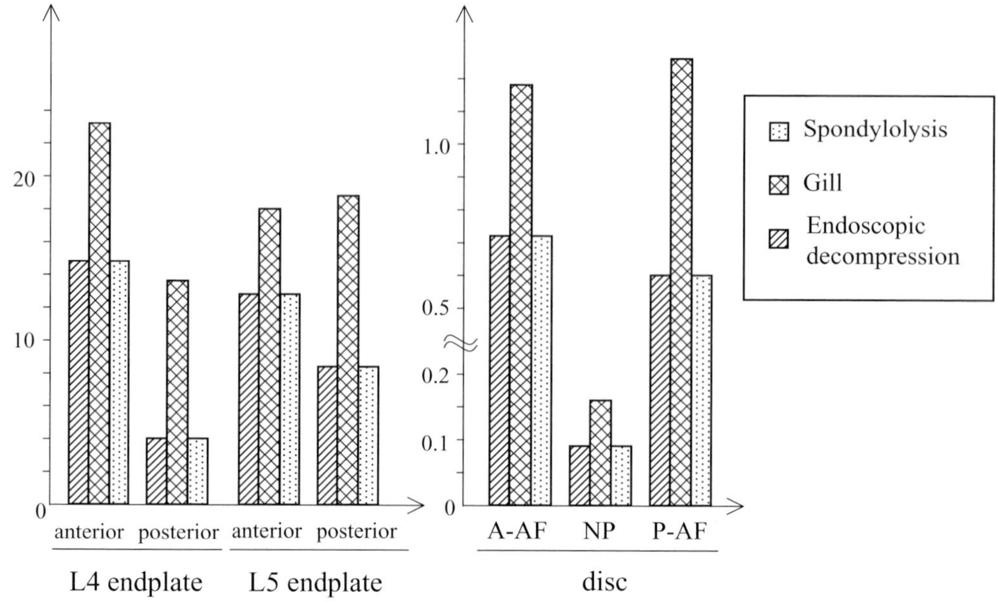

FIG. 3.6. Von Mises Stress values at various structures in all three models. Stresses increase after Gill's laminectomy; however, after the endoscopic surgery, stresses do not change.

experiment using baboon immature spines (12). The results were similar. Based on the clinical study using MRIs of patients showing isthmic slippage, Ikata et al. (20) proposed that the slippage may occur after the separation between osseous and cartilaginous endplates. This proposed slippage site is anatomically the growth plate.

We hypothesized further that the growth plate, being the weakest link, is always more stressed at the lytic vertebra when compared to intact. The increased mechanical stress may weaken the growth plate leading to slippage. To prove this, we created models of the

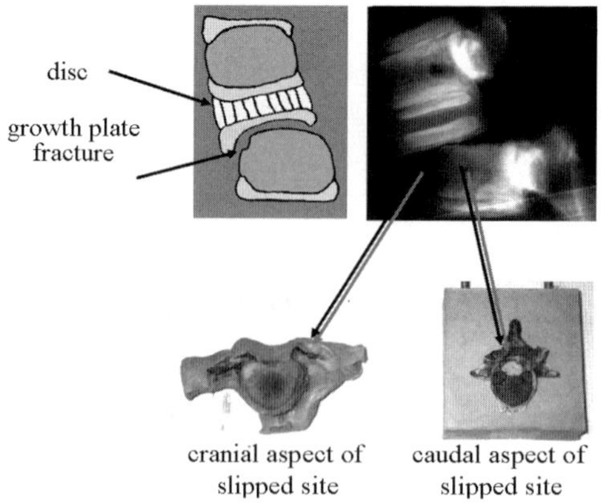

FIG. 3.7. Slippage site. On the radiograph, the cranial vertebral body slips forward following the growth plate fracture of the caudal vertebral body.

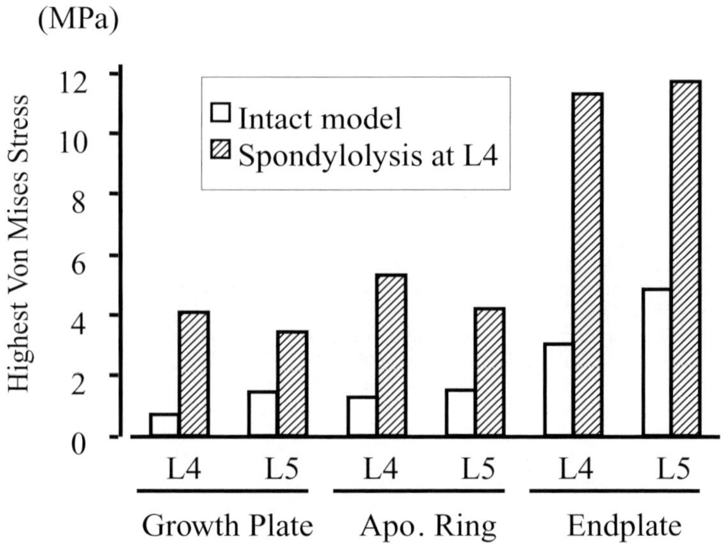

FIG. 3.8. Stresses at various structure during lumbar extension in intact and spondylolysis model. At any structure, stresses are higher in the spondylolysis model when compared to intact.

pediatric intact spine (L3–L5) and L4 spondylolytic lumbar spine. The pediatric lumbar spine model included the growth plate and apophyseal bony ring. During all lumbar motions, the stresses at the growth plate increased in the spondylolytic spine. During extension, increase in stress was much greater than other motions, and stress increased sixfold compared to the intact (Fig. 3.8).

Sakamaki et al. (24) created a rat model showing forward vertebral slippage with epiphyseal separation. Using this model, Sairyo et al. (3) found that the separation did occur after stress fracture of the growth plate. This in vivo animal model further lends support that the growth plate becomes the weakest link following pars defect.

From these clinical and in vitro and in vivo biomechanical studies, we concluded that isthmic spondylolisthesis occurs at the growth plate not at the disc. Thus, we propose the following mechanism for the isthmic spondylolisthesis. First, the spondylolysis in the pediatric spines occurs due to overloading in extension and/or rotation (in sports activities, for example). This leads to an increase in the mechanical stress at the growth plate, the weakest link. Finally, the stress fracture of the growth plate occurs, and it causes forward slippage of the spondylolytic vertebra.

CONCLUSION

In this chapter, we have briefly described biomechanical investigations dealing with lumbar spondylolysis and spondylolisthesis with reference to their etiology, diagnosis, treatment, and slippage. Besides the biomechanical factors, these disorders have genetic predispositions. Thus, biological and genetic investigations are needed as well as biomechanical consideration.

ACKNOWLEDGMENT

Several studies were supported in part by a fellowship grant from DePuy Spine, Inc., Raynham, Massachusetts. The authors wish to thank Miranda N. Shaw, MS, for her editorial assistance.

REFERENCES

1. Sairyo K, Katoh S, Sakamaki T, et al. A new endoscopic technique to decompress lumbar nerve roots affected by spondylolysis: technical note. *J Neurosurg* 2003;98 (3 suppl):290–293.
2. Sairyo K, Katoh S, Sakamaki T, et al. Three successive stress fractures at the same vertebral level in an adolescent baseball player. *Am J Sports Med* 2003;31:606–610.
3. Sairyo K, Katoh S, Sakamaki T, et al. Slippage occurs following epiphyseal separation in immature spine and its occurrence is unrelated to disc degeneration. *Spine* 2004;29:524–527.
4. Sairyo K, Katoh S, Takata Y, et al. MRI signal changes of the pedicle as an indicator for early diagnosis of spondylolysis in children and adolescents: a clinical and biomechanical study. The 31st Annual meeting of ISSLS, Porto, Portugal, May 31–June 5, 2004.
5. Sairyo K, Katoh S, Sasa T, et al. Athletes with unilateral spondylolysis are at risk of stress fracture at the contralateral pedicle and pars interarticularis: a clinical and biomechanical study. *Am J Sports Med* 2005;33:583–590.
6. Wiltse LL, Widell EH Jr, Jackson DW. Fatigue fracture: the basic lesion is isthmic spondylolisthesis. *J Bone Joint Surg Am* 1975;57:17–22.
7. Fredrickson BE, Baker D, McHolick WJ, et al. The natural history of spondylolysis and spondylolisthesis. *J Bone Joint Surg Am* 1984;66:699–707.
8. Saraste H. Spondylolysis and spondylolisthesis. *Acta Orthop Scand* 1993;(suppl):251:84–86.
9. Goel VK, Monroe BT, Gilbertson LG, et al. Interlaminar shear stresses and laminae separation in a disc: finite element analysis of the L3–4 motion segment subjected to axial compressive loads. *Spine* 1995;20:689–698.
10. Goel VK, Ramirez SA, Kong WZ, et al. Cancellous bone Young's modulus variation within the vertebral body of a ligamentous lumbar spine—application of bone adaptive remodeling concepts. *J Biomech Eng* 1995; 117:266–271.
11. Kong WZ, Goel VK. Ability of the finite element models to predict response of the human spine to sinusoidal vertical vibration. *Spine* 2003;28:1961–1967.
12. Konz RJ, Goel VK, Grobler LJ, et al. The pathomechanism of spondylolytic spondylolisthesis in immature primate lumbar spines in vitro and finite element assessments. *Spine* 2001;26:E38–E49.
13. Seitsalo S, Antila H, Karrinaho T, et al. Spondylolysis in ballet dancers. *J Dance Med Sci* 1997;1:51–54.
14. Soler T, Calderón C. The prevalence of spondylolysis in the Spanish elite athlete. *Am J Sports Med* 2000;28:57–62.
15. Fujii K, Katoh S, Sairyo K, et al. Union of defects in the pars interarticularis of the lumbar spine in children and adolescents. *J Bone Joint Surg-B* 2004,86:225–231.
16. Buck JE. Direct repair of the defect in spondylolisthesis: preliminary report. *J Bone Joint Surg* 1970;52-B:432–437.
17. Gill GG, Manning JG, White HL. Surgical treatment of spondylolisthesis without spine fusion. *J Bone Joint Surg* 1955;37-A:493–520.
18. Osterman K, Lindholm TS, Laurent LE. Late results of removal of the loose posterior element (Gill's operation) in the treatment of lytic lumbar spondylolisthesis. *Clin Orthop* 1976;117:121–128.
19. Farfan HE, Osteria V, Lamy C. The mechanical etiology of spondylolysis and spondylolisthesis. *Clin Orthop* 1976;117:40–55.
20. Ikata T, Miyake R, Katoh S, et al. Pathomechanism of sports-related spondylolisthesis in adolescents: radiographic and magnetic resonance imaging study. *Am J Sports Med* 1996;24:94–98.
21. Kajiura K, Katoh S, Sairyo K, et al. Slippage mechanism of pediatric spondylolysis: biomechanical study using immature calf spines. *Spine* 2001;26:2208–2212.
22. Sairyo K, Goel VK, Grobler LJ, et al. The pathomechanism of isthmic lumbar spondylolisthesis: a biomechanical study in immature calf spines. *Spine* 1998;23:1442–1446.
23. Sairyo K, Katoh S, Ikata T, et al. Development of spondylolytic olisthesis in adolescents. *Spine J* 2001;1: 171–175.
24. Sakamaki T, Sairyo K, Katoh S, et al. The pathogenesis of slippage and deformity in the pediatric lumbar spine: a radiographic and histologic study using a new rat in vivo model. *Spine* 2003;28:645–650.

4
Mechanics of Neurological Impingement

Brian J. C. Freeman

Anatomical stenosis of the lumbar spinal canal was first suggested as a cause for spinal stenosis syndromes by Sarpyener (1) and Verbiest (2,3). It is necessary to review the basic anatomy before discussing the classification of lumbar spinal stenosis and in particular the mechanics of neurological impingement in lumbar spondylosis, spondylolysis, and spondylolisthesis.

ANATOMY

The vertebral column houses osseoligamentous spaces that accommodate, protect, and transmit the delicate neurovascular structures. It is essential to define clearly what is meant by the terms *spinal canal*, *nerve root canal*, and *intervertebral foramen.*

Spinal Canal

The spinal canal is formed behind the articulated vertebral body by the posterior elements of the vertebral column. The normal lumbar spinal canal varies in shape as it descends. In the normal state it is circular in cross section in the upper part of the lumbar spine and trefoil in shape at the lower part. The lumbar spinal canal can be divided into a *central* portion and two *lateral* portions. The central portion is occupied by the thecal sac. Hoffman ligaments sequentially attach the thecal sac to the anterior wall of the vertebral canal and posterior longitudinal ligament especially at the disc level.

Nerve Root Canal

The nerve root canal is a tubular conduit that starts in the spinal canal at the point where the nerve root sheath comes off the dural sac and ends where the nerve root emerges from the intervertebral foramen (Fig. 4.1). The length of the canal varies, depending on the site of origin of the root sleeve from the dural sac. The L5-S1 root canal is considerably longer than those running at higher lumbar levels. The *roof* or posterior aspect of the canal is formed by the ligamentum flavum and contiguous borders of the superior articular process and superior margin of the lamina corresponding in number to the nerve root. Further laterally, the roof is formed by the pars interarticularis of this lamina and the ligamentum flavum related to it. The *floor* or anterior aspect is formed by the annulus fibrosus of the intervertebral disc, the posterior surface of the vertebral body, and their soft tissue coverings. The *medial "wall"* of the canal is formed by the dural sac and soft tissues of the epidural space including fat, blood vessel, and nerve. The *lateral wall* is formed first by the medial side and then by the inferior aspects of the pedicle.

The nerve root canal contains the nerve root bundle, radicular arteries, veins, and lymphatic vessels. The nerve root generally occupies the cranial portion of the foramina. The nerve root

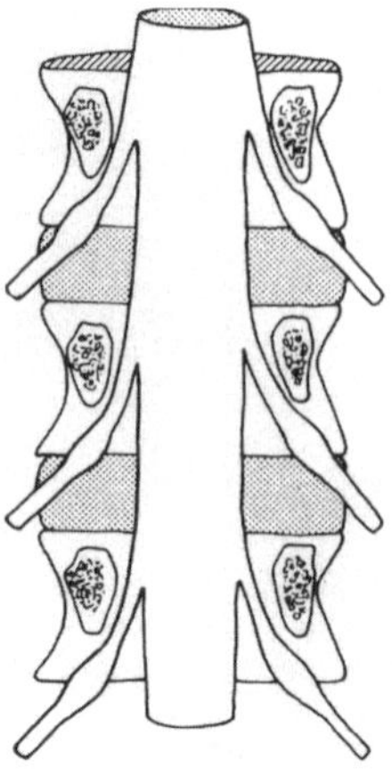

FIG. 4.1. Posterior view of the nerve root canals showing relationship of the nerve root to the pedicles.

canal has been compartmentalized by several authors into the entrance zone, the midzone, the exit zone, and the extraforaminal zone (4–6). These will now be described in detail:

1. The *entrance zone* lies medial to the pedicle and the superior articular process. It is infundibular in shape and accommodates the root sleeve and the unsheathed nerve roots.
2. The *midzone*, also called the subpedicular or pedicle zone, extends from the medial to the lateral pedicle edge, is cylindrical in shape, and contains the nerve root and dorsal root ganglion.
3. The *exit zone,* also known as the foraminal zone or foramen proper, is a shallow annular hiatus, which Crock has compared to a doorway at the end of a passage (6).
4. The *extraforaminal zone*, or postcanal zone, is where far lateral disc herniations, extraforaminal ligaments, and membranes or bony structures such as the transverse process may compress, kink, or constrict lumbar nerves.

Intervertebral Foramen

The intervertebral foramen has the shape of an inverted teardrop. The superior boundary is the pedicle of the vertebra above. The inferior boundary is the pedicle situated caudal to the nerve root. The anterior wall is formed by the posterior aspect of the vertebral body, the intervertebral disc, and the body below. The posterior wall (or roof) is formed by the pars interarticularis, the ligamentum flavum attached to it, and the apex of the superior articular process of the vertebra situated at the inferior aspect of the foramen (Fig. 4.2).

DYNAMIC CHANGES

Dynamic radiographic studies such as flexion/extension radiographs and functional myelography have shown that the dimensions of the spinal canal change dramatically in flexion, extension, and rotation of the spine (7).

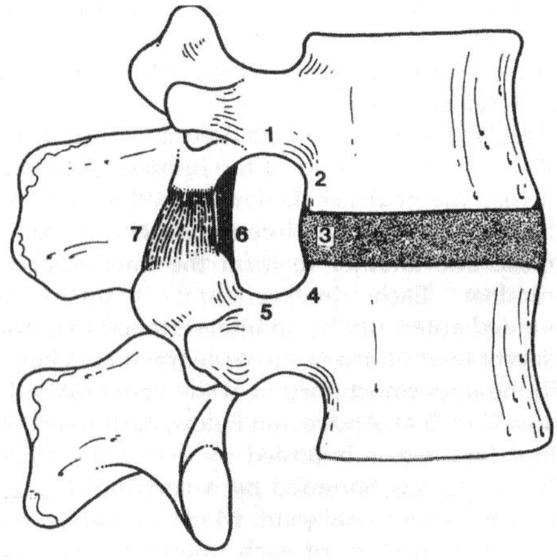

FIG. 4.2. Boundaries of the intervertebral foramen: 1, superior pedicle; 2, posterior vertebral body; 3, intervertebral disc; 4, posterior vertebral body; 5, inferior pedicle; 6, ligamentum flavum; 7, facet joint.

Rauschning has studied cadaveric lumbar spines frozen-in-situ in different functional positions (8). The sagittal dimensions of the *spinal canal* increase in flexion and decrease in extension. During flexion, the vertebral body moves closer anteriorly and farther apart posteriorly, stretching the posterior portion of the annulus fibrosis. The opposite occurs in extension of the spine: the ligamentum flava shorten, become thicker, and buckle and the annulus fibrosus bulges posteriorly causing a decrease of the sagittal dimension of the canal at the intervertebral level. The changes in size and shape of the vertebral canal that occur in flexion or extension are mainly caused by thickening and retraction of the ligamentum flava, and they involve the central spinal canal with the thecal sac undergoing constriction at the intervertebral level.

Dynamic changes in the nerve root canal do occur. They are caused by bulging of the posterolateral region of the disc into the subarticular portion of the nerve root canal and buckling of the anterior capsule of the facet joint. Rotational deformation of the vertebral canal affects the subarticular portion of the root canal. Torsion of a vertebra results in increased posterior bulging of the disc on the side *toward* which torsion occurs. On this side, the nerve root canal decreases in width.

Rauschning reported on 10 lumbar spines with slight to moderate *degenerate* changes frozen in postures known to cause neural compression (9). In specimens with normal intervertebral disc height, *extension* caused the superior articular process to slide superiorly and anteriorly pulling the thick capsular ligamentum flavum anteriorly, compressing and flattening the posterior aspect of the dorsal root ganglion. In this regard the L4/L5 motion segment displays the greatest mobility. In the presence of disrupted intervertebral discs, a vacuum phenomenon was observed in two facet joints when the specimen was frozen in rotation. The root sleeves were compressed and flattened by the bulging annulus fibrosus and the medial portion of the superior articular process and by infolding of the ligamentum flavum.

In most instances, the vertebral canal has a sufficient reserve space to accommodate the neural structures. If this reserve space is limited by pre-existing stenosis of the vertebral canal, even minor additional narrowing causes compression of nervous and vascular structures.

SPINAL STENOSIS

Spinal stenosis may be defined as a narrowing of the central spinal canal, the nerve root canal, or the intervertebral foramen. It may be local, segmental, or generalized. It may be caused by bone or by soft tissue, and the narrowing may involve the bony canal alone or the dural sac or both. Central canal stenosis presents with bilateral symptoms; lateral recess stenosis commonly presents with unilateral symptoms.

Normal canal size has been reported as a midsagittal diameter of greater than 11.5 mm and a cross-sectional area of greater than 1.45 cm^2 (10,11). *Absolute stenosis* is said to occur when the midsagittal diameter of the canal is less than 10 mm, and *relative stenosis* is said to occur when the midsagittal diameter of the canal is between 10 mm and 13 mm (12). The natural history of spinal stenosis remains unclear. There are few longitudinal prospective studies documenting the cause in untreated patients. Existing literature would suggest that symptoms progress in approximately 20% to 33% of nonoperated patients (13).

Lumbar spinal stenosis has been classified by Arnoldi in 1976 (14) (Table 4.1). In primary stenosis, the narrowing of the lumbar spinal canal is caused by congenital malformation (congenital stenosis) or a defective postnatal development of the lumbar vertebra (developmental stenosis) such as achondroplasia or constitutional stenosis. In secondary stenosis, where the spinal cord is developmentally normal, neural compression is due to an *acquired* condition. In this category is spondylotic change possibly associated with degenerative spondylolisthesis. Other possibilities include late sequelae of fractures or infection or systemic bone diseases like Paget disease.

Degeneration in the three-joint complex typically starts the process of spinal stenosis. Synovitis commencing in the facet joints leads to the thinning of articular cartilage and loosening of the joint capsule (15). This leads to greater spinal motion accelerating degeneration in the disc. Disc height is lost leading to a reduction in the size of the neural foramina (so-called up–down stenosis). The ligamentum flavum becomes redundant with infolding, further contributing to a reduction in canal dimensions. Osteophytes on the superior articular facet narrow the lateral recess. Osteophytes on the inferior articular facet narrow the central canal. At the level of the disc, ballooning of the disc and marked

TABLE 4.1. *Classification of lumbar spinal stenosis according to Arnoldi et al. (14)*

1. *Congenital/Developmental Stenosis*
    - a. Idiopathic
    - b. Achondroplastic
2. Acquired
    - a. Degenerative
        - i. Central canal stenosis
        - ii. Peripheral canal stenosis
        - iii. Degenerative spondylolisthesis
    - b. Combined congenital and/or disc herniation
    - c. Spondylolytic or spondylolisthetic
    - d. Iatrogenic
        - i. Postlaminectomy
        - ii. Postfusion
        - iii. Postchemonucleolysis
    - e. Posttraumatic
    - f. Miscellaneous (e.g., Paget disease)

thickening of the ligamentum flavum in combination with hypertrophy of the superior articular process leads to compression of the vertebral canal such that a small triangular conduit is produced. Reduction in canal volume can compromise vascular supply to the neural elements leading to an ischemic neuritis, and direct compression of nerve roots may lead to demyelination, causing unremitting pain.

The *midzone* of the foramen (subpedicular) may be encroached upon by osteophytes at the insertion of the ligamentum flavum. Neural compromise occurs as a result of disc protrusion anteriorly and large facet joint osteophytes posteriorly. At the level of the posterior wall of the vertebral body, the spinal canal may be narrow, but it is never stenotic. Degenerative changes of the superior articular process are responsible for narrowing the root canals. The hypertrophied inferior articular process narrows the posterior portion of the central spinal canal.

SPONDYLOLYSIS

A defect of the pars interarticularis is unique to human beings, who by virtue of being bipedal, transfer considerable weight through this part of the lumbar spine. The incidence of spondylolysis is approximately 4.5% during the first year of school and is more common in boys than girls (16). However, the incidence of symptomatic pars defects in the young, athletic population is much higher and is variously estimated at between 15% and 47% (17).

With increasing age, the inevitable instability in spondylolysis leads to early and severe disc degeneration. This allows translatory and rotatory movement. The "beak" of the pars interarticulares is dislodged anteriorly and inferiorly plunging into the interlamina ligamentum flavum, pushing it anteriorly against the upper endplate of the vertebra below and the posterior annulus fibrosus with resultant nerve root compression (Fig. 4.3 A). Edelson and Nathan in 1986 identified a hooklike projection in the proximal lamina at the inlet to the intervertebral foramen in 32% of specimens with spondylolysis (18). The authors state that this hooklike projection may be responsible for the nerve root compromise in spondylolysis. The authors also comment on fibrocartilaginous tissues in the area of the lysis, together with bony excrescences commonly found on the proximal and distal ends of the neural arch, leading to aggravation of the neural entrapment (Fig. 4.3 B)

Dynamic instability caused by the fracture may irritate the nerve root further. The tissue occupying the defect has been studied by Wiltse (19). He described a well-developed "ligamentous" structure. Soft tissue from this defect has subsequently been shown to contain nerve endings possibly accounting for back pain (20).

SPONDYLOLYTIC SPONDYLOLISTHESIS

Spondylolisthesis is present in 4% of the general adult population (21). Spondylolytic spondylolisthesis is almost never associated with central spinal stenosis; in fact, the anteroposterior diameter of the spinal canal is actually widened. True herniation of the disc at the level of the spondylolytic spondylolisthesis is extremely rare (22)

The neural foramen is narrowed most commonly by the forward shift of L5 on S1. Reduction in disc height can lead to further foraminal stenosis (so-called up–down stenosis) leaving little room for the exiting L5 nerve root. Magnetic resonance imaging is reasonably sensitive in discriminating between nerve roots that are associated with a radiculopathy and those that are not (23). Typically MR image shows circumferential or pincerlike entrapment of the nerve root with obliteration of the perineural fat. For an L5-S1 lytic

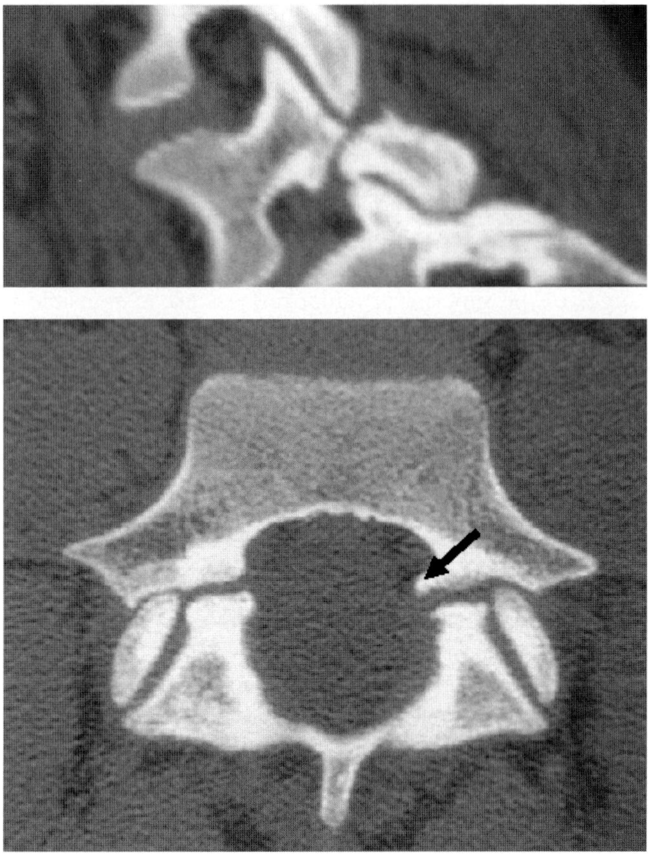
A
B

FIG. 4.3. A: Sagittal reconstruction computed tomography showing spondylolysis of L5 vertebra. The exiting L5 nerve root is just in contact with the "beak." **B:** Reverse gantry CT scan on same patient showing bilateral spondylolysis of L5. Note bony spur on the patient's left side (arrow).

spondylolisthesis, it is the L5 nerve root that is entrapped. This is best shown on the parasagittal T1-weighted MR image (Fig. 4.4).

DEGENERATIVE SPONDYLOLISTHESIS

Degenerative spondylolisthesis occurs when a vertebra is displaced in relation to that immediately below it *without* disruption of the neural arch and in the presence of degenerative changes. Often this condition is associated with central spinal stenosis and hypertrophic changes of the facet joints that result in narrowing of one or both neural foramina. Degenerative changes in the superior articular process lead to nerve root canal stenosis, and hypertrophy of the inferior articular process of the olisthetic vertebra narrows the posterior portion of the *central* canal. The dural sac follows the slipped vertebra as it is tightly held by Hoffman ligaments. Most of the compression occurs between the intervertebral disc and the superior articular process and posterior arch of the slipped vertebra. Inevitably, disc degeneration occurs, resulting in posterior disc bulge into the canal, which contributes further to central stenosis.

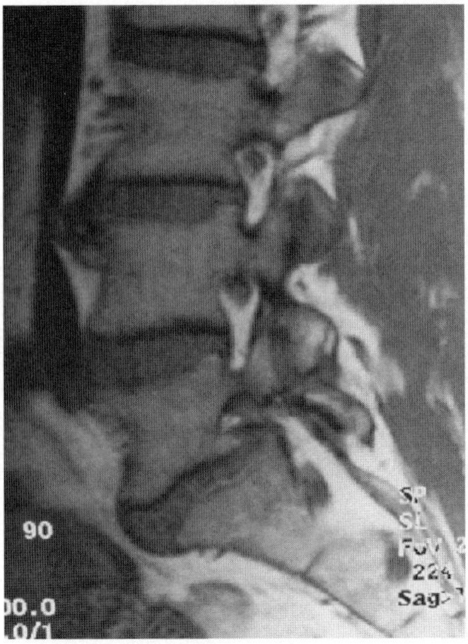

FIG. 4.4. T1-weighted parasagittal MRI. Grade 1 spondylolytic spondylolisthesis with entrapment of the right L5 nerve root. Note the change in shape of the lowermost foramen.

REFERENCES

1. Sarpyener MA. Congenital stricture of the spinal canal. *J Bone Joint Surg* 1945;27:70.
2. Verbiest H. A radicular syndrome from developmental narrowing of the lumbar vertebral canal. *J Bone Joint Surg* 1954;36-B:230–237.
3. Verbiest H. Further experiences on the pathological influence of a developmental narrowness of the bony lumbar vertebral canal. *J Bone Joint Surg* 1955;37-B:576–583.
4. Jenis LJ, An HS. Spine update: lumbar foraminal stenosis. *Spine* 2000;25:389–394.
5. Lee CK, Rauschning W, Glenn W. Lateral lumbar spinal canal stenosis: classification, pathological anatomy and surgical decompression. *Spine* 1988; 13:313–320.
6. Crock H. Normal and pathologic anatomy of the lumbar spinal nerve root canals. *J Bone Joint Surg Br* 1981;63:487–490.
7. Kirkaldy-Willis WH, Wedge JH, Yong-Hing K, et al. Pathology and genesis of lumbar spondylosis and stenosis. *Spine* 1978;3:319–328.
8. Rauschning W. Pathoanatomy of lumbar disc degeneration and stenosis. *Acta Orthop Scand* 1993;64 (suppl 251):3–12.
9. Rauschning W. Normal and pathological anatomy of the lumbar root canals. *Spine* 1987;12:1008–1019.
10. Aryanpur J, Ducker T. Multi-level lumbar laminotomies: an alternative to laminectomy in the treatment of lumbar stenosis. *Neurosurgery* 1990;26:429–433.
11. Ullrich CG, Binet EF, Sanecki MG, et al. Quantitative assessment of the lumbar spinal canal by computed tomography. *Radiology* 1980;137–143.
12. Eisenstein S. The morphology and pathological anatomy of the lumbar spine in South African Negroes and Caucasians with specific reference to spinal stenosis. *J Bone Joint Surg Br* 1977;59:173.
13. Freeman BJC. Laminectomy for spinal stenosis. In: Herkowitz HN, ed. *The Lumbar Spine.* 3rd edition. Official publication of the International Society for the Study of the Lumbar Spine. Philadelphia: Lippincott, Williams & Wilkins, 2004:501–508.
14. Arnoldi CC, Brodsky AE, Cauchoix J, et al. Lumbar spinal stenosis and nerve root entrapment syndromes: definition and classification. *Clin Orthop Relat Res* 1976;115:4–5.
15. Yong-Hing K, Kirkaldy-Willis WH. The pathophysiology of degenerative disc disease of the lumbar spine. *Orthop Clin North Am* 1983;14:491–504.
16. Sales de Gauzy J, Vadier F, Cahuzac JP. Repair of lumbar spondylolysis using Morscher material: 14 children followed for 1–5 years. *Acta Orthop Scand* 2000;71:292–296.

17. Rossi F, Dragoni S. Lumbar spondylolysis: occurrence in competitive athletes: updated achievements in a series of 390 cases. *J Sports Med Phys Fitness* 1990;30:450–452.
18. Edelson JG, Nathan H. Nerve root compression in spondylolysis and spondylolisthesis. *J Bone Joint Surg* 1986;68-B:596–599.
19. Wiltse LL. The etiology of spondylolisthesis. *J Bone Joint Surg* 1962:44-A:539–560.
20. Eisenstein SM, Ashton IK, Roberts S, et al. Innervation of the spondylolysis "ligament." *Spine* 1994;19:912–916.
21. Bail W. Observations on the etiology and frequency of spondylolisthesis and its precursors. *Radiology* 1947;48: 107–102.
22. Wiltse LL. Spondylolisthesis: classification and etiology. In: *American Academy of Orthopaedic Surgery Symposium on the Spine.* St. Louis: CV Mosby; 1969:143–167.
23. Jinkins JR, Rauch A. Magnetic resonance imaging of entrapment of lumbar nerve roots in spondylolytic spondylolisthesis. *J Bone Joint Surg* 1994;76-A:1643–1648.

5

Isthmic and Degenerative Spondylolisthesis: When Does it Hurt and Why?

Tommy Hansson

Spondylolisthesis is frequently regarded as one of the very few specific diagnoses of low back pain and often also sciatica. Spondylolisthesis is defined as a forward displacement of a vertebra relative to the vertebra below. Less frequent and with more indistinct clinical significance, retrolisthesis can be defined as the opposite, a backward displacement of a vertebra relative to the vertebra below. Andre described lumbosacral spondylolisthesis as "the hollow back" as early as the 16th century, and Kilian in 1854 was the first to introduce the term *spondylolisthesis* from the Greek name for vertebra, *spondylos*, and *olisthesis* being a slip.

According to Wiltse et al., the two main types of spondylolisthesis are the isthmic and the degenerative types (1). Much more unusual are the dysplastic, traumatic, and pathological types.

The two main pathophysiological causes or prerequisites of a spondylolisthesis are a defect in the neural arch (the isthmic type) and degenerative changes (the degenerative type). The latter usually is associated with advanced changes in all components of the intervertebral three-joint complex.

DEVELOPMENT AND PROGRESSION

Most investigators favor the opinion that the neural arch defect develops in a congenitally weakened pars, most probably as a fatigue failure. The incidence in newborns has in repeat studies been found to be zero (2–5). In their 45-year follow-up of 30 subjects out of an initial cohort of 500 children, Beutler et al. found that 4.4% had uni- or bilateral pars defects of the lumbar spine at the age of 6 years and that another eight subjects developed a defect between the ages of 12 and 25 years (6). Only one of the women (n = 10) in this unique sample reported back problems in relation to childbearing, but only during one of her pregnancies. A single pain episode during childhood and adolescence was reported, by just one of the 30 subjects, and none reported any severe pain episodes during all the follow-up years. Although only recorded during the last years of the study, the health-related quality of life (SF-36) did not differ from that of age-matched controls (6).

BIOMECHANICS AND RISK FACTORS

It has been noted that when the lumbosacral spine has been subjected to loading, the pars region is quite resistant to tensile bending and shearing stresses but is likely to fail relatively early when loaded repetitively (submaximal loading = fatigue failure). In subjects with a weakened pars region, the stresses caused during normal walking have been assumed to be enough to cause a fatigue failure. Whether the greatest stress on the pars occurs with the spine in flexion or in extension is still not settled.

The shape of the lumbar lordosis has long been related to the occurrence of a lysis or olisthesis. It has not been possible to confirm such a relation when the size of the lordosis was compared in children with spondylolisthesis and normal controls.

Although the size of the lordosis has not been found to strongly influence the risk for an isthmic type of olisthesis, a lot of interest has been focused on the sagittal alignment of the spine as a significant risk factor for a lysis and especially for a slip. For the lumbosacral region, parameters measurable on radiographs, like lumbosacral joint angle, sagittal rotation, sacral inclination and/or rounding, wedging of the vertebral body, and others, have not been shown to increase the risks for either the development of a lysis or the progression of a slip (7,8). In retrospective studies, factors influencing the risk for a progression have been slip percentage, high-grade olisthesis, and slip angle (9–11). Studies have also shown that the measuring error in determining the degree of slip is large, which adds to the difficulty of finding prognostic factors (9–11).

Recently it has been suggested that a more pronounced pelvic incidence appears to be a risk factor for the development of an olisthesis (12). This measure has been described as specific and constant for each individual and is also said to determine the orientation of the pelvis and to be essential for the shape of the lumbar lordosis. The final importance of this measure has to be validated in future prospective studies.

More general factors proposed as risks for the development or progression of a slip, like gender and rapid growth, have never been solidly established.

PAIN MECHANISMS

As stated in the beginning of this chapter, typical symptoms due to a spondylolisthesis are varying degrees of back pain and sciatica. While some with a light or moderate slip have no symptoms at all, others—usually with a larger slip—might exhibit increasing deformity and sometimes severe symptoms.

Whether the spondylolisthesis is of an isthmic or a degenerative type, there are two main pathomechanisms in the generation of pain. The first one is the slip, or the forward translation of the vertebra, itself. At a certain point, the translation compromises the available space for the nerve roots in the cauda to such an extent that direct compression of the nerve roots typically elicits symptoms and signs of neurogenic claudication. A secondary effect of an advanced slip might be a direct stretching of the nerve roots at the actual vertebral level. A third effect of the vertebral translation might be stretching of the back muscles due to the elongation that occurs as a result of the translation.

The compression of the nerve roots in the cauda is likely to cause symptoms when the compression due to translation creates a pressure among the roots that obstructs circulation. In spinal stenosis, the pressure among the nerve roots builds when the available space for the roots, the cross-sectional area of the cauda, is reduced below around 75 mm^2 (13,14). This so-called critical size (CS) was determined on the L3–L4 and L4–L5 levels and not on the L5-S1. It is likely that the CS on this level is less than on the more proximal vertebral levels. As far as known, no studies have tried to define the minimum available space in the spinal canal at the site of the olisthesis.

Forward Translation

It has long been known that the degree of slip does not necessarily relate to the presence of symptoms from the lower back. Longitudinal studies over many years have also shown that, with very few exceptions, patients with spondylolysis or low-grade olisthesis are asymptomatic (15). In spite of these findings, it has long been assumed that a spondylolysis or olisthesis indicates a vulnerable spine.

OLISTHESIS AND WORK-RELATED BACK PROBLEMS

As early as 1929, Bohart suggested that certain radiographic findings, including spondylolysis and spondylolisthesis, indicated a frail spine (16). That suggestion initiated, especially in the United States, the use of preemployment roentgenographs of job applicants' spines. Numerous studies involving tens of thousands of subjects have analyzed the prognostic effects of a lot of different radiographically visible changes in the human spine on the occurrence of work-related back problems. Spondylolysis and olisthesis irrespective of isthmic or degenerative have usually been two of the visible changes found in studies of that type.

A unique opportunity to evaluate the relevance of a lysis or olisthesis for the development of acute and/or more long-lasting back problems leading to back disability occurred when the x-ray archives at an occupational clinic became available (17). The films from 615 sets of spinal examinations were studied. The films consisted of 208 preemployment screening radiographs of longshoremen. Two hundred seven of the films were taken at the time of acute back injury claims by longshoremen whose employers did not use preemployment radiographic screening. Two hundred were selected among longshoremen disabled by back problems for more than half a year. Since most of the longshoremen were men, the study was restricted to men. All three groups were randomly selected from the files except 50 subjects in the group with long-lasting disability. To avoid skewed age distribution between this group and the other two groups, these 50 were instead randomly selected among subjects below the age of 30 years with long-term back disability.

The x-ray examinations of all participants were made during the same 9-month period. The examinations included anteroposterior and lateral projection of the lumbosacral spine, including spot views of the L5-S1 region.

All the roentgenograms were scrutinized for the presence or absence of:

- Spondylolysis, including whether bilateral or unilateral pars defects, but with no displacement over the neighboring vertebra.
- Spondylolisthesis, as a forward displacement of one vertebral body in relationship to the underlying vertebral body. No attention was given in spondylolisthesis cases to the presence or absence of lysis.

The study showed that in spite of the selection used, those in the chronic disabled group tended to be somewhat older than those in the control and the acute groups. As can be seen in Table 5.1, there was no difference between the incidence of either lysis or olisthesis in the control, acute, or chronic groups. Since the same finding has been made in several other studies, it seems shown beyond most objections that neither lysis or olisthesis will increase the risk for either acute or long-lasting work-related back problems.

TABLE 5.1. *The relative incidence of spondylolysis and spondylolisthesis on radiographs of subjects without (controls) and with acute or chronic low back problems.*

	Control	Acute	Chronic	p-value
Spondylolysis	9.1	4.4	7.5	> 0.5
Spondylolisthesis	4.3	2.9	4.0	> 0.5

INSTABILITY

Instability resulting from motions either in the pars defect or possibly due to the degenerative processes in the intervertebral joint is, besides the nerve compression effects of the slip, a source of pain and symptoms in spondylolisthesis. Irrespective of the direct cause of the instability, its significance is still heavily debated. A lot of different methods have been used to study the intervertebral motions in both the isthmic and the degenerative types of spondylolisthesis. Examples of such methods used are flexion–extension and biplanar radiography, videofluoroscopy, and stereophotogrammetry.

When eight patients with isthmic spondylolysis or olisthesis were studied with roentgen stereophotogrammetry and their results were compared with those from a control group, no significant differences were found in the intervertebral mobility along the sagittal or the vertical axis of motion. The transverse translations were found to be negligible in both the groups (18,19).

MRI

During the last years, open magnetic resonance imaging (MRI) has become available and has allowed imaging with the lumbosacral spine in different positions. Comparison of subjects with and without olisthesis has revealed no signs of instability or hypermobility of the lumbar spine (20,21). It must be remembered that techniques like radiostereophotogrammetry and open MRI without cine function still represent a static examination technique although they allow comparisons of different positions.

Cineradiography makes it possible to study the kinematics. When that was done in subjects with symptomatic degenerative olisthesis at the L4 level and comparisons were made with asymptomatic volunteers, considerable differences in motion patterns were found (22). In the nondegenerated spines, flexion–extension of the lumbar spine occurred as a harmonic motion. In the subjects with a degenerative olisthesis at the L4–L5 level, less than 15% showed a large flexion–extension motion and what the authors called a disordered motion pattern. Those with a slip greater than 15% demonstrated, on the other hand, less motion in translation but also a disordered motion pattern of the lumbar spine throughout the flexion.

Intervertebral Motion Device (IMD)

Some years ago we introduced a device for dynamic determination of the motion between adjoining vertebrae. We called it the intervertebral motion device (IMD) (23). The IMD is rigidly fixed to the vertebrae through metal pins inserted around 15 to 20 mm into the spinous processes of two adjacent vertebrae (Fig. 5.1). The device consists of a linkage transducer system that permits the measurement of the sagittal plane. The system

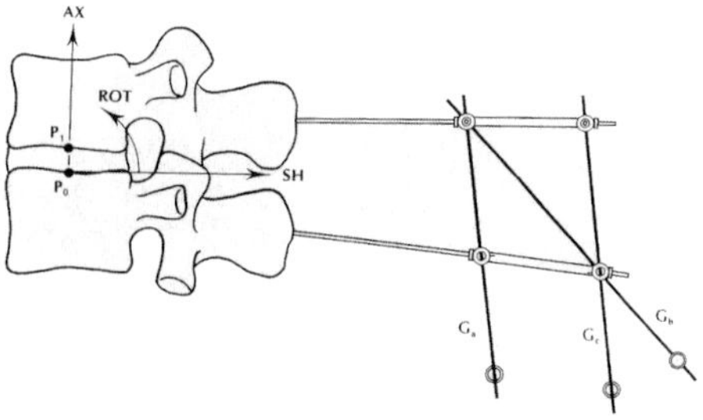

FIG. 5.1. A schematic drawing of the IMD, or intervertebral motion device, for dynamic measurement of intervertebral motions.

is highly repeatable and has accuracy (root mean square, or RMS, error) of 0.4 degrees and 0.14 mm for rotary and translatory movements, respectively (23). Three displacement transducers detect the motion, which occurs between the pins during flexion–extension (Fig. 5.2).

When the IMD is used for measuring motions in a human spinal segment, a goniometer fixed to the body records the total trunk flexion–extension simultaneously. Studies with the IMD in back patients with assumed segmental instability indicated that the total flexion–extension motion in the tested intervertebral joint usually was very small. That led us to believe that the *pattern of motion* was of greater interest than just determining the achieved angle at the end of a motion (24–26).

The stability of the spine is based on both active and passive systems (27,28). The vertebrae, the intervertebral discs, and the ligaments are the main elements of the passive

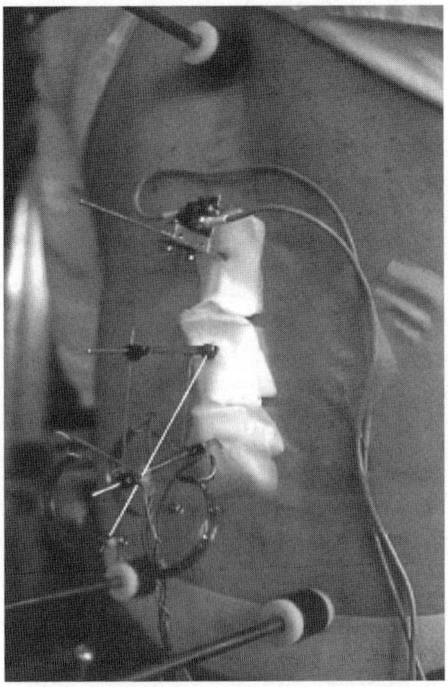

FIG. 5.2. The IMD implanted in the spinous processes of two adjacent vertebrae in the lumbar spine.

system, while the muscles and tendons surrounding the spine constitute the active system. Panjabi has postulated that impairments in any of these components can result in changes like functional compensation by another system, compensation by changes (like hypertrophy) in the other systems, or impairment of other systems. It was further postulated that decreased function in one of those systems would be accompanied by typical clinical symptoms (27,28). As strongly suggested by the IMD findings in subjects with, for example, supposed segmental instability, function and stability of the spine might to a large extent be upheld by compensatory mechanisms (24).

Movements like flexion–extension in the lumbar spine are directed by an intrinsic neuromuscular system that involves passive structures like the intervertebral disc, ligaments, bone, and active structures like muscles and their tendons inclusive. A disorder or injury might disturb the neuromuscular balance and cause dysfunction and/or pain. In back-healthy subjects flexion–extension is a pain-free movement. It is accomplished by appropriately timed excitation of all the involved muscles.

During the deeper part of flexion of the lumbar spine, several studies have shown that there is a spontaneous reduction in electric activity of the erector spinae muscles (29,30). This reduction in myoelectric activity was referred to as a "flexion–relaxation" phenomenon. It was suggested that the muscular activity was shut off by signals from receptors in the spinal ligaments stimulated through stretching of them during deep trunk flexion (30). More recent studies in our group have made this explanation the most plausible for the decreased muscular activity during deep flexion of the lumbar spine (31).

One of many structures stretched during deep flexion is the facet joint capsules, known to contain proprioceptors (31,32). Experimental studies on our pig model have demonstrated that stretching of those joint capsules elicit inhibitory responses in the lumbar paraspinal muscles (31).

It is reasonable to assume that structures like the disc, posterior ligaments, and fascia, as well as stretched but electrically silent muscles, provide stability during "the flexion–relaxation" period (29,33). It has been also shown that the more lateral lumbar muscles, the quadratus lumborum and the iliocaostalis, were activated, whereas the more medial muscles (multifidus) were inactivated during deep and progressive flexion (29,33). In other words, the spine is not only guarded by passive structures during deep flexion but by muscles as well, albeit they are more laterally located than previously thought.

Absence of the flexion–relaxation is a common finding in chronic low back pain. Since a continuous back muscle activity during deep trunk flexion has been found closely correlated with ongoing pain, the presence of the phenomenon can be used as such a pain indicator. It seems reasonable to assume that absence of flexion–relaxation is an indicator of current back pain irrespective of whether the problems are acute, subacute, or chronic in nature.

IMD and the Pattern of Intervertebral Motion

The pattern of motion, the muscular activity, and the overall trunk motion were determined during dynamic flexion–extension in seven patients with chronic low back pain (24). Their pain was supposedly caused by changes that might affect the stability of at least one intervertebral joint in the lumbar spine. All of the subjects had an olisthesis of degenerative type with the largest slip of less than 20%. Their supposed segmental instability diagnosis was based on pain history, clinical findings, and the pronounced radiographic change, greater than in one of the L2–L3, L3–L4, L4–L5, or L5-S1 intervertebral joints. The pain history included sudden stabbing pain episodes, especially during certain movements of the spine and typically when the spine was not "guarded." The patients also had difficulty flexing the lumbar spine or rising from a flexed position. All the patients had at least two of the four following radiographic criteria on the suspected level.

1. Anterior–posterior translation >3 mm on lateral view static standing radiographs.
2. Angulatory disc space collapse accompanied by translation of the affected vertebra on flexion–extension radiographs
3. Pronounced disc space narrowing (>50% lowering of disc height compared to the nearest disc of normal height).
4. Apparent traction spurs on both sides of the disc.

In all but one patient, there was just one supposed unstable intervertebral joint. One patient had two possible unstable segments. Both levels were studied in this patient (24). The suspected levels were three L2–L3, two L3–L4, and three L4–L5. Two adjacent motion segments were studied in half of the controls.

Using continuous measuring techniques, the muscular behavior could be precisely defined in relation to the segmental motion throughout the flexion–extension movement the subjects performed (Fig. 5.3). An identical protocol was used in the control group of six volunteers without any recent back problems. The patient group consisted o four men and three women (mean age 51.4, range 46–56 years). The control group consisted of three men and three women with a mean age of 40.5, range 38–48 years (24).

Human in Vivo IMD

In the study, Steinmann pins (2.6 mm diameter) were rigidly fixed under surgical conditions to the neighboring spinous processes on the actual vertebral level. The IMD was then secured to the pins (Fig. 5.1). In subjects in whom two segments were tested, the caudal

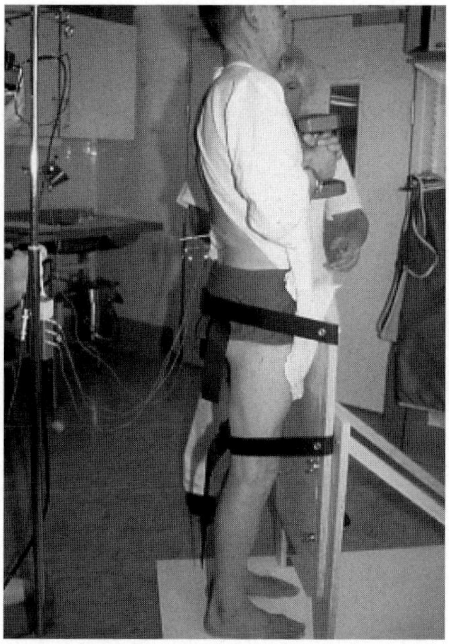

FIG. 5.3. Kinematic measurements of a patient with symptomatic degenerative olisthesis.

motion segment was tested first (24). The trunk flexion–extension angle was simultaneously measured during the flexion–extension protocol using a goniometer attached to the side of the upper right arm of the subject. During testing the subject was instructed to hold the arms and hands firmly against the chest and to maintain a constant position during the flexion–extension.

EMG

Electromyographic (EMG) activity of the lumbar erector spinae muscles was recorded during the flexion–extension from two sets of surface electrodes placed bilaterally to the L3–L4 inter space and 3 cm lateral to the spinous process recording signals from the lumbar part of the longissimus thoracis lumbar fibers.

Flexion–Extension of the Trunk

When performing the flexion–extension protocol, the subjects were asked to maintain sagittal plane symmetry of the body. Beginning from an erect standing posture, the subject bent forward as deep as possible, after which the subject reversed the direction of the movement, passing through the neutral position, and continued until maximum extension was reached and then returned to the neutral position.

Kinematics in Experimental Clinical Study

For all three kinematic variables, sagittal rotation, axial translation, and shear translation, the ranges of motion were significantly *less*, at least 50%, among the patients than among the controls. The controls also flexed and extended their trunks more than the patients. As in the animal models, the maximum range of motion did not necessarily occur at the endpoints and the maximum range not always was equal to the end range of motion. This was especially pronounced for the axial translation and here more for the patients than for the controls.

There were many differences in the pattern of motion between patients and controls. Overall, it was found that the patients displayed *less* intervertebral motion than the controls and especially so in flexion. Even the axial translation, motion was less in the patients (24).

EMG Behavior

For the controls under forward flexion, the EMG activity increased to a maximal value. After that maximum value, a progressive decrease in myolelectric activity occurred to full trunk flexion, that is, the flexion–relaxation phenomenon. From full flexion, the EMG activity increased dramatically to a maximal value and therefore decreased to practically no activity in full extension.

In the patients, the EMG activity increased but not as much or to a peak value as in the controls. This meant that there was no flexion–relaxation. From full flexion, the pattern in the patients was similar to that in the controls.

Pattern of Motion in Degenerative Olisthesis

This study showed that intervertebral motion was significantly *less*, by at least 50% in the patients with a symptomatic degenerative olisthesis/segmental instability. Trunk flexion and extension were also significantly reduced in the patients. In the control group, flexion–relaxation was demonstrated by a 78% increase in EMG activity. In contrast, most of the patient-subjects demonstrated absolutely no flexion–relaxation. Flexion–relaxation in the controls occurred in those in whom intervertebral rotation had reached a stage of completion before maximum trunk flexion was achieved (24).

Compensatory Muscular Activity and Back Pain in Degenerative Olisthesis

Experimental studies have shown that reflex activity causing contraction of the paraspinal muscles will be elicited upon injury to the annulus fibrosus or mechanical deformation of the supraspinal ligament (34–36). That reflex activity will result in a stiffening of the motion segments. We interpreted the findings in the symptomatic patients measured with IMD as most probably having a "segmental instability" instability, however compensated for by an increased continuous back muscle activity, stiffening (24,25). Presently we cannot decide whether the muscular activity is caused by a postural or pain-elicited reflex activity or a combination of both. Since long-lasting pain usually is modulated by higher centers, psychological factors might play an important role at least hypothetically facilitating for the central connections and thus amplifying the muscular activity and the stiffening of the back.

The extent to which this muscular activity contributes to the back pain is not known. Several pain mechanisms are possible, such as accumulation of metabolites, impaired blood supply, and even the development of compartment syndrome (37).

Muscular Pathology in Degenerative Olisthesis

When biopsies from the paravertebral muscles were taken from patients undergoing surgery for symptomatic monosegmental olisthesis, histology including immune and enzyme histochemistry and electron microscopy revealed several severe pathological alterations (38). A marked higher than normal frequency of Type 1 muscle fibers indicated that the muscles in this patients had been subjected to an extreme increase in static strain.

Most other disturbances of the normal muscle found in this group of patients were less specific, indicating myopathy, aging, severe metabolic disorders, etc.

REFERENCES

1. Wiltse LL The etiology of spondylolisthesis. *Am J Orthop* 1962;44-A:539–560.
2. Fredrickson BE, Baker D, McHolick WJ, et al. The natural history of spondylolysis and spondylolisthesis. *J Bone Joint Surg Am* 1984; 66(5):699–707.
3. Hensinger RN. Spondylolysis and spondylolisthesis in children and adolescents. *J Bone Joint Surg Am* 1989;71(7):1098–1107.
4. Wiltse LL, Newman PH, Macnab I. Classification of spondylolisis and spondylolisthesis. *Clin Orthop Relat Res* 1976;117:23–29.
5. Newman PH. A clinical syndrome associated with severe lumbo-sacral subluxation. *J Bone Joint Surg Br* 1965;47:472–481.
6. Beutler WJ, Fredrickson BE, Murtland A, et al. The natural history of spondylolysis and spondylolisthesis: 45-year follow-up evaluation. *Spine* 2003;28(10):1027–1035.
7. Legaye J, Duval-Beaupere G, Hecquet J, et al. Pelvic incidence: a fundamental pelvic parameter for three-dimensional regulation of spinal sagittal curves. *Eur Spine J* 1998;7(2):99–103.
8. Huang RP, et al. Predictive value of pelvic incidence in progression of spondylolisthesis. *Spine* 2003;28(20): 2381–2385.
9. Frennered AK, Danielson BI, Nachemson AL. Natural history of symptomatic isthmic low-grade spondylolisthesis in children and adolescents: a seven-year follow-up study. *J Pediatr Orthop* 1991;11(2):209–213.

10. Danielson B, Frennered K, Irstam L Roentgenologic assessment of spondylolisthesis. I. A study of measurement variations. *Acta Radiol* 1988;29(3):345–351.
11. Danielson B, Frennered K, Selvik G, et al. Roentgenologic assessment of spondylolisthesis. II. An evaluation of progression. *Acta Radiol* 1989;30(1):65–68.
12. Labelle H, Roussouly P, Berthonnaud E, et al. Spondylolisthesis, pelvic incidence, and spinopelvic balance: a correlation study. *Spine* 2004;29(18):2049–2054.
13. Schonstrom N, Bolender NF, Spengler DM, et al. Pressure changes within the cauda equina following constriction of the dural sac: an in vitro experimental study. *Spine* 1984;9(6):604–607.
14. Schonstrom N, Hansson T. Pressure changes following constriction of the cauda equina. An experimental study in situ. *Spine* 1988;13(4):385–388.
15. Saraste H. Long-term clinical and radiological follow-up of spondylolysis and spondylolisthesis. *J Pediatr Orthop* 1987;7(6):631–638.
16. Bohart WH. Anatomic variations and anomalies of the spine. *JAMA* 1929;92:698–704.
17. Bigos SJ, Hansson T, Castillo RN, et al. The value of preemployment roentgenographs for predicting acute back injury claims and chronic back pain disability. *Clin Orthop Relat Res* 1992;283:124–9.
18. Axelsson P, Johnsson R, Stromqvist B. The spondylolytic vertebra and its adjacent segment: mobility measured before and after posterolateral fusion. *Spine* 1997;22(4):414–417.
19. Axelsson P, Johnsson R, Stromqvist B. Is there increased intervertebral mobility in isthmic adult spondylolisthesis? A matched comparative study using roentgen stereophotogrammetry. *Spine* 2000;25(13):1701–1703.
20. McGregor AH, Anderton L, Gedroyc WM, et al. Assessment of spinal kinematics using open interventional magnetic resonance imaging. *Clin Orthop Relat Res* 2001;392:341–348.
21. McGregor AH, Anderton L, Gedroyc WM, et al. The use of interventional open MRI to assess the kinematics of the lumbar spine in patients with spondylolisthesis. *Spine* 2002;27(14):1582–1586.
22. Takayanagi K, Takahashi K, Yamagata M, et al. Using cineradiography for continuous dynamic-motion analysis of the lumbar spine. *Spine* 2001;26(17):1858–1865.
23. Kaigle AM, Pope MH, Fleming BC, et al. A method for the intravital measurement of interspinous kinematics. *J Biomech* 1992;25(4):451–456.
24. Kaigle AM, Wessberg P, Hansson TH. Muscular and kinematic behavior of the lumbar spine during flexion-extension. *J Spinal Disord* 1998;11(2):163–174.
25. Kaigle AM, Holm SH, Hansson TH. Experimental instability in the lumbar spine. *Spine* 1995;20(4):421–430.
26. Kaigle AM, Holm SH, Hansson TH. 1997 Volvo Award winner in biomechanical studies. Kinematic behavior of the porcine lumbar spine: a chronic lesion model. *Spine* 1997;22(24):2796–2806.
27. Panjabi MM. The stabilizing system of the spine. Part I. Function, dysfunction, adaptation, and enhancement. *J Spinal Disord* 1992;5(4):383–389.
28. Panjabi MM. The stabilizing system of the spine. Part II. Neutral zone and instability hypothesis. *J Spinal Disord* 1992;5(4):390–397.
29. Andersson E, Oddsson L, Grundstrom H, et al. The role of the psoas and iliacus muscles for stability and movement of the lumbar spine, pelvis and hip. *Scand J Med Sci Sports* 1995;5(1):10–16.
30. Sihvonen T, Partanen J, Hanninen O, et al. Electric behavior of low back muscles during lumbar pelvic rhythm in low back pain patients and healthy controls. *Arch Phys Med Rehabil* 1991;72(13):1080–1087.
31. Indahl A, Kaigle A, Reikeras O, et al. Electromyographic response of the porcine multifidus musculature after nerve stimulation. *Spine* 1995;20(24):2652–2658.
32. Cavanaugh JM, Ozaktay AC, Yamashita HT, et al. Lumbar facet pain: biomechanics, neuroanatomy and neurophysiology. *J Biomech* 1996;29(9):1117–1129.
33. Andersson EA, Oddsson LI, Grundstrom H, et al. EMG activities of the quadratus lumborum and erector spinae muscles during flexion-relaxation and other motor tasks. *Clin Biomech* (Bristol, Avon) 1996;11(7):392–400.
34. Solomonow M, Zhou BH, Harris M, et al. The ligamento-muscular stabilizing system of the spine. *Spine* 1998;23(23):2552–2562.
35. Stubbs M, Harris M, Solomonow M, et al. Ligamento-muscular protective reflex in the lumbar spine of the feline. *J Electromyogr Kinesiol* 1998;8(4):197–204.
36. Indahl A, Kaigle AM, Reikeras O, et al. Interaction between the porcine lumbar intervertebral disc, zygapophysial joints, and paraspinal muscles. *Spine* 1997;22(24):2834–2840.
37. Styf J, Lysell E. Chronic compartment syndrome in the erector spinae muscle. *Spine* 1987;12(7):680–682.
38. Ramsbacher J, Theallier-Janko A, Stoltenburg-Didinger G, et al. Ultrastructural changes in paravertebral muscles associated with degenerative spondylolisthesis. *Spine* 2001;26(20):2180–2185.

6

Imaging of Lumbar Spondylolisthesis

Jean-Louis Dietemann, Adriana Bogorin, Robertson Correia Bernardo, and Georg Zöllner

Radiological investigations using plain films, multidetector row helical computed tomography (CT) with multiplanar reformations, magnetic resonance imaging (MRI), and lumbar myelography may recognize the type of spondylolisthesis, evaluate the degree and progression of the slip, explain the clinical presentation, and help the physician to choose the appropriate treatment.

SPONDYLOLISTHESIS

Diagnosis of spondylolisthesis is obtained on lateral plain films of the lumbar spine performed in upright position, CT with sagittal reformations, or sagittal MR imaging of the lumbar spine. Lumbar spondylolisthesis may decrease, even disappear in supine position.

Measurement of the slip degree, using lateral plain radiographs obtained in upright position, is based on Meyerding's classification, Taillard's index, or Wiltse-Winter index. Meyerding's classification describes five slip grades: grade 1 = 25%, grade 2 = 25% to 50%, grade 3 = 50% to 75%, grade 4 = 75% to 100%, and grade 5 = more than 100% corresponding to a complete dislocation, called spondyloptosis. Using Taillard's index or Wiltse-Winter index, the degree of slip is expressed as a percentage (1–3) (Fig. 6.1).

CLASSIFICATION OF SPONDYLOLISTHESIS

Lumbar spondylolisthesis is classified into five main types (1–3):

Type 1: Dysplastic or Congenital Spondylolisthesis

Dysplastic spondylolisthesis occurs at birth or early in life and is related to dysplasia of the upper sacrum (absence or dysplasia of the superior articular facets of S1 or elongated pars of L5). The slip is marked (grade 5 or spondyloptosis); the L5 vertebra may be displaced in front of S1 (Fig. 6.2). Hypoplasia and wedging of the L5 vertebral body is noted. Sacral rounding involving the upper aspect of S1 is usually observed. CT confirms absence or dysplasia of articular facets or bilateral elongated pars interarticularis; CT with sagittal reformations and MR imaging evaluate the degree of slip and foraminal and central canal stenosis (Fig. 6.3). There is usually an important central canal stenosis with compression of the dural sac and nerve roots between the neural arch of L5 and the posterior part of the S1 body (4).

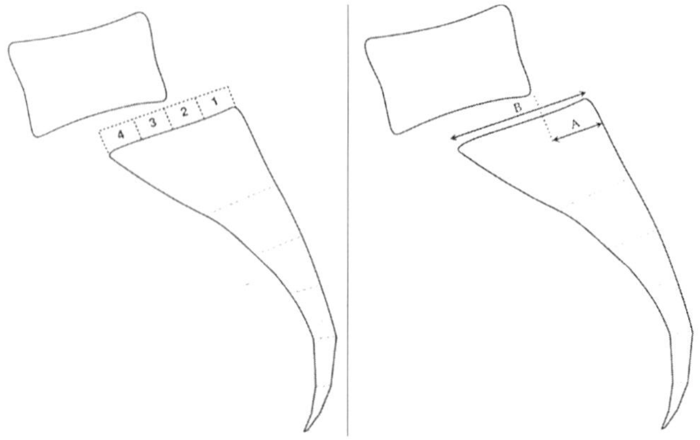

A B

FIG. 6.1. Slip grades. **A:** Meyerding's slip grades. **B:** Taillard's index (A/B X 100).

Type 2: Isthmic Spondylolisthesis

Three subtypes are described: subtype A is related to a stress fracture of the pars interarticularis. In subtype B there is no defect but the pars interarticularis appears elongated; repeated healed microfractures are probably the cause of pars elongation. Subtype C corresponds to an acute fracture related to severe trauma.

Isthmic spondylolisthesis (subtype A) related to a stress or fatigue fracture (spondylolysis) involves the pars interarticularis of L5 in 90% of cases and usually occurs between the ages of 5 and 7. The spondylolisthesis appears between the ages of 10 and 15 and rarely increases after age 20 (2).

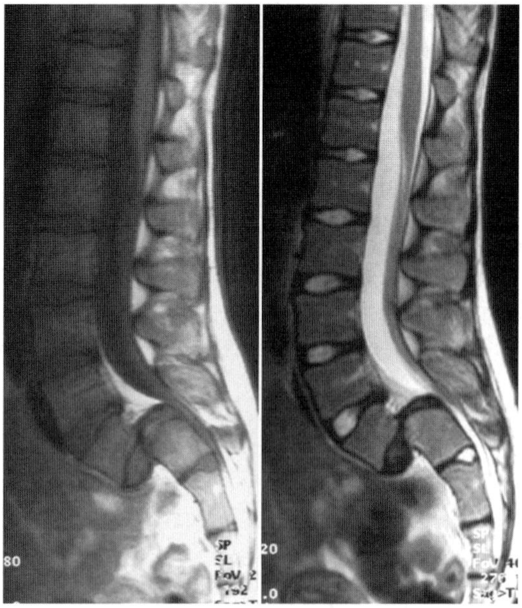

A B

FIG. 6.2. Dysplastic L5-S1 spondylolisthesis. **A:** Sagittal MR imaging with T1 and (**B**) T2 weighted imaging. Grade 5 spondylolisthesis severe stenosis of the dural sac at the level of the listhesis.

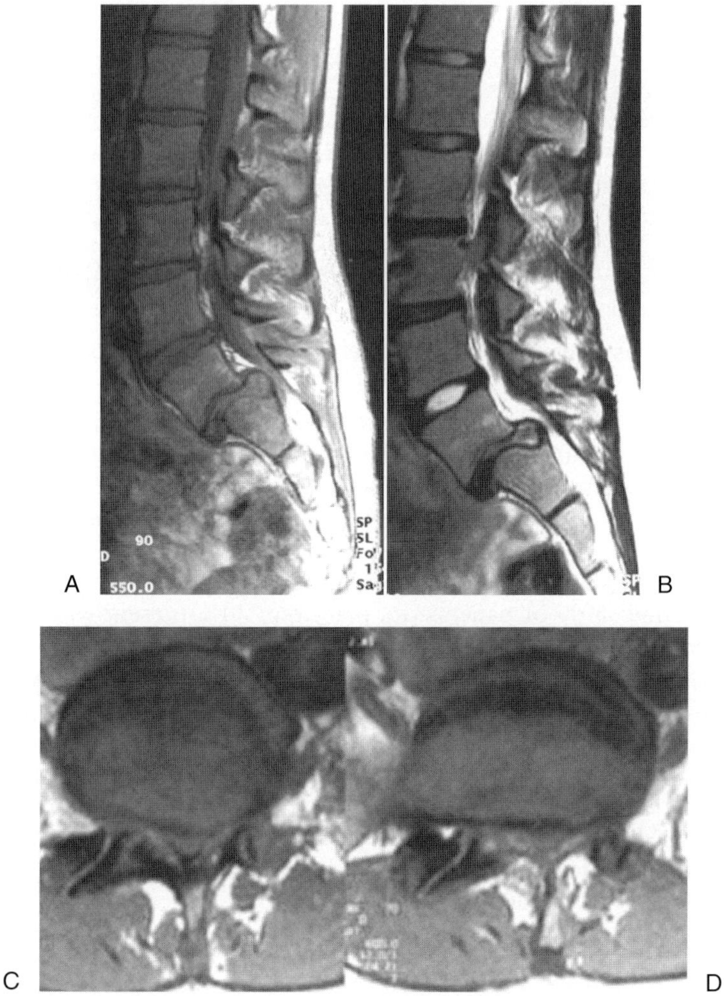

FIG. 6.3. Dysplastic L5-S1 spondylolisthesis demonstrated on sagittal T1 (**A**) and T2 (**B**) sagittal MR weighted imaging related to agenesis of the left articular process of S1 and dysplasia of the right articular process of S1 demonstrated on axial T1 weighted imaging (**C,D**).

Plain films and CT demonstrate the defect involving the pars interarticularis. Spondylolysis associated with spondylolisthesis is best identified on coned lateral, anteroposterior with 30 degrees cranial angulation, and oblique plain radiographic projections (5) (Fig. 6.4). Visualization of the spondylolysis may be difficult on plain radiographs in the earliest stages before spondylolisthesis occurs. Multidetector helical CT with multiplanar reformations using thin section and reverse plane axial angulation allows precise analysis of the neural arch and appears superior to MR imaging for confirmation of the spondylolysis (5). However, improved visualization of the pars interarticularis is possible by using thin (3 mm) reverse-angle oblique axial T1W images (6,7). Axial CT may recognize recent and old stress fractures. However, CT may appear normal in the earliest stage of spondylolysis, before the fracture appears. At this stage, bone scan may reveal unilateral or bilateral increased activity involving the neural arch. MR imaging may demonstrate at the earliest stage of the stress fracture, low signal on T1 weighted imaging (WI), high signal on T2 WI, particularly on T2-STIR WI, and enhancement involving the pars interarticularis

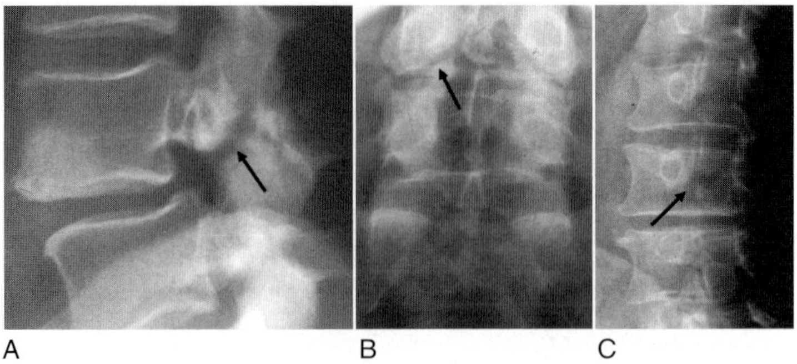

FIG. 6.4. Spondylolysis demonstrated on lateral (**A**), frontal (**B**), and oblique (**C**) plain radiographs of the lumbar spine (*arrows*).

but also the adjacent pedicles and the soft tissues surrounding the neural arch; these abnormalities are related to edema and increased vascularization (8,9) (Fig. 6.5).

Unilateral spondylolysis may induce hypertrophy and bone sclerosis within the contralateral neural arch (Fig. 6.6). Rarely, the stress fracture involves the pedicle or the lamina (Fig. 6.7).

The clinical presentation of patients with spondylolysis with or without spondylolisthesis appears varied: 50% of patients are pain-free, 30% present with back pain, and 20% present with radicular pain. Radicular pain is rarely related to disc herniation located at the level of the listhesis; the disc herniation presents usually an ascending migration (Fig. 6.8). Disc herniation may sometimes occur at the level above the slippage. False disc herniation may be related to hypoplasia and posterior wedging of L5 (Fig. 6.9). Radicular pain is mainly caused by stenosis of the foramen related to the slip, the disc space narrowing and to the bulging disc (Fig. 6.10). Traction osteophytes may develop laterally and posteriorly with the possibility of nerve root compression within the foramen; sagittal CT reformations are needed for the visualization of the osteophyte (Fig. 6.11). A fibrocartilagenous mass (Gill's node) arising on the margins of the pars defect may develop medially and compress the dural sac (10) (Fig. 6.12). Narrowing of

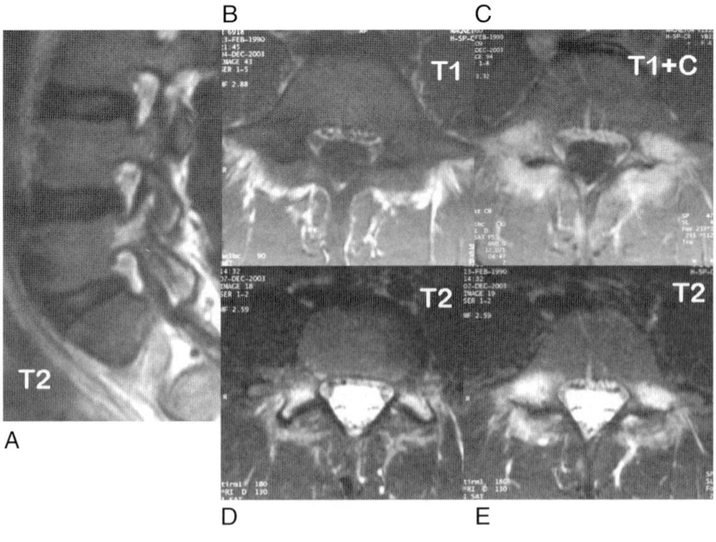

FIG. 6.5. Bilateral spondylolysis at the early stage. Note the hyperintense signal on T2 WI involving the neural arch (**A,D,E**). On T1 WI, this area appears hypo-intense (**B**) and enhancement is demonstrated on postcontrast T1 WI (**C**).

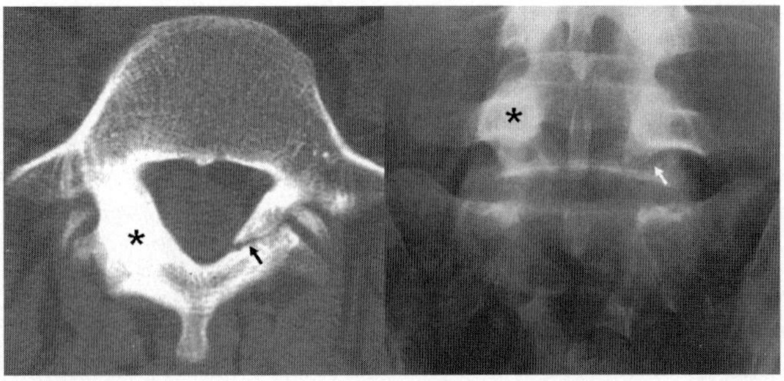

A B

FIG. 6.6. Unilateral spondylolysis involving the left neural arch of L5 demonstrated by axial CT (**A**) and frontal view (**B**) (*arrow*). Note hypertrophy and bone sclerosis of the right neural arch (*star*).

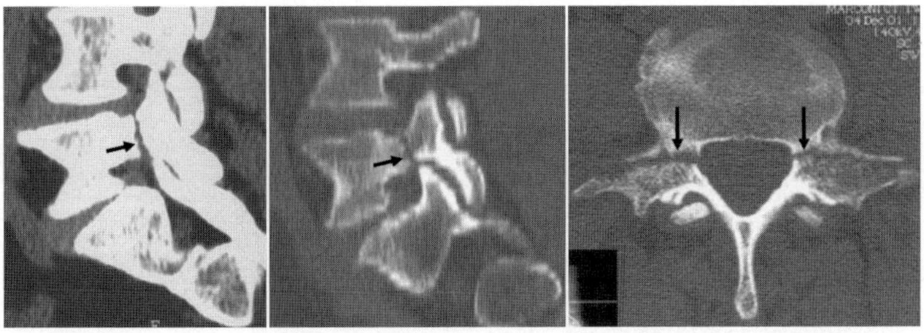

A B C

FIG. 6.7. Bilateral stress fracture involving the pedicles of L5 (*arrow*).

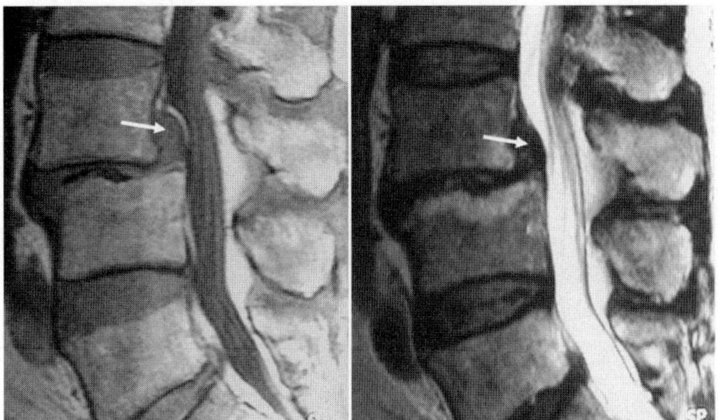

A B

FIG. 6.8. Grade 2 L3–L4 spondylolisthesis. Sagittal T1 WI (**A**) and T2 WI (**B**) visualize median ascending disc herniation (*arrow*).

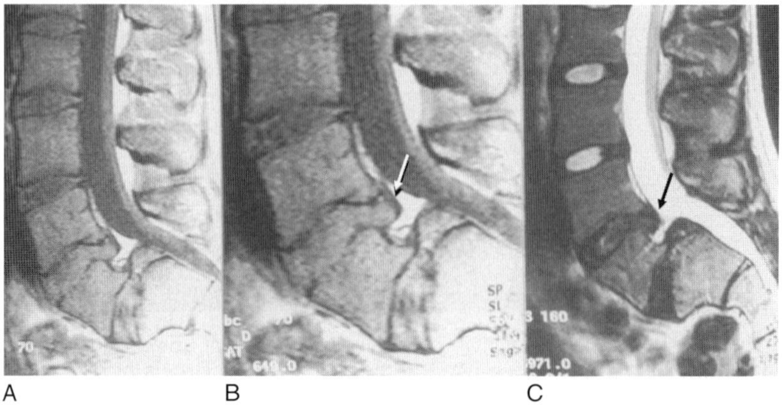

FIG. 6.9. False L4–L5 disc herniation on T1 WI (**A,B**) and T2 WI (**C**). The posterior bulging of the L4–L5 disc (*arrow*) is related to hypoplasia and posterior wedging of L5 (the "kissing discs").

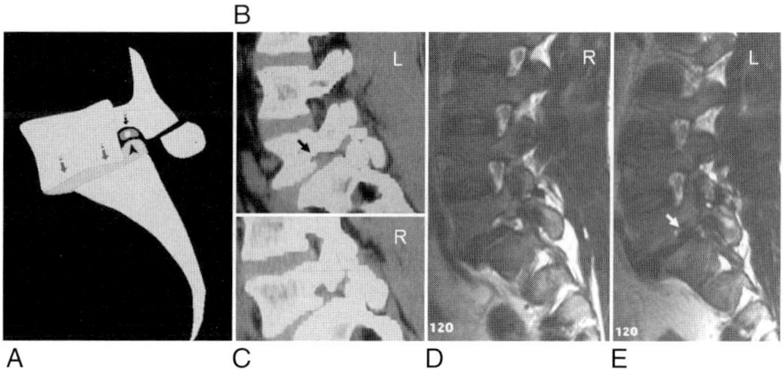

FIG. 6.10. L5-S1 spondylolisthesis related to spondylolysis. Narrowing of the left foramen (*arrow*).

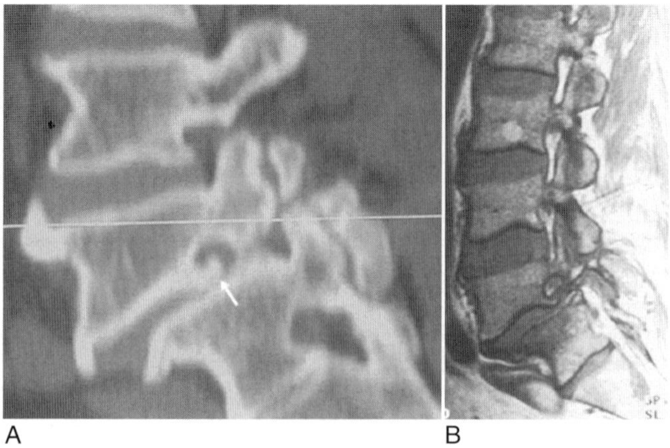

FIG. 6.11. L5-S1 spondylolysthesis. Sagittal CT reformation (**A**) and sagittal T1 WI (**B**) demonstrating foraminal stenosis related to traction osteophyte (*arrow*).

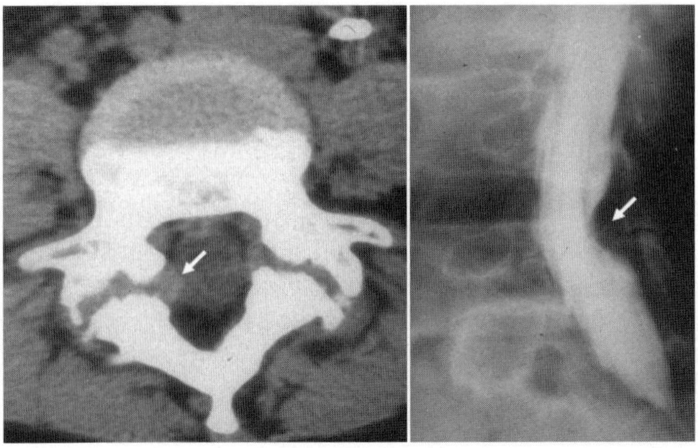

A B

FIG. 6.12. Bilateral L5 spondylolysis. The fibrocartilagenous mass (Gill's node) arising from the pars interarticularis defect is demonstrated on CT (**A**) and myelography (**B**) and may compress the dural sac (*arrow*).

the transverse diameter of the spinal canal related to Gill's node is possible, but sagittal narrowing is only observed with degenerative spondylolisthesis; spondylolisthesis related to spondylolysis is associated with an increased anteroposterior diameter (11).

Back pain may sometimes be explained by inflammatory changes involving end plates at the level of spondylolisthesis with Modic type 1 changes on MR imaging (Fig. 6.13).

Type 3: Degenerative Spondylolisthesis (or Spondylolisthesis with Intact Neural Arch, or Pseudospondylolisthesis)

Degenerative spondylolisthesis is related to degenerative changes involving the apophyseal joints and intervertebral disc. CT and MR imaging evaluate the degree of slip, central canal, lateral recess, and foraminal stenosis related to degenerative changes;

A 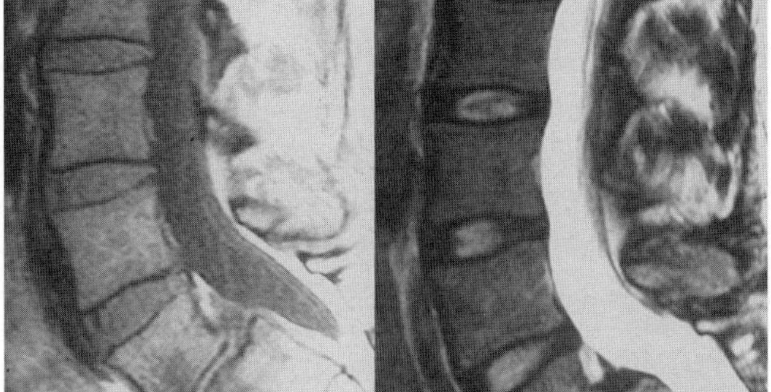 B

FIG. 6.13. L5-S1 spondylolisthesis with Modic type 1 changes involving the adjacent end-plates.

lumbar myelography or open MR imaging may help to appreciate the degree and extent of the stenosis and radicular compression particularly in upright position and during dynamic studies.

Patients with degenerative spondylolisthesis may present with back pain, radicular pain, bilateral neurogenic claudication, or cauda equina syndrome. Back pain is related to degenerative disc disease, degenerative facet joints, and instability with subluxations (Fig. 6.14). Osteoarthritis of the apophyseal joints may lead to hypertrophy of the joints and to the development of synovial cysts with central canal, lateral recess, and foraminal stenosis responsible for nerve root entrapment (Fig. 6.15). Multidetector helical CT with multiplanar reformations and MR imaging may clearly identify these changes and evaluate compression of the dural sac and nerve roots. MR imaging using T2-STIR WI and postcontrast T1 WI may demonstrate inflammatory changes involving the apophyseal joints (Fig. 6.16). However, CT and MR imaging are performed in supine position leading to an underestimation of the degree of stenosis and nerve root entrapment and of the extent of the stenosis (Fig. 6.17). Information from myelography or MR imaging performed on an open MR system obtained in upright position with dynamic studies may be required (12,13) (Fig. 6.18).

Type 4: Traumatic Spondylolisthesis

Traumatic spondylolisthesis related to fracture involving the pars interarticularis or posterior elements other than pars interarticularis is rare and results from major trauma (14). Iatrogenic spondylolisthesis may be observed after surgery with ablation of the joint for spinal stenosis related to apophyseal joint osteoarthritis. Multidetector helical CT

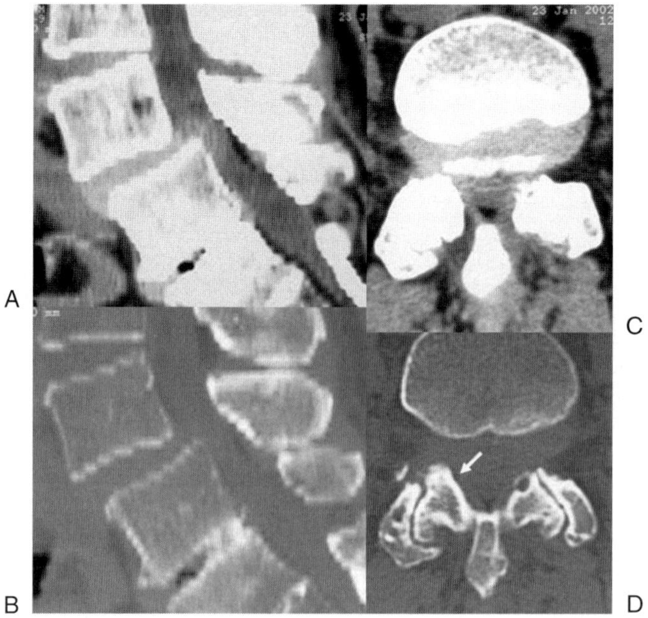

FIG. 6.14. Degenerative spondylolisthesis. Sagittal reformations (**A,B**) show grade 1 L4–L5 spondylolisthesis. Axial CT (**C,D**) demonstrate hypertrophy of apophyseal joints and subluxation on the right side (*arrow*).

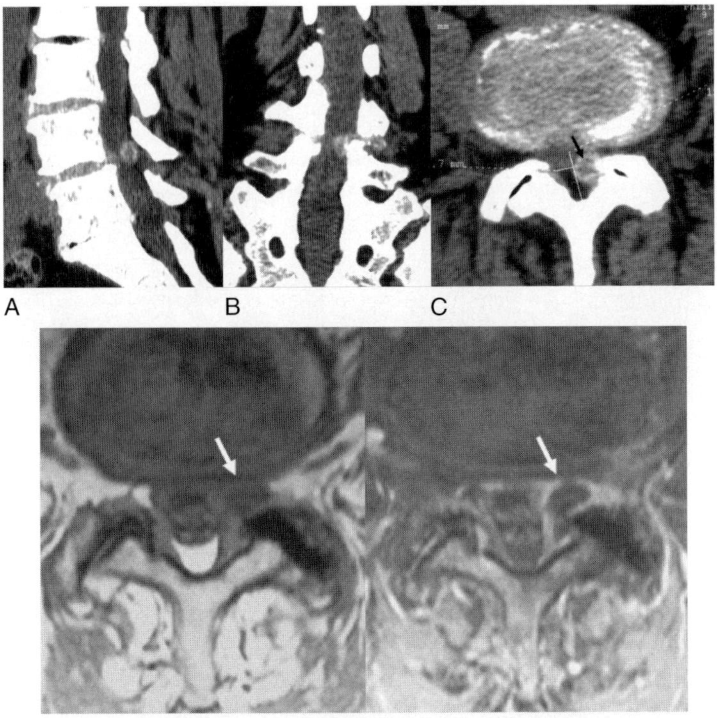

FIG. 6.15. L4–L5 degenerative spondylolisthesis. Sagittal (**A**), frontal (**B**), and axial CT scans (**C**) show a left synovial cyst (*arrows*). Axial MR scans with T1 WI (**D**) and postcontrast T1 WI (**E**) demonstrate enhancement of the wall of the cyst (*arrows*).

with multiplanar reformations may demonstrate the fractures involving the neural arch. MR imaging is required if neurologic signs are noted.

Type 5: Pathologic Spondylolisthesis

Pathologic spondylolisthesis is related to generalized bone disease (osteogenesis imperfecta, osteomalacia, achondroplasia) or localized bony changes (Paget disease,

A 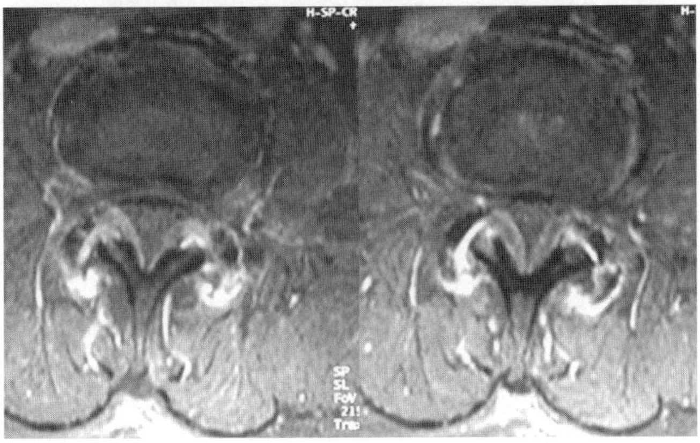 B

FIG. 6.16. Degenerative changes involving L4–L5 apophyseal joints. Postcontrast T1 WI show enhancement within the joint and involving the surrounding soft tissues.

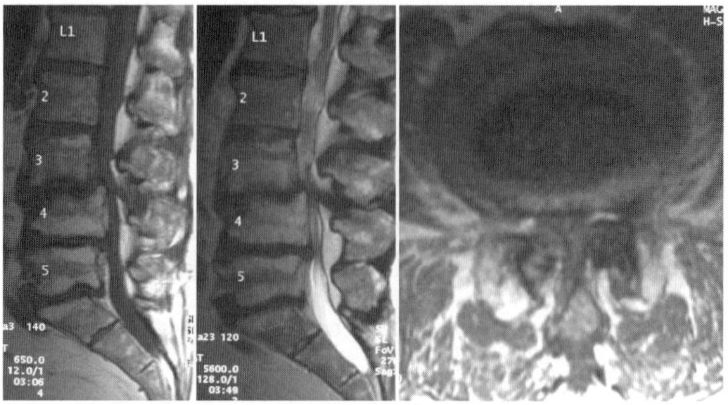

A B C

FIG. 6.17. Degenerative L3–L4 spondylolisthesis. MR imaging with sagittal T1 (**A**), T2 (**B**), and axial T1 (**C**) weighted images demonstrate severe canal stenosis involving L3–L4 and L4–L5 levels.

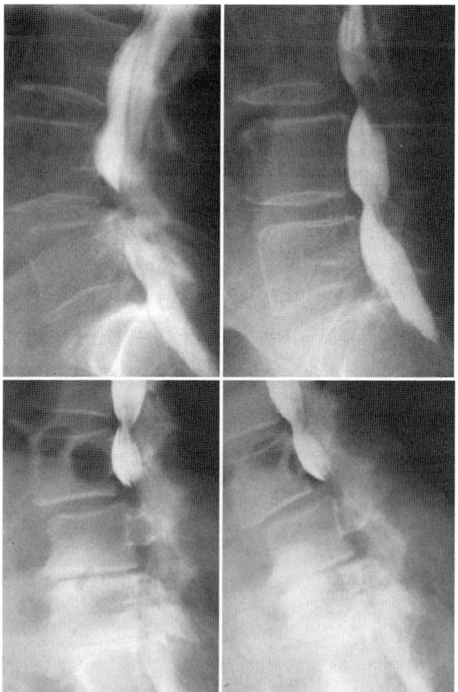

A B C D

FIG. 6.18. Myelography of degenerative spondylolisthesis in three different patients. **A:** Grade 1 L4–L5 spondylolisthesis with severe central canal stenosis. **B:** Mild spondylolisthesis involving the L3–L4 and L4–L5 levels with severe stenosis related to bulging disc. **C:** Complete stop at the L3–L4 level. **D:** Same patient as in (C); the dynamic study with flexion shows instability.

metastasis) (2). Neurofibromatosis type 1 may induce thinning of the neural arch and vertebral scalloping related to dilatation of the dural sac and may induce fatigue fracture involving the pars interarticularis, the pedicle or the lamina (15). CT and MR imaging allow precise evaluation of bony changes.

CONCLUSION

Plain radiographs and multidetector helical CT with multiplanar reformations may demonstrate the spondylolisthesis and define the type. MR imaging and sometimes dynamic myelography are required for the evaluation of dural sac and nerve roots compression.

REFERENCES

1. Dietemann JL, Dosch JC, Steib JP. *Imagerie des Spondylolisthésis.* Paris: Masson; 1994.
2. McCulloch JA, Transfeldt EE. *Macnab's Backache.* 3rd edition. Baltimore: Williams & Wilkins; 1997.
3. Wiltse LL, Winter RB. Terminology and measurements of spondylolisthesis. *J Bone Joint Surg* 1983;65-A:768–772.
4. Leone LD, Lamont DW. Diagnosis and treatment of severe dysplastic spondylolisthesis. *J Am Osteopath Assoc* 1999;99:326–328.
5. Harvey CJ, Richenberg JL, Saifuddin A, et al. The radiological investigation of lumbar spondylolysis. *Clin Radiol* 1998;53:723–728.
6. Campbell RS, Grainger AJ. Optimization of MRI pulse sequences to visualize the normal pars interarticularis. *Clin Radiol* 1999;54:63–68.
7. Udeshi UL, Reeves D. Routine thin slice MRI effectively demonstrates the lumbar pars interarticularis. *Clin Radiol* 1999;54:615–619.
8. Stabler A, Paulus R, Steinborn M, et al. Spondylolysis in the developmental stage: diagnostic contribution of MRI. *Röfo* 2000;172:33–37.
9. Ulmer JL, Elster AD, Mathews VP, et al. Lumbar spondylolysis: reactive marrow changes seen in adjacent pedicles on MR images. *AJR Am J Roentgenol* 1995;164:429–433.
10. Major NM, Helms CA, Richardson WJ. MR imaging of fibrocartilaginous masses arising on the margins of spondylolysis defects. *AJR Am J Roentgenol* 1999;173:673–676.
11. Ulmer JL, Elster AD, Mathews VP, et al. Distinction between degenerative and isthmic spondylolisthesis on sagittal MR images: importance of increased anteroposterior diameter of the spinal canal ("wide canal sign"). *AJR Am J Roentgenol* 1994;163:411–416.
12. Nizard RS, Wybier M, Laredo JD. Radiologic assessment of lumbar intervertebral instability and degenerative spondylolisthesis. *Radiol Clin North Am* 2001;39:55–71.
13. Wildermuth S, Zanetti M, Duewell S, et al. Lumbar spine quantitative and qualitative assessment of positional (upright flexion and extension) MR imaging and myelography. *Radiology* 1998;207: 391–398.
14. Tsirikos AI, Saifuddin A, Noordeen MH, Tucker SK. Traumatic lumbosacral dislocation: report of two cases. *Spine* 2004;29:E164–E168.
15. Bensaid AH, Dietemann JL, Kastler B, et al. Neurofibromatosis with dural ectasia and bilateral symmetrical pedicular clefts: report of two cases. *Neuroradiology* 1992;34: 107–109.

7

The Value of Bone Scintigraphy and CT Scan in Diagnosis and Treatment of Active Spondylolysis in Elite Athletes

J. Sys and J. Michielsen

Low back pain accounts for 5% to 8% of athletic injuries (1). Spondylolysis is one of the major causes of low back pain in young athletes (1–6). Incidences of spondylolysis of over 40% have been reported in studies among female gymnasts, football players, weightlifters, wrestlers, and divers (7–10). In these studies, no distinction was made between acute and chronic spondylolysis. Micheli and Wood found spondylolytic stress fractures or acute spondylolysis of the pars interarticularis in 47% of 100 adolescent athletes (11). In adolescent and young adult athletes, special attention should be given to fatigue fractures of the pars interarticularis because of their possible evolutive nature (4,11–15).

Although genetic and racial factors may predispose an individual to spondylolysis (16–18), the most generally favored theory is that spondylolysis is a fracture caused by mechanical stress and that the mode of failure is fatigue (19–27). In general, the prevalence of spondylolysis is not higher in athletes than it is in nonathletes, although participation in sports involving large stress reversals in the pars interarticularis appears to be associated with disproportionately higher rates of spondylolysis (3). The mechanical etiology of this fatigue fracture is controversial, and many experimental studies have been carried out to determine the fatigue strength of the pars interarticularis and to delineate the movements causing failure (12,28–32). Experiments on cadaveric lumbar motion segments have shown that full flexion and extension movements bend the inferior articular process sufficiently to cause a fatigue fracture of the pars interarticularis (33). The likelihood of fatigue failure would be greater in activities that require alternating flexion and extension of the lumbar spine, because this would involve large stress reversals in the pars interarticularis (22,33,34). Movements of this type occur in gymnastics, volleyball, tennis, pole vaulting, cricket, etc. Also, the clinical outcome of nonoperative treatment seems to be unfavorable in athletes participating in these high-risk sports (35)

Athletes with spondylolysis present with pain during certain performance activities. The onset of pain can be either acute or progressive. The pain may become more chronic and dull with time. Clinical examination frequently reveals paraspinal muscle spasm and hamstring tightness (13).

TERMINOLOGY

It may be assumed that a stress reaction, a microfracture, a macrofracture, and spondylolisthesis can be the consecutive stages of the same overuse injury at the pars interarticularis (4,13,15,36–38) (Fig. 7.1). No single imaging or scintigraphic technique allows

Stages of spondylolysis

Stress-reaction
↓
Microfracture
↓
Macrofracture
↓
Nonunion

FIG. 7.1. Stages of spondylolysis.

differentiation between these stages. Several authors have discerned early, progressive, and terminal stages, either with standard radiography (x-ray) (15), computed tomographic (CT) scan (4), or magnetic resonance imaging (MRI) (37,39,40). Rather than using the terms *acute* or *chronic*, *early* or *late*, we prefer using the terms *active* and *inactive*, with reference to the appearance on bone scintigraphy.

Sys et al. have advocated differentiation between bilateral and *pseudobilateral spondylolysis* (Fig. 7.2) according to the scintigraphic appearance (41). When tracer uptake is present on both sides of one vertebra and uptake is clearly asymmetrical, the lesion is called pseudobilateral. In pseudobilateral spondylolysis, only the fracture with a highly increased uptake on bone scintigraphy is considered recent or *active*. The fracture on the other side is an older or scintigraphically less active lesion. The terms *active* and *inactive* provide a better understanding of the true nature of the lesion. The term *acute spondylolysis* is related to the appearance of symptoms rather than to the age of the lesion(s). From this study, we know that these do not always correlate.

Lesions can be classified as unilateral, bilateral, or pseudobilateral, according to their scintigraphic appearance (41). The relative number of counts at one side of a lesion needs to be compared with the number of counts on the other side. The average count from 10 transverse cuts is calculated for each side with the center of the vertebral body as a reference. When the ratio of the most active side to the least active side is between 0.8 and 1.19, the lesion is considered bilateral; when the ratio is more than 2.0, the lesion is considered unilateral. Lesions with a ratio between 1.2 and 2.0 are considered pseudobilateral.

DIAGNOSIS AND FOLLOW-UP

Early radiographic features of spondylolysis and prespondylolytic stress reactions such as vertebral anisocoria have been described extensively (42,43). Nevertheless, the sensitivity of different lumbosacral radiographic views in the detection of spondylolysis is limited (4,36,41,44,45). Bone scintigraphy is the most sensitive tool for early diagnosis of acquired spondylolysis in young athletes (4,19,36,38,46–49). With single photon emission computed tomography (SPECT), spatial separation of overlapping bony structures is possible: The anatomic localization of a hot spot is improved and sensitivity is increased (8,38,44,46). A scintigraphic active pars interarticularis defect is associated with a healing process, which may elicit pain, whereas a normal bone scan in the presence of a radiographically demonstrable pars defect is consistent with a healed (fibrous), pain-free nonunion or pseudarthrosis (27,38,44,46,47).

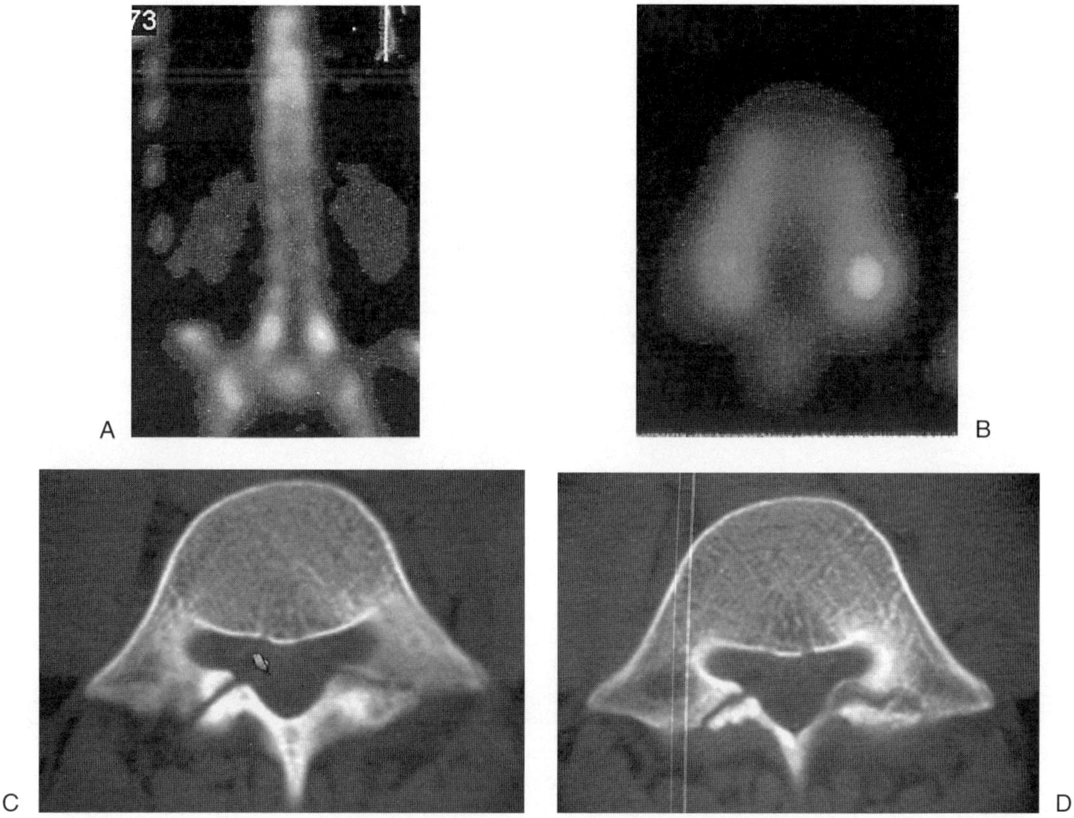

FIG. 7.2. Example of a pseudobilateral spondylolysis. **A:** Coronal SPECT bone scan. The hot spot at the left side is more pronounced. **B:** Axial SPECT bone scan. The hot spot at the left side is more pronounced. **C:** CT-scan shows chronic spondylolysis on the right side and a recent stress fracture on the left side. **D:** CT scan 3 months after the onset of treatment. Lysis has increased at the left fracture site, and there are no signs of bony healing.

A bone scan is believed to show increased uptake for about 1 year after occurrence of the fracture, although firm data is lacking. It is impossible to determine the exact onset of a lesion and to really define a recent lesion, but one may assume that lesions detectable on bone scintigraphy but not detectable on x-rays are recent, either prespondylolytic stress reactions (Fig. 7.3A) or microfractures (Fig. 7.3B). The value of MRI for early diagnosis of these early stages of active spondylolysis seems to be promising but is yet to be determined (39,40).

Information as to when a young athlete should stop bracing and return to competition could be provided by means of a scintigram (41,46), but CT scan remains the only tool to evaluate the completeness of healing and to show bridging trabecular bone across a fracture line (4,50).

DISCUSSION

Participation in sports involving large stress reversals in the pars interarticularis appears to be associated with higher rates of spondylolysis (3). With an increase in the number of skeletally immature athletes competing at more demanding levels of competition, an associated increase in the number of such cases may be seen (6).

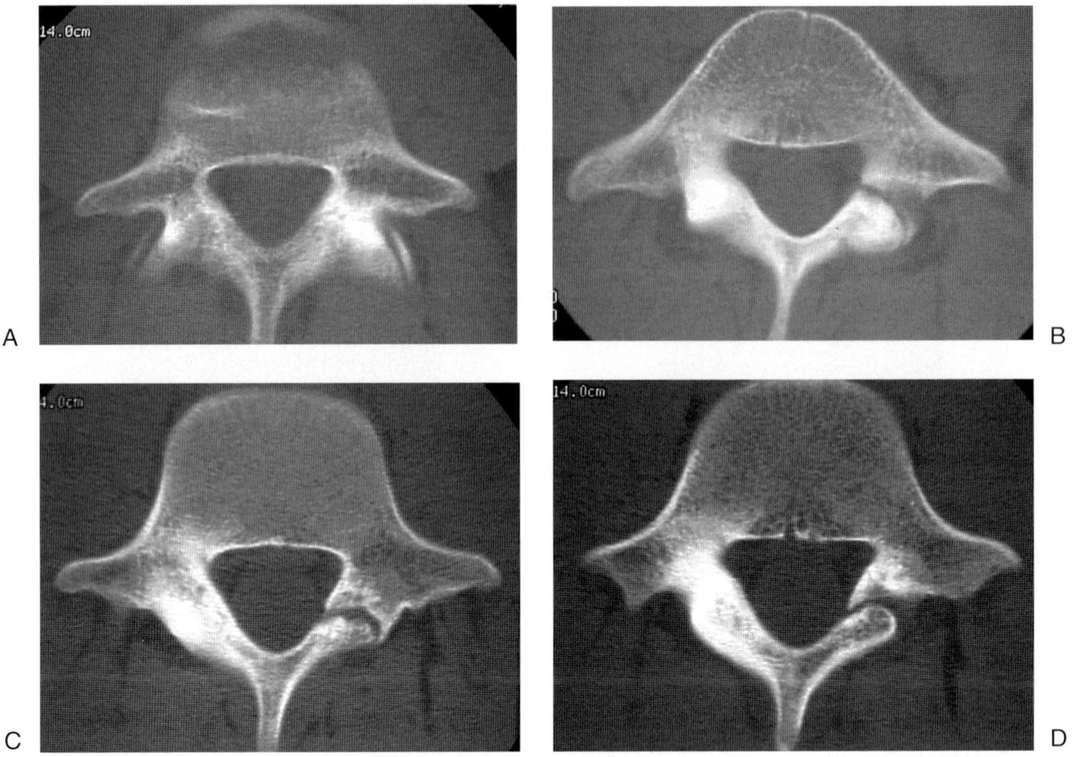

FIG. 7.3. Stages of spondylolysis. **A:** Example of a unilateral prespondylolytic stress reaction. There is slight hyperostosis at the left pars interarticularis, but no cortical defect can be noted. X-ray was negative. Bone scan showed increased uptake at the left pars interarticularis. **B:** Example of a unilateral microfracture. There is a thin fracture line at the left pars interarticularis. X-ray was negative. Bone scan showed increased uptake at the left pars interarticularis. **C:** Example of a unilateral macrofracture. At the left pars interarticularis is an overt fracture line that was visible on x-ray. Bone scan showed increased uptake at the left pars interarticularis. **D:** Example of a unilateral pseudarthrosis or nonunion: At the left pars interarticularis is an old fracture that was visible on x-ray. Bone scan showed no increased uptake at the left pars interarticularis.

Early diagnosis of active spondylolysis in young athletes is important. Congeni et al. reported that after nonoperative treatment of those athletes with symptoms for longer than 6 months, 80% were classified as chronic fractures on CT scan (4). Athletes with a shorter duration of symptoms had chronic as well as acute and incomplete fractures. Blanda et al. found healing in 73% of early stage defects, in 39% of progressive stage defects, and in none of the terminal-stage defects (36). Both Blanda et al. (36) and Ciullo and Jackson (51) found that the longer the symptoms were present before treatment, the more likely that surgical intervention was needed.

Sys et al. suggest that osseous healing is more likely to occur in unilateral active spondylolysis as compared to bilateral and pseudobilateral active spondylolysis (41). Blanda et al. found that healing was achieved in 87% of athletes with unilateral lesions and that 87% of the athletes in whom nonunion was diagnosed had bilateral defects (36). Miller et al. found that the bilaterality of a defect is more important than the stage of apparent healing on early CT scans for predicting bony union (50). Chances for osseous healing decrease when the fracture is bilateral, probably because one of the fractures is less recent and thus less liable to healing (32,41,50).

Bone scintigraphy is the most sensitive tool for early diagnosis of active spondylolysis in young athletes (4,19,36,38,46–49). No single imaging or scintigraphic technique allows differentiation of the different stages of this overuse injury of the pars interarticularis: a stress reaction, a microfracture, a macrofracture (Fig. 7.3C), a pseudarthrosis (Fig. 7.3D), and eventually spondylolisthesis. Bone scintigraphy in combination with x-ray and CT scan allows differentiation among a stress reaction, a microfracture, and an overt macrofracture as well as differentiation between an active lesion and an inactive lesion or pseudarthrosis. Once an inactive fracture is present, consecutive x-rays are sufficient for exclusion or diagnosis of spondylolisthesis. MRI's value for early diagnosis of active spondylolysis seems promising, but its value for differentiation among the different stages of spondylolysis still needs to be determined (39,40).

Rest, bracing (11,35,41,52), physiotherapy (53), and electrical stimulation (54) are the most common nonoperative treatment modalities for active spondylolysis. Their effectiveness has not been shown in prospective studies, and therefore further research is warranted.

Bone scintigraphy is helpful for follow-up of active spondylolysis: Determination of the time of bracing and return to competition could be provided with the use of a scintigram, but CT scan remains the only tool to evaluate the completeness of healing (4,41,50). If both bone scintigraphy and CT scan were to be performed for diagnosis and follow-up of pars interarticularis defects however, the cost/benefit ratio would be high and very unattractive.

Nonoperative treatment of active spondylolysis results in successful pain relief in approximately 80% of athletes, independent of radiographic evidence of defect healing (3,41,50). Nonunion of a pars interarticularis defect apparently does not mean that the segment is unstable. Fibrous healing occurs and may lead to a good clinical result (8,22,51). Our study shows that most adolescent athletes treated nonoperatively for symptomatic spondylolysis achieve a good functional outcome at 13 months after the onset of treatment, regardless of bony healing of the defect (41). In a recent study, Miller et al. showed that this good functional outcome persists up to 11 years after the onset of treatment (50).

Once inactive spondylolysis is noted, sports can be resumed, but it is unclear whether or not repetitive activities with high demands of the lumbar spine should be avoided (55,56). Moderate low back pain can be treated with rehabilitation of abdominal muscles (56,57) and local infiltration of anesthetics and/or steroids at the site of nonunion.

Surgical intervention may be considered in athletes who have unremitting symptoms despite 6 months of conservative treatment (13,36,55). Several methods of fixation have been described (23,24,58–62). The past 3 years, high success rates have been reported in several studies: High-level athletes returned to their same level of activity in over 80% of cases (23,24,58,60,61). In most studies, however, the successful return to sport is not detailed.

CONCLUSION

Although early radiographic signs of fractures of the pars interarticularis have been described, it is recommended that athletes with stress-related symptoms be screened using planar and SPECT scintigraphy in order to diagnose fatigue fractures in the presence of normal radiographs. When it is combined with a CT scan, bone scintigraphy is valuable in both staging and follow-up of this overuse injury. Nonoperative treatment of active spondylolysis leads to excellent results and sports resumption within 6 months in the majority of athletes.

Bony healing is most likely to occur in unilateral spondylolysis. Chances for osseous healing diminish when the fracture is bilateral and even more when it is pseudobilateral. Nonunion does not seem to compromise the overall outcome or sports resumption in the short term and middle term. One can assume that the stability obtained by fibrous healing is considerable and mostly sufficient for sports activities in the first 10 years after the onset of treatment. This finding confirms that conservative treatment is primarily indicated in elite adolescent athletes with acquired active spondylolysis. However, the equal success rates of surgical treatment reported in recent studies may change our strategy in the future.

REFERENCES

1. Harvey J, Tanner S. Low back pain in young athletes: a practical approach. *Sports Med* 1991;12:394–406.
2. Alexander MJL. Biomechanical aspects of lumbar spine injuries in athletes: a review. *Can J Appl Sport Sci* 1985;10:1–20.
3. Bono CM. Low-back pain in athletes. *J Bone Joint Surg* 2004;86-A(2):382–396.
4. Congeni J, McCulloch J, Swanson K. Lumbar spondylolysis: a study of natural progression in athletes. *Am J Sports Med* 1997;25:248–253.
5. Sward L. The thoracombular spine in young elite athletes. *Sports Med* 1992;13:357–364.
6. Wimberly RL, Lauerman WC. Spondylolisthesis in athletes. *Clin Sports Med* 2002;21:133–145.
7. Ferguson RJ, McMaster JH, Stanitski CI. Low back pain in college football linemen. *J Sports Med* 1974; 2:63–69.
8. Jackson DW, Wiltse LL, Ciricione RJ. Spondylolysis in the female gymnast. *Clin Orthop* 1976;117:68–73.
9. Jackson DW. Low back pain in athletes: evaluation of stress reaction and discogenic problems. *Am J Sports Med* 1979;7:364–366.
10. Rossi F, Dragoni S. Lumbar spondylolysis: occurrence in competitive athletes. *J Sports Med Phys Fitness* 1990;30:450–452.
11. Micheli LJ, Wood R. Back pain in young athletes: significant differences from adults in causes and patterns. *Arch Pediatr Adolesc Med* 1995;149:15–18.
12. Cyron BM, Hutton WC, Troup JDG. Spondylolytic fractures. *J Bone Joint Surg* 1976;58-B:462–466.
13. Garry JP, McShane J. Lumbar spondylolysis in adolescent athletes. *J Fam Pract* 1988;46:145–149.
14. Grobler LJ, Wiltse LL. Classification, non-operative and operative treatment of spondylolistheses. In: Frymoyer JW, ed. *The Adult Spine. Principles and Practice.* New York: Raven Press; 1991:1655–1700.
15. Morita T, Ikata T, Miyake R. Lumbar spondylolysis in children and adolescents. *J Bone Joint Surg* 1995;77-B:620–625.
16. Eisenstein S. Spondylolysis: a skeletal investigation of two population groups. *J Bone Joint Surg* 1978;60-B:488–492.
17. Frederickson BE, Baker D, McHolick WJ, et al. The natural history of spondylolysis and spondylolisthesis. *J Bone Joint Surg* 1984;66-A:699–707.
18. Porter RW, Park W. Unilateral spondylolysis. *J Bone Joint Surg* 1982;64-B:344–348.
19. Commandre FA, Gagnerie G, Zakarian M, et al. The child, the spine, and sport. *J Sports Med Phys Fitness* 1988;28:104–107.
20. Commandre FA, Taillan B, Gagnerie F, et al. Spondylolysis and spondylolisthesis in young athletes: 28 cases. *J Sports Med Phys Fitness* 1988;28:11–19.
21. Hulkko A, Orava S. Diagnosis and treatment of delayed and non-union stress fractures in athletes. *Ann Chir Gynaecol* 1991;80:177–184.
22. Letts M, Smallman T, Afanasiev R, et al. Fracture of the pars interarticularis in adolescent athletes: a clinical-biomechanical analysis. *J Pediatr Orthop* 1986; 6:40–46.
23. Reitman CA, Esse SI. Direct repair of spondylolytic defects in young competitive athletes. *Spine* 2002; 2:142–144.
24. Reitman CA, Gertzbein SD, Francis WR. Lumbar isthmic defects in teenagers resulting from stress fractures. *Spine* 2002;4:303–306.
25. Riel KA, Bernett P. Ermudungsbruche im Sport. Eigene Erfahrungen und Literaturüberblick. *Z Orthop* 1991; 129:471–476.
26. Weir MR, Smith DS. Stress reaction of the pars interarticularis leading to spondylolysis: a cause of adolescent low back pain. *J Adolesc Health Care* 1989;573–577.
27. Wiltse L, Widell EH, Jackson DW. Fatigue fracture: the basic lesion in isthmic spondylolisthesis. *J Bone Joint Surg* 1975;57-A:17–22.

28. Adams MA, Dolan P, Hutton WC. The lumbar spine in backward bending. *Spine* 1988;13:1019–1026.
29. Cyron BM, Hutton WC. The fatigue strength of the lumbar neural arch in spondylolysis. *J Bone Joint Surg* 1978;60-B:234–238.
30. Dunlop RB, Adams MA, Hutton WC. Disc space narrowing and the lumbar facet joints. *J Bone Joint Surg* 1984;66-B:706–710.
31. Lafferty JF, Winter WG, Gambaro SA. Fatigue characteristics of posterior elements of vertebrae. *J Bone Joint Surg* 1977;59-A:154–158.
32. Mazel CH. Le spondylolisthesis du sportif. *Presse Med* 1991;20:596–600.
33. Green TP, Allvey JC, Adams MA. Spondylolysis: bending of the inferior articular processes of lumbar vertebrae during simulated spinal movements. *Spine* 1994;19:2683–2691.
34. Chosa E, Totoribe K, Tajima N. A biomechanical study of lumbar spondylolysis based on a three-dimensional finite element method. *J Orthop Res*2004;158–163.
35. D'Hemecourt PA, Zurakowski D, Kriemler S, et al. Spondylolysis: returning the athlete to sports participation with brace treatment. *Orthopedics* 2002;25:653–657.
36. Blanda J, Bethem D, Moats W, et al. Defect of the pars interarticularis in athletes: a protocol for nonoperative treatment. *J Spinal Disord* 1993;6:406–411.
37. Ikata T, Miyake R, Katoh S, et al. Pathogenesis of sports-related spondylolisthesis in adolescents: radiographic and magnetic resonance imaging study. *Am J Sports Med* 1996;24:94–98.
38. Itoh K, Hashimoto T, Shigenobu K, et al. Bone SPET of symptomatic lumbar spondylolysis. *Nucl Med Commun* 1996;17(5):389–396. Erratum in *Nucl Med Commun* 1996;17(8):732–734.
39. Lim MR, Yoon SC, Green DW. Symptomatic spondylolysis: diagnosis and treatment. *Curr Opin Pediatr* 2004;16:37–46.
40. Sairyo K, Takata T, Katoh S, et al. Early diagnosis of pediatric spondylolysis: significance of MRI and its biomechanical corroboration. *Spine* 2004;5:S69.
41. Sys J, Michielsen J, Bracke P, et al. Nonoperative treatment of active spondylolysis in elite athletes with normal x-ray findings: literature review and results of conservative treatment. *Eur Spine J* 2001;10:498–504.
42. Maldague B, Malghem J. Aspects radiologiques dynamiques de la spondylolyse lombaire. *Acta Orthop Belg* 1981;47:441–457.
43. Sherman FC, Wilkinson RH, Hall JE. Reactive sclerosis of a pedicle and spondylolysis in the lumbar spine. *J Bone Joint Surg* 1977;59-A:49–54.
44. Harvey CJ, Richenberger JL, Saifuddin A, et al. Pictorial review: the radiological investigation of lumbar spondylolysis. *Clin Radiol* 1998;53:723–728.
45. Pierce ME. Spondylolysis: what does it mean? A review. *Australas Radiol* 1987;31:391–394.
46. Bellah RD, Summerville DA, Treves ST, et al. Low-back pain in adolescent athletes: detection of stress injury to the pars interarticularis with SPECT. *Radiology* 1991;180:509–512.
47. Kanstrup IL. Bone imaging in sports medicine: a review. *Scand J Med Sci Sports* 1997;7:322–330.
48. Papanicolaou N, Wilkinson RH, Emans JB, et al. Bone scintigraphy and radiography in young athletes with low back pain. *AJR Am J Roentgenol* 1985;145:1039–1044.
49. Rosen PR, Micheli LJ, Treves S Early scintigraphic diagnosis of bone stress and fractures in athletic adolescents. *Pediatrics* 1982;70:11–15.
50. Miller SF, Congeni J, Swanson K. Long-term functional and anatomical follow-up of early detected spondylolysis in young athletes. *Am J Sports Med* 2004;32:928–933.
51. Ciullo JV, Jackson DW. Pars interarticularis stress reaction, spondylolysis and spondylolisthesis in gymnasts. *Clin Sports Med* 1985;4:95–110.
52. Micheli LJ. Back injuries in female gymnasts. *Clin Sports Med* 1998;4:85–93.
53. McNeely ML, Torrance G, Magee DJ. A systematic review of physiotherapy for spondylolysis and spondylolisthesis. *Man Ther* 2003;2:80–91.
54. Stasinopoulos D. Treatment of spondylolysis with external stimulation in young athletes: a critical literature review. *Br J Sports Med* 2004;38:352–354.
55. Crielaard JM, Reginster JY, Franchimont P. Spondylolyse et spondylolisthesis: contre-indications á la pratique sportive? *Rev Med Liege* 1985;40:215–219.
56. Lindh M. Biomechanics of the lumbar spine. In: Nordin M, ed. *Basic Biomechanics of the Musculoskeletal System.* Philadelphia: Lea and Febiger; 1989:183–203.
57. Norris CM. Abdominal muscle training in sport. *Br J Sports Med* 1993;27:19–27.
58. Debnath UK, Freeman BJ, Gregory P, et al. Clinical outcome and return to sport after the surgical treatment of spondylolysis in young athletes. *J Bone and Joint Surg* 2003;85–B:244–249.
59. Kip PC, Esses SI, Doherty BI, et al. Biomechanical testing of pars defect repairs. *Spine* 1994;19:2692–2697.
60. Nozawa S, Schmizu K, Miyamoto K, et al. Repair of pars interarticularis defect by segmental wire fixation in young athletes with spondylolysis. *Am J Sports Med* 2003;3:359–364.
61. Ranawat VS, Dowell JK, Heywood-Waddington MB. Stress fractures of the lumbar pars interarticularis in athletes : a review based on long-term results of 18 professional cricketers. *Injury* 2003;12:915–919.
62. Salib RM, Pettine KA. Modified repair of a defect in spondylolysis or minimal spondylolisthesis by pedicle screw, segmental wire fixation, and bone grafting. *Spine* 1993;18:440–443.

8

Dynamic MRI Using the Upright or Positional MRI Scanner

F. W. Smith, M. H. Pope, and D. Wardlaw

Clinical symptoms in many spinal syndromes such as lumbar spinal stenosis are posture related. Pain and numbness in the buttock and leg are provoked either by walking or by prolonged standing. On the contrary, lying and sitting can obtain symptomatic relief. Not only spinal canal area but also intervertebral foraminal space can decrease with extension (1). The nerve root is constrained in the intervertebral foramen (IVF) and may be easily compressed or mechanically irritated under unfavorable conditions of degeneration and movement.

FINDINGS OF PREVIOUS STUDIES

Kinematic Change of Intervertebral Foramen

Panjabi et al. (1) performed an in vitro study providing data about the three-dimensional movements of the IVF. In nondegenerated specimen, the average height, width, and area of the IVF were 20.9 mm, 10.2 mm, and 185.0 mm. The height of the IVF increases about 7% during flexion and decreases about 6% decrease during extension. The width of the IVF increases about 15% during flexion and decreases about 12% decrease during extension.

Nowicki et al. (2) examined cadaveric lumbar motion segments with computed tomography (CT) and magnetic resonance imaging (MRI). They examined the effect of extension, flexion, lateral bending, and axial rotation on the anatomical relationship of the spinal nerves in the neural foramen to the ligamentum flavum and the intervertebral disc. The neural foramina were classified as having no evident stenosis, as being stenotic, as having occult stenosis, or as showing resolved stenosis on the basis of the images and sections before and after loading. Extension loading produced the most cases of nerve root contact. Nowicki et al. demonstrated intermittent stenosis of the neural foramina.

Axial Loading of the Spine in Patients with Lumbar Spinal Stenosis

To determine the mechanical effects on the lumbar spinal canal in a simulated upright position, Willen et al. used a portable device for axial loading of the lumbar spine in CT and MRI (3). They found a statistically significant reduction of the dural sac cross-sectional area in at least one site during axial compression. Narrowing of the lateral recess and deformation of nerve roots could be estimated in the MRI study but not measured.

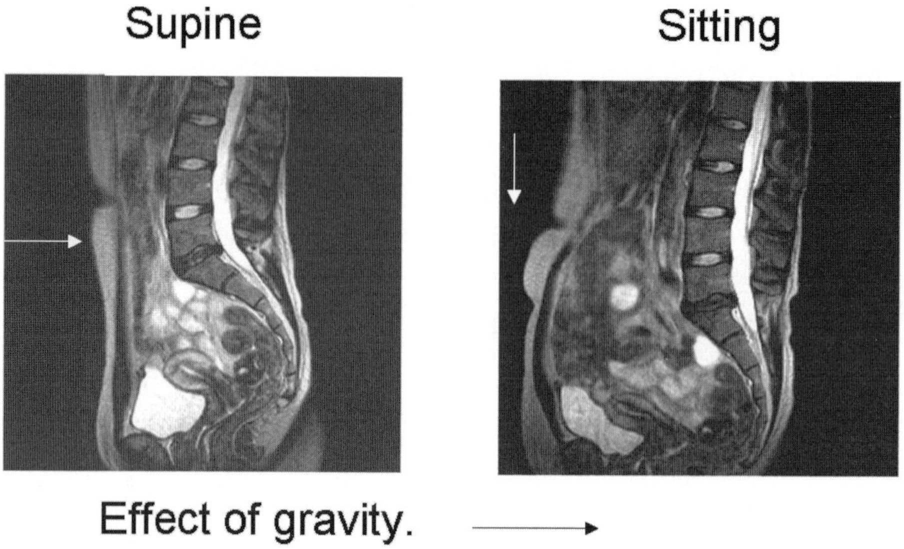

FIG. 8.1. Effect of gravity: supine versus erect.

Positional MRI

A newly developed positional MRI (pMRI) machine (Indomitable from FONAR) allows patients to simply walk in and be scanned while standing up and sitting down. Using this MRI, we can get the image of lumbar standing position, flexion, and extension position. The new stand-up MRI machine at the University of Aberdeen allows patients to walk in and be scanned while lying down, standing up, or sitting down. The gravity vector is roughly parallel to the spine in the erect or seated posture rather than at right angles in the supine posture. This changes the configuration of the spine (Fig. 8.1). The signs and symptoms of much of spinal conditions (i.e., spinal stenosis) are often posture related.

Jinkins and Dworkin (4) demonstrated the general utility of the pMRI unit in enabling upright, weight-bearing positional evaluation of the spinal column during various dynamic-kinetic maneuvres in patients with degenerative conditions of spine.

Intervertebral Relationships and Lumbar Posture

The study reported below was performed to assess the relationship between intervertebral relationships and lumbar posture in patients using pMRI.

Materials and Methods

Subjects

Fifty-eight patients with the signs and symptoms of spinal stenosis were studied. All gave informed consent. Grampian Research Ethics Committee approved this study, and informed consent was obtained from all participants.

Imaging

The MRI examination was performed using the 0.6-tesla Indomitable MRI system manufactured by FONAR of New York. This stand-up or positional open MRI system incorporates a patient-scanning table with tilt, translation, and elevation functions. It

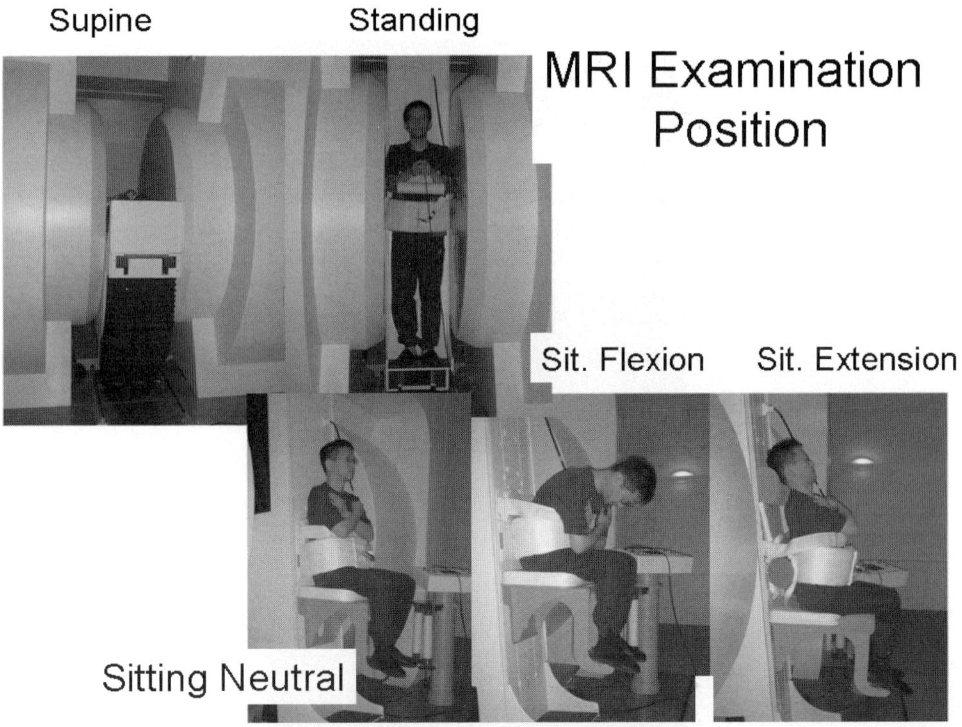

FIG. 8.2. MRI examination positions.

allows for upright, weight-bearing, and recumbent position. For the sitting position, a specially made seat was fixed on the examination table. The removable bars can be inserted at virtually any position within the magnet gap to provide supplementary support when the patient is being scanned in atypical positions or positions involving flexion or extension (Fig. 8.2).

All patients were examined with sagittal T2 images. Each had images made using T2 weighted spin echo sequences in the supine, erect standing, and seated posture. In the seated position, the spine was examined in neutral, flexion, and extension. The pulse sequences used were repetition time (TR)/echo time (TE) = 3,262/140 for T2 weighted sequences. Slice thickness was 4.5 mm, and field of view was 30 cm for sagittal images. The imaging matrix was 256 × 256 for the sagittal sequences.

Protocol

Each MRI examination was performed early in the morning before the subject's daily work. First, each subject was studied in the supine position with a cushion below the knees (conventional psoas-relaxed position). Then each was studied in the standing position with his or her hands on a bar in front of the body and fixed by a belt to reduce movement (Fig. 8.2). The last series was in the sitting position. The seated series consist of three positions: sitting neutral, sitting flexion, and sitting extension. For sitting neutral, the subject was simply seated on the chair with hands on the bar. For sitting flexion, the subject was requested to bend forward as much as possible and the subject's head and

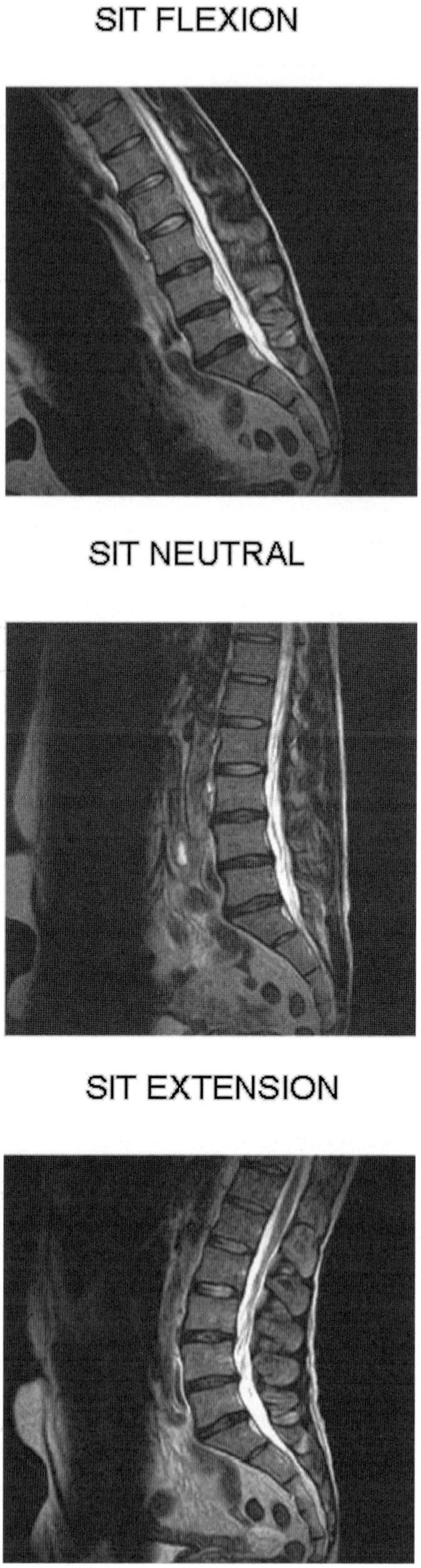

FIG. 8.3. Degenerate discs.

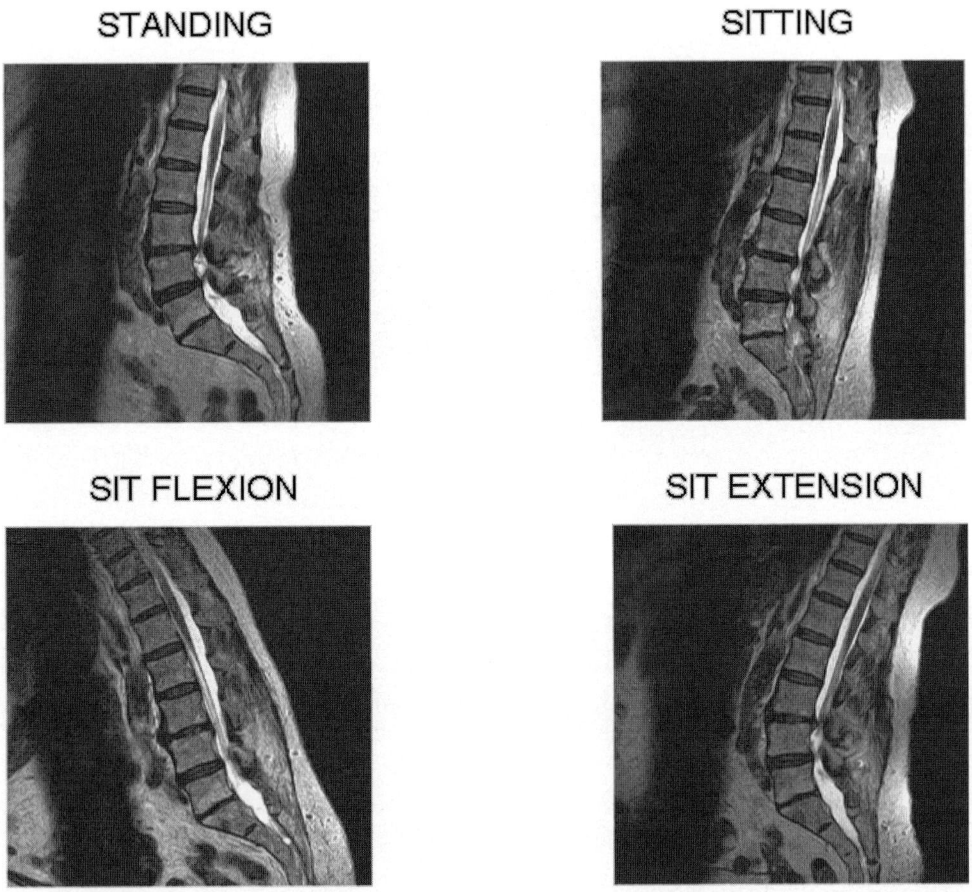

FIG. 8.4. Differences as a function of posture.

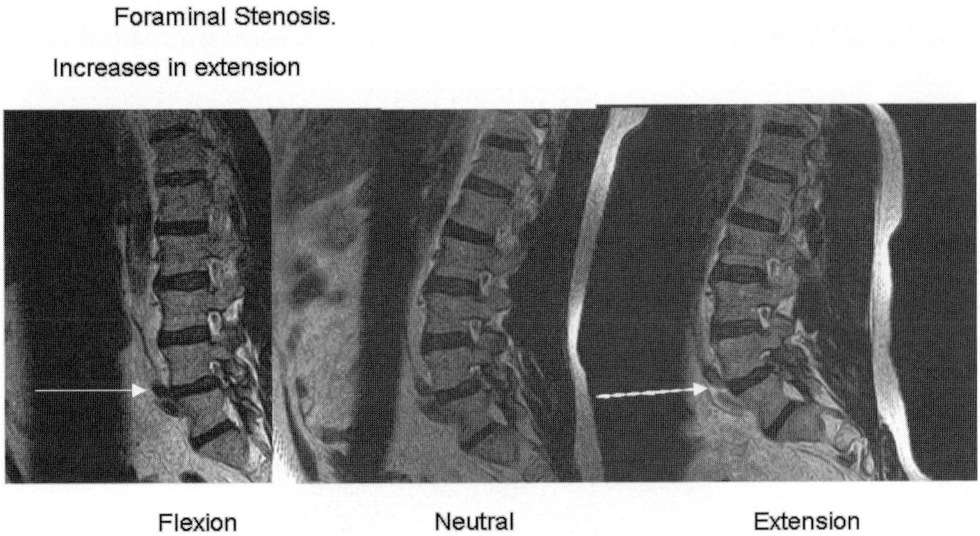

FIG. 8.5. Foraminal stenosis increases in extension.

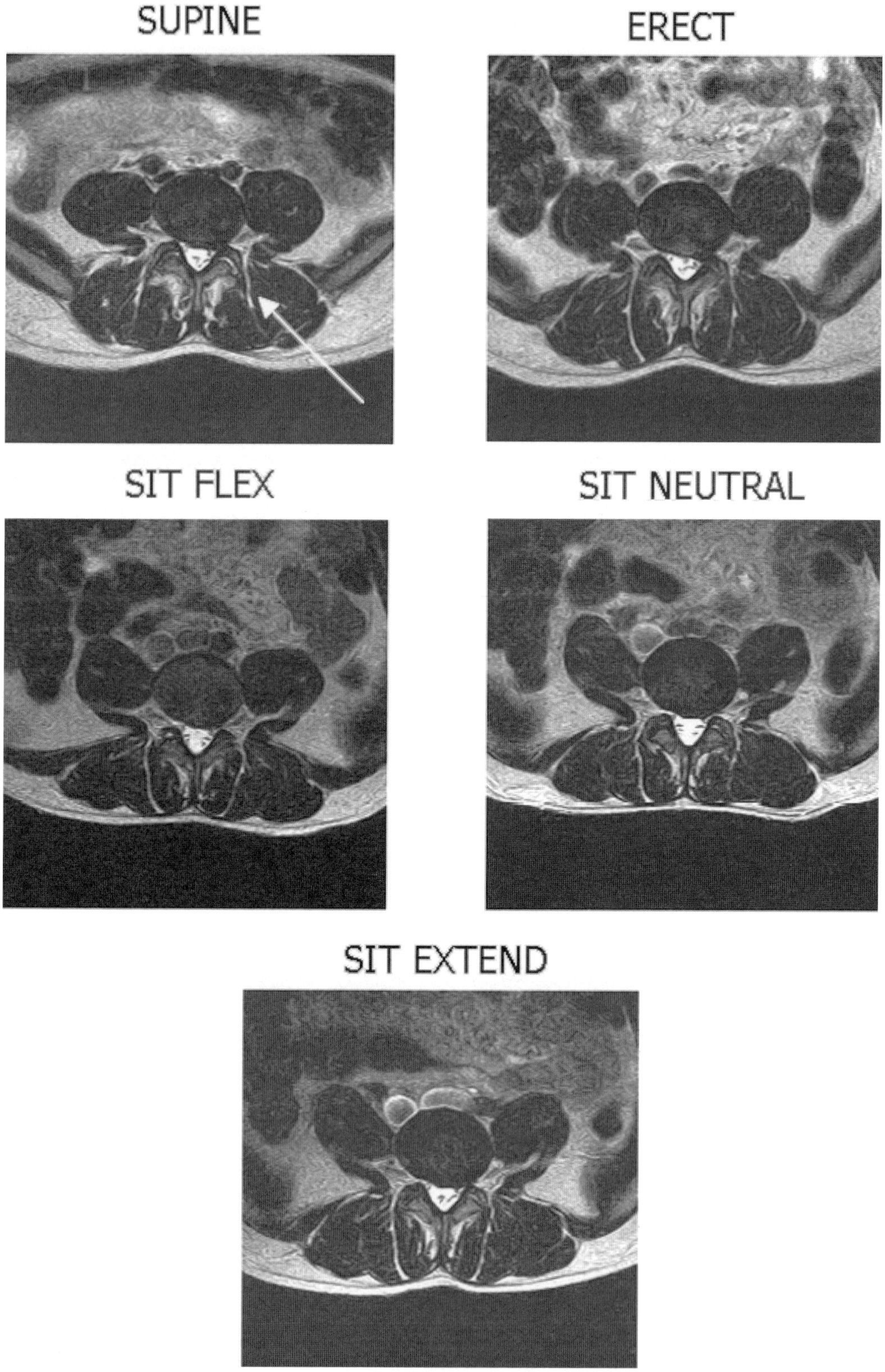

FIG. 8.6. Axial views.

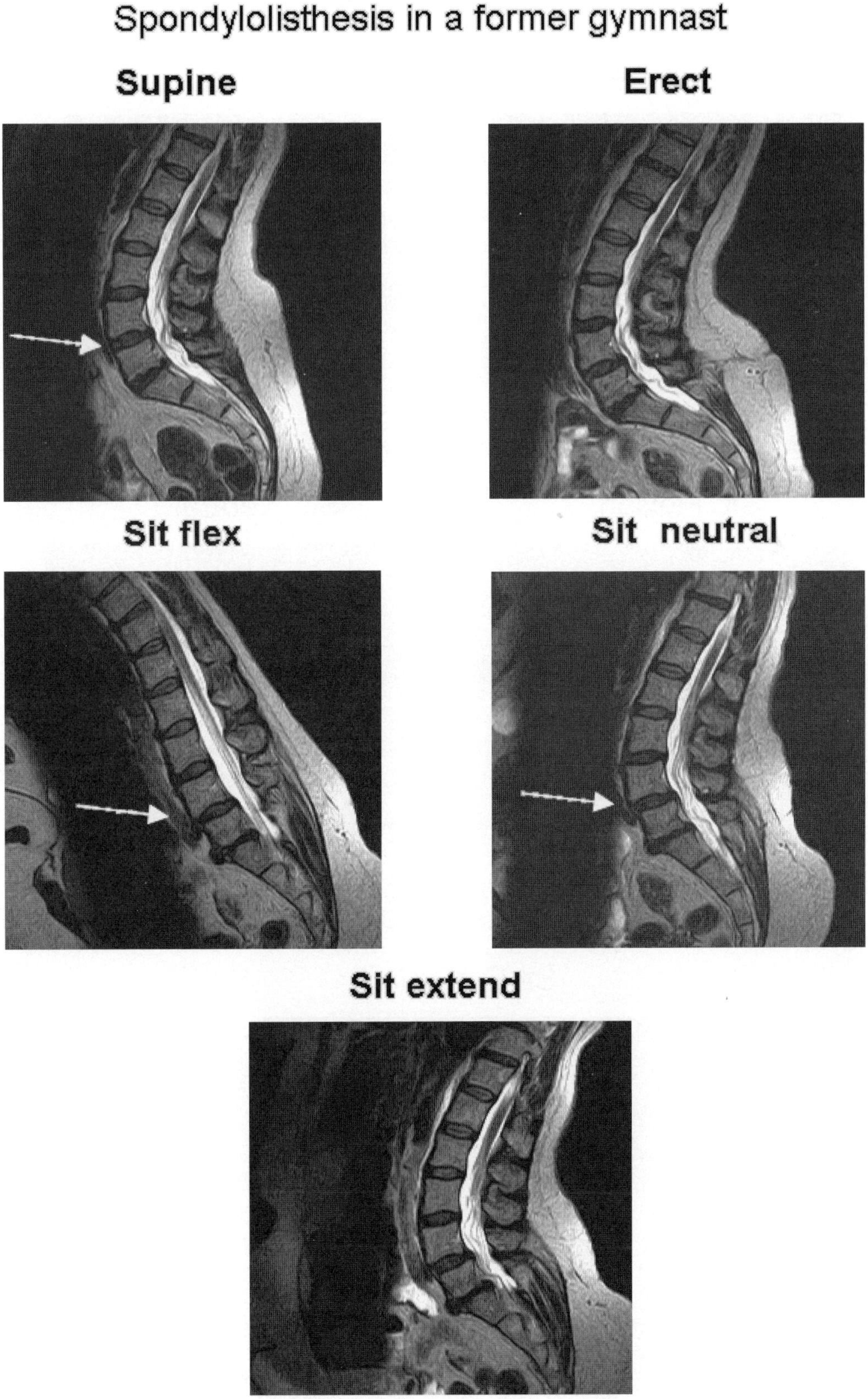

FIG. 8.7. Spondylolysthesis in various postures.

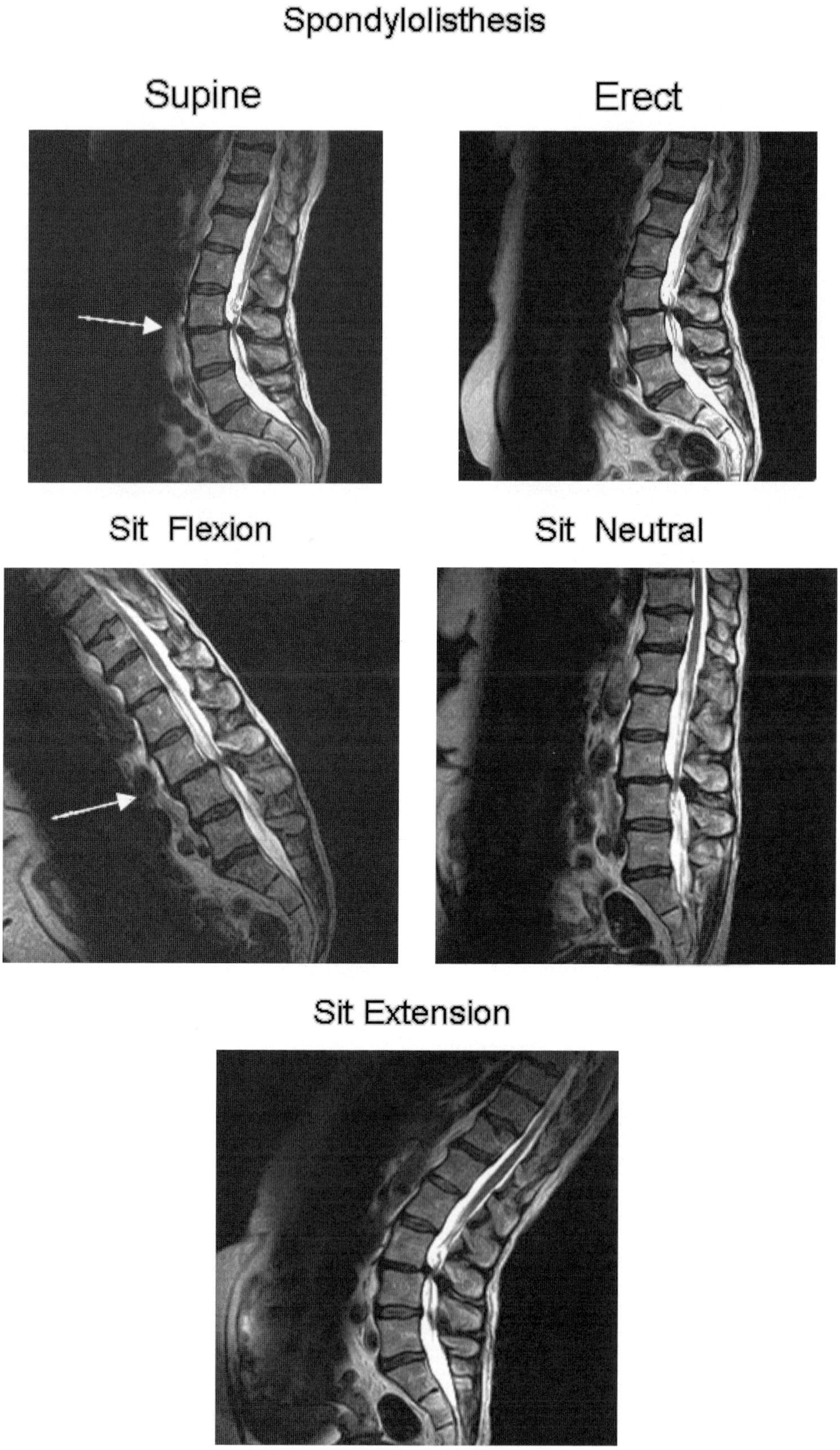

FIG. 8.8. Spondylolysthesis in various postures.

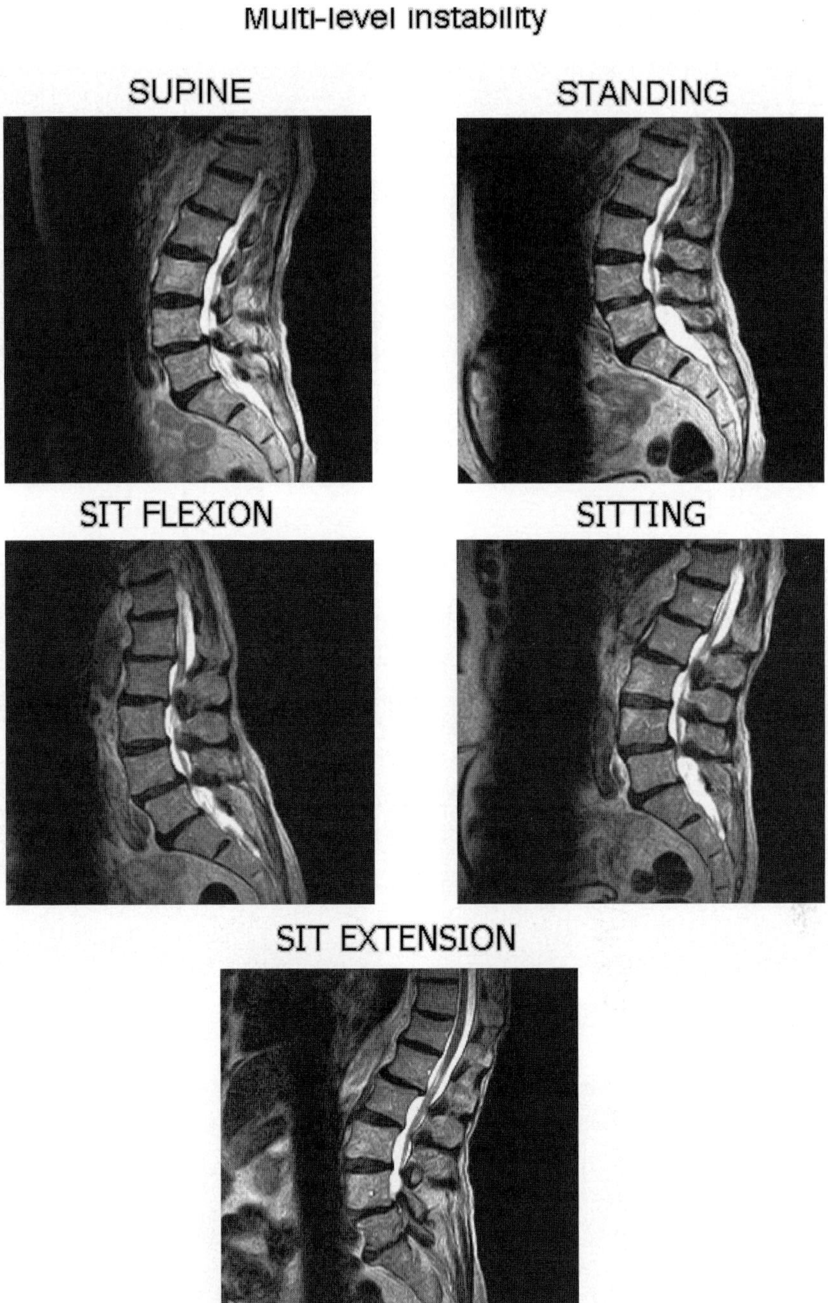

FIG. 8.9. Multilevel instability in various postures.

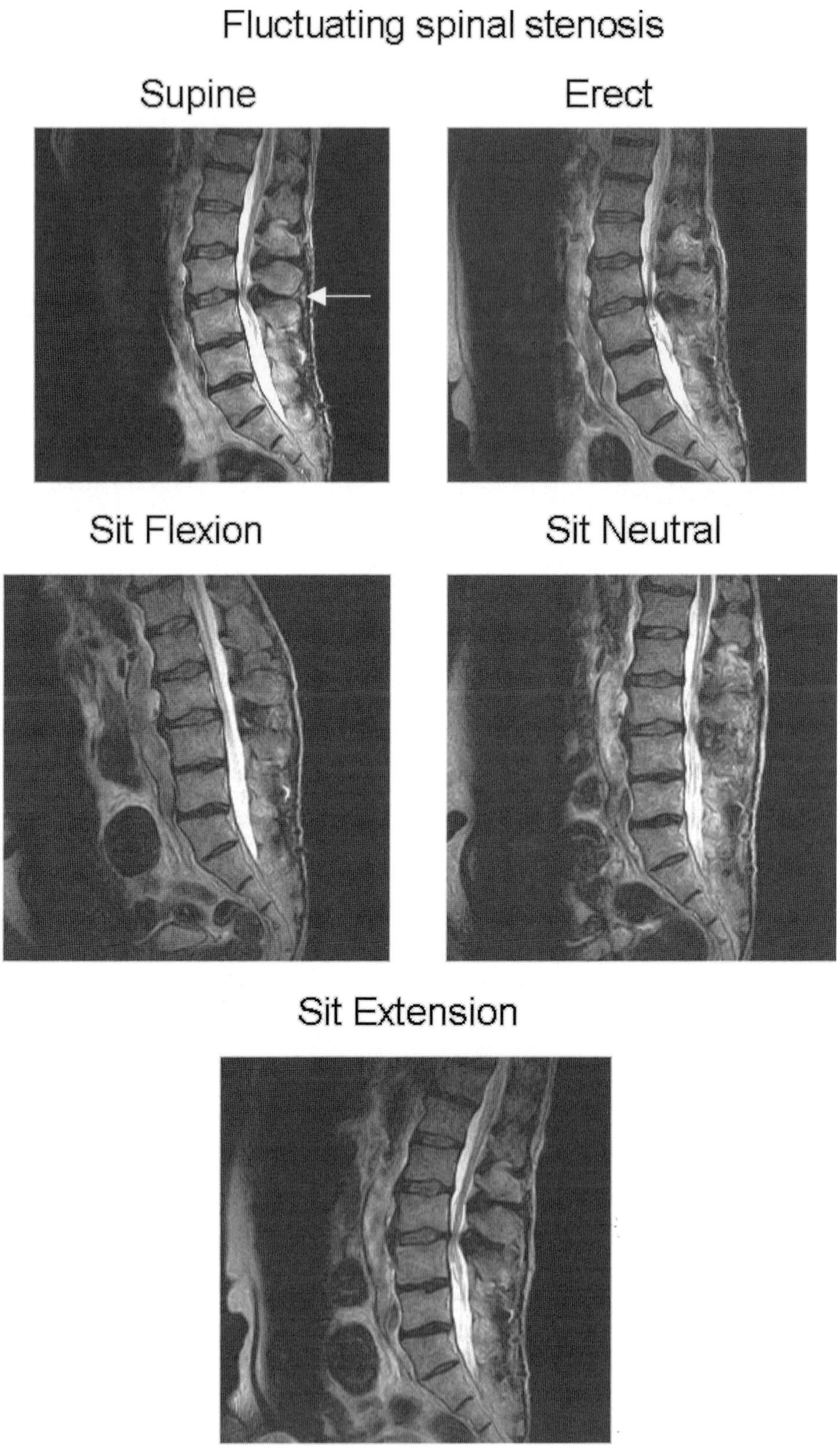

FIG. 8.10. Fluctuating spinal stenosis in various postures.

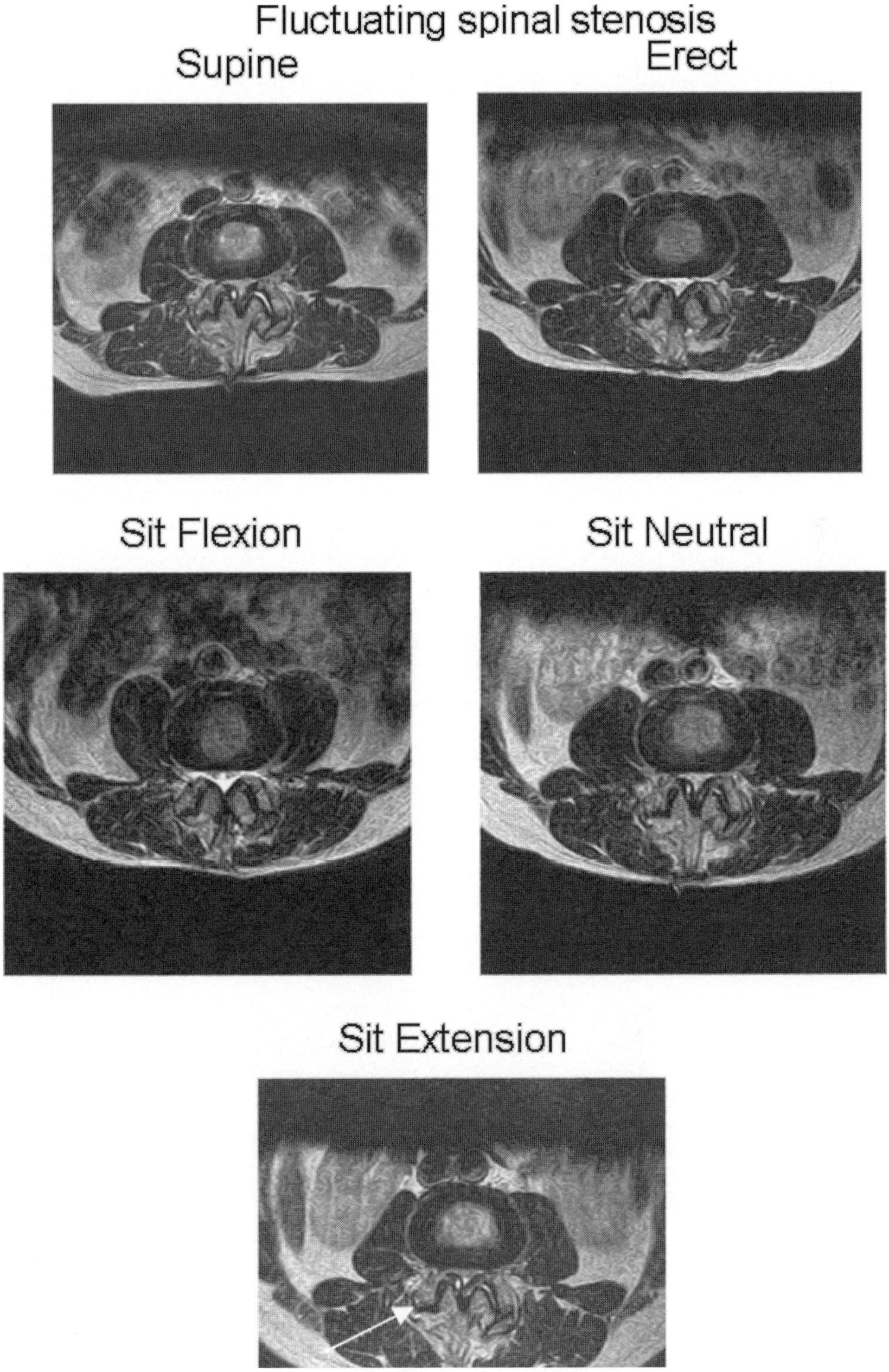

FIG. 8.11. Axial views.

forearms were supported by two bars to increase stability. For sitting extension, a cushion was placed behind the lumbar spine and the subject was requested to bend backward as much as possible and the forearms were supported with the bar.

Image Analysis

The measurements were made using a personal computer (CPU Pentium 4, 2.4 GHz) using the Osiris software (Digital Imaging Unit, University Hospital of Geneva). The setting of the measurement software was such that 1 pixel was equal to 1.18 mm on sagittal image.

Results

Healthy discs show less than 2 mm difference in height between supine and seated postures. In 80% of cases, discs showing degenerative changes (Figs. 8.3 and 8.4) decrease in height by more than 2 mm, especially anteriorly on flexion (3–4 mm). Thirty-eight patients with posterior prolapsed disc showed an increase in the degree of prolapse when seated. In 30 of the 38, the amount of prolapse decreased on flexion and increased on extension. In 67% with lateral disc prolapse, the prolapse was more prominent when seated and decreased on flexion and increased on extension.

In foraminal stenosis, there was an increase in extension (Figs. 8.5 and 8.6). In 14 cases with Grade 1 spondylolisthesis, the anterolisthesis was more evident in the seated posture (Figs. 8.7 and 8.8). In 10 of the 14 cases, the degree of spondylolisthesis increased on flexion and was seen in association with tears of the interspinous ligament.

Important changes were also seen as a function of posture in cases of multilevel instability (Fig. 8.9) and in fluctuating spinal stenosis (Figs. 8.10 and 8.11).

Discussion

The ability to image the spine in different postures adds significantly to the diagnostic accuracy of the MRI examination. For more than 50% of the patients examined in our study, a better understanding of the condition of the spine was obtained, resulting in improved management.

REFERENCES

1. Panjabi MM, Takata K, Goel VK. Kinematics of lumbar intervertebral foramen. *Spine* 1983;8:348–357.
2. Nowicki BH, Haughton VM, Schmidt TA, et al. Occult lumbar lateral spinal stenosis in normal foramina subjected to physiologic loading. *AJNR Am J Neuroradiol* 1996;17:1605–1614.
3. Willen J, Danielson B, Gaulitz A, et al. Dynamic effects on the lumbar spinal canal. *Spine* 1997;22:2968–2976.
4. Jinkins JR, Dworkin J. Upright, weight-bearing, dynamic-kinetic MRI of the spine: pMRI/kMRI. *Asian Oceanian J Radiol* 2002;7(3):135–152.

9

Classification of Spondylolysis and Spondylolisthesis

Michael Sullivan

The condition of slippage of the fifth lumbar vertebra on the sacrum has been known for many years, by obstetricians particularly. The condition was described by Herbeneaux in France at the end of the 18th century and then by two other people at almost the same time: Rokitansky in Vienna and Kilian in Britain in about 1853. However, it was Neugebauer, working as a gynecologist and obstetrician in Warsaw, who coined the modern term by combining the Greek words *spondylo,* meaning spine, and *olisthesis*, meaning slippage, to form the word *spondylo-olisthesis*. Of course, this was well before the days of x-rays, and so he described the physical characteristics. His original papers, in fact, show patients with what is now called dysplastic spondylolisthesis, typified by shortening of the trunk and a crease across the abdomen.

Junghauns in 1930 then proposed the term "pseudo" spondylolisthesis for what we now call degenerative spondylolisthesis. However, immediately after World War II, three surgeons independently introduced classifications, which were not very dissimilar. The three surgeons were MacNab in 1950, Wiltse in 1957, and Newman in 1963.

The International Society for the Study of the Lumbar Spine (ISSLS) had its first meeting in Montreal in 1974. Harry Farfen was the host, Leon Wiltse was made the first president, and I was made the first secretary. The outcome of this was that the second meeting in 1975 was held in London at The Royal College of Surgeons; I was privileged to host the meeting. The same three surgeons, namely MacNab, Wiltse, and Newman, presented three papers at that meeting. All three gave their expert opinion on classification of spondylolisthesis. At the end of the meeting, the committee asked these three eminent spinal surgeons to unite to produce a common classification to be presented at the following year's ISSLS meeting in Bermuda. It is their classification that is most widely accepted around the world. When anything is done through a committee, there has to be some compromise and this is the case in their classification.

They classified spondylolisthesis into five types, with three subtypes in Type 2:

Type 1. Dysplastic
Type 2. Isthmic
Type 3. Degenerative
Type 4. Traumatic
Type 5. Pathological

The three subgroups of Type 2, Isthmic, are

2A. Lytic fatigue fracture of the pars
2B. Elongation but intact pars
2C. Acute fracture

DYSPLASTIC SPONDYLOLISTHESIS

Type 1 spondylolisthesis is associated with congenital dysplasia of the upper sacrum and neural arch, which Newman classified as "congenital type." There is a weakness of the posterior elements and therefore a gradual sliding forward of the fifth lumbar vertebra on the sacrum. This weakness of the posterior elements allows L5 to slide forward, and as it slides forward, it slowly compresses the neural elements. When 25% slippage occurs, either the posterior elements must give way with elongation or fracture; or if neither of these situations occurs and the slip continues, the slippage transects or certainly completely compresses the cauda equina. The fundamental feature of dysplastic spondylolisthesis is the presence of the dysplastic posterior elements. Fracture into the pars interarticularis occurs in the isthmic type, and this is where confusion tends to occur. The presentation of dysplastic spondylolisthesis is quite different from the other types. It occurs during the adolescent growth spurt. The children with this condition have a short trunk compared to the length of the lower limbs. As the pelvis tilts, they acquire: a crease across the front of the abdomen (Fig. 9.1), a strange gait because of the marked hamstring

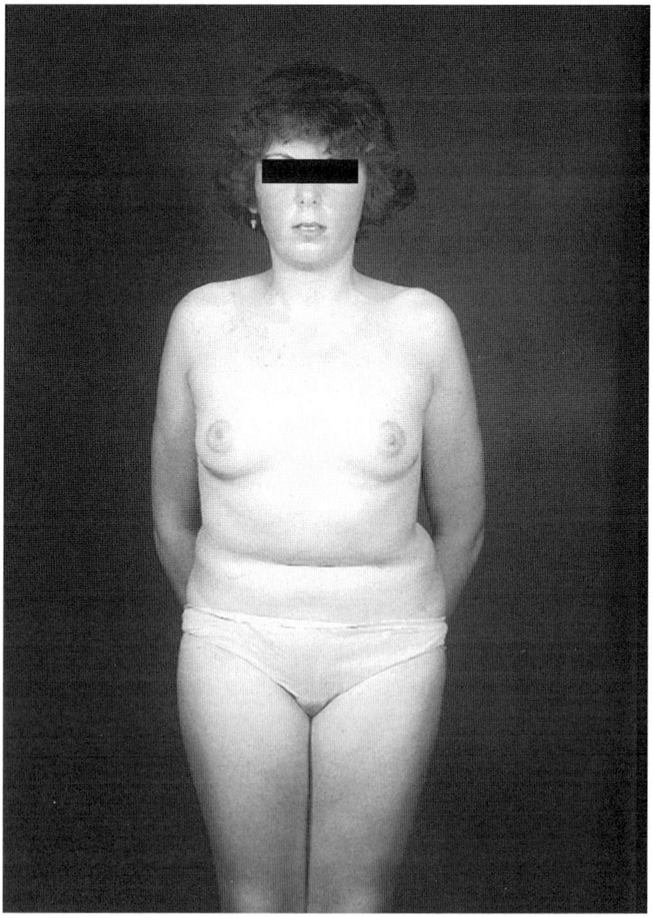

FIG. 9.1. Dysplastic spondylolisthesis showing the typical short trunk compared to lower limbs and showing anterior skin.

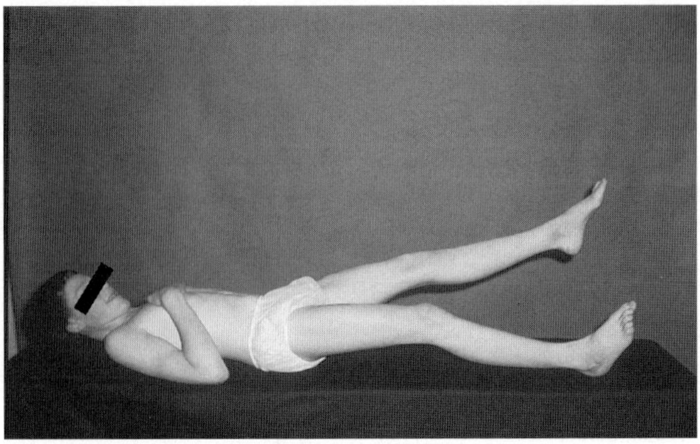

FIG. 9.2. Dysplastic spondylolisthesis with marked muscle spasm.

spasm, and also the inability to bend (Fig. 9.2). The slippage is often eccentric and therefore leads to an apparent scoliosis.

ISTHMIC

In the case of Type 2, isthmic spondylolisthesis, the posterior elements are not dysplastic. The lesion is in the isthmus.

Subtype 2A

In the first subtype of isthmic spondylolisthesis, there is lysis of the pars interarticularis, which is essentially a fatigue fracture. It occurs without any symptoms in the vast majority of children with this condition, and the incidence in children over the age of 10 varies from 5% in British and North American children to 50% in Inuit children. The vast majority never proceed to listhesis and are completely symptom free. If symptoms do occur, then it is usually in late adolescence and early adult life and the symptoms proceed to slippage.

Subtype 2B

The second subtype of isthmic spondylolisthesis is marked by elongation of the pars interarticularis without separation. Its etiology is assumed to be the same as for Subtype 2A; that is to say, micro–fatigue fractures that lead to elongation. Practically, on x-rays it is quite difficult to distinguish between dysplastic spondylolisthesis and Subtype 2B of the isthmic type (Fig. 9.3). They present in a different way clinically, however; the tilting of the pelvis seen in the dysplastic type is not present in the isthmic subtype, nor is the acute hamstring spasm. As the pars extends, it thins out and looks like pulled-out chewing gum. The microfractures are not visible on x-ray.

Subtype 2C

This subtype is associated with an acute fracture of the pars interarticularis, which occurs only in acute trauma, such as a motor vehicle accident. It is uncommon and not

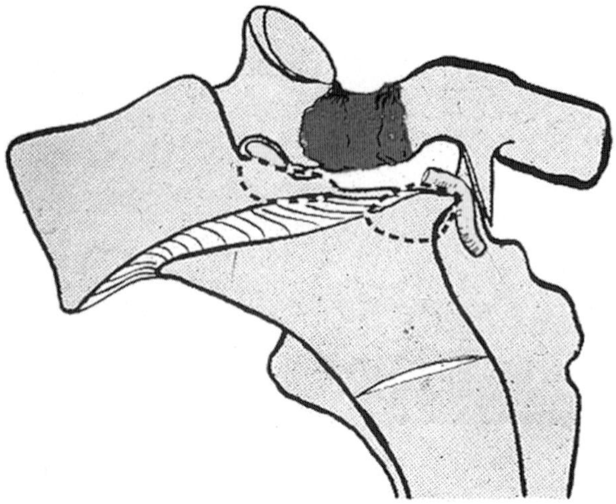

FIG. 9.3. Isthmic Subtype 2B spondylolisthesis very similar to dysplastic.

dissimilar to Type 4, traumatic spondydolisthesis. It is not slowly progressive in the same way as Subtype 2A and Subtype 2B can be. In any case, the fractures unite like any other fracture if reduced properly.

DEGENERATIVE

Type 3, degenerative spondydolisthesis, occurs in motion segments that have had long-standing degenerative change with dysfunction of the disc, and with it wear occurs in the facet joints posteriorly. This allows the mortice formed by the facet joints to become loose and therefore the vertebra to slip forward. One would expect this to occur in older patients, and that is the case. It seldom occurs before the age of 50. It is four times more common in females than in males, and 90% of the slips are at the L4–L5 motion segment. The slippage is not gross and it is essentially stable and therefore presents with back pain and occasional root stenosis (Fig. 9.4).

TRAUMATIC

Type 4, traumatic spondylolisthesis, is very similar to Subtype 2B in that it is an acute traumatic fracture, but the fracture is not in the pars interarticularis. It can be in any part of the posterior elements except the pars. The fracture allows the vertebra above to slide forward on the vertebra below. This type is also very uncommon but will unite if immobilized properly even without internal fixation.

PATHOLOGICAL

Type 5, pathological spondylolisthesis, is the slippage of one vertebra forward on the other due to pathological abnormality of the bone. The bone gives way under the shear effect of gravity. The pathological process may be either generalized or localized. Generalized diseases such as arthrogryphosis and Albers-Schonberg can give rise to this condition. These are extremely rare diseases. Local causes can be primary tumors or more

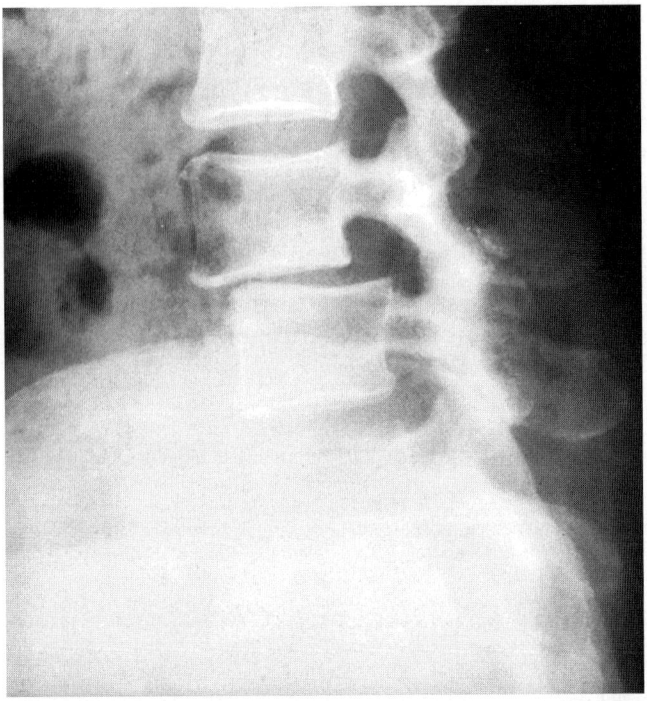

FIG. 9.4. Degenerative spondylolisthesis at L4–L5.

commonly secondary deposits in the posterior elements. Paget disease can soften the bone and allow slippage and, with it, local spinal stenosis. In the Wiltse, MacNab, and Newman 1976 classification of spondylolisthesis, "aquisita" is included in pathological spondylolisthesis. (But some textbooks call this Type 6.) It is best to stick to the original classification. In spondylolisthesis aquisita, there is a spondylolisthesis above a previous fusion. It is iatrogenic due to either excess stripping of muscle and thus damage to the blood supply or direct damage to the penosteum. The lysis can, of course, lead to a slip. Spondylolisthesis aquisita can also occur after excessive decompression for stenosis for these same reasons. The classification of MacNab, Wiltse, and Newman has remained the gold standard now for 30 years. There have been numerous attempts to reclassify this original classification. We have just seen spondylolisthesis aquisita given its own type. It has been suggested that it might be more efficacious to classify spondylolisthesis according to the degree of stability. There is no doubt that some forms of spondylolistheses are highly unstable and others are essentially stable. Some classifications would divide on this basis. This is a spurious classification because with the passage of time the indications for surgery have varied and because different surgeons take different views as to what should and should not be operated upon.

At the Royal National Orthopaedic Hospital, we tried to form a subgroup [Isthmic Type 2A (Lytic)] based on the observation that spondydolisthesis that occurs above the lumbosacral level behaves differently from spondydolisthesis at the lumbosacral level. There is no doubt that higher-level isthmic spondylolisthesis behaves differently from that at the lumbosacral level. It leads predominantly to radicular pain rather than back pain and occurs in a much older age group. This classification has never been accepted, and most clinicians remain with the original classification. The degrees of slippage have also been classified by numerous people, but Meyerding's scale is usually accepted as the best. It allows a way of comparing one physician's treatment with another. Meyerding graded the slippage on a scale of 1 to 4:

Grade 1. Less than 25%
Grade 2. 25%–50%
Grade 3. 50%–75%
Grade 4. 75%–100%

Spondyloptosis is part of the Grade 4 slip, although some would make it Grade 5. Hopefully, no one will attempt any further reclassification in the foreseeable future.

REFERENCES

1. Jackson A, Kirwan E, Sullivan M. Lytic spondylolisthesis above the lumbo-sacral level. *J Bone Joint Surg* 1978; 60-B:439–440.
2. Junghauns H. Spondylolisthesis. *Klin Chir* 1929;158:554.
3. MacNab I. Spondylolisthesis with an intact neural arch. *J Bone Joint Surg* 1950;32:325–333.
4. Newman PH. Etiology of spondylolisthesis. *J Bone Joint Surg* 1963;45-B:39–59.
5. Newman PH. 1975. Spondylolisthesis paper. ISSLS Meeting, London, 1975.
6. Neugebauer FL. Neur beitag zur aetiology und casuistic der spondyl-olisthesis. *Arch Gynak* 1895;25:182
7. Wiltse LL. Classification and etiology of spondylolisthesis. In: *Symposium on the Spine.* St. Louis: Mosby; 1969:143–167.
8. Wiltse LL. 1975. Spondylolisthesis paper. ISSLS Meeting, London, 1975.
9. Wiltse LL, Newman PH, MacNab I. Classification of spondylolysis and spondylolisthesis. *Clin Orthop Rel Res* 1976;117:23.

10
Children

F. Balagué and J. Dudler

Most review articles claim that the majority of spondylolysis and olisthesis cases in children are asymptomatic (1,2). However, a fundamentally contrary view is defended by Österman et al., who argue that "spondylolisthesis is the most important cause of back pain in children and adolescents..." (3). Such controversy is not without any impact on our clinical practice. If indeed children are asymptomatic, we have to rely on large prospective general population cohort studies for information on the disease. The implication is also that diagnosis will heavily rely on sophisticated radiological studies applied to a large, more and less selected population. On the opposite side, if the majority of patients seek medical attention, we should focus on the appropriateness of the history and clinical examination and their respective sensitivity and specificity for the populations at hand. A rather unique radiographic study including 500 unselected first-graders and their families demonstrated that the incidence of spondylolysis increased with age (4). In the several subjects where a pars interarticularis defect developed while under observation, it seems that none complained of discomfort or pain. Similarly, progression of olisthesis was found to be quite unusual, particularly after adolescence, and never symptomatic in this population from age 6 to age 25. This study supports the notion that both pathologies are frequently asymptomatic, at least at the young age when they initially appear (4). However, spondylolysis in children is considered to have a genetic predisposition, while lesions occurring in adolescents, particularly athletes, are considered to be stress fractures due to excessive load of the spine without predisposition (5). Such differences may also have an impact on clinical presentation and explain the opposite claims previously mentioned. Therefore, children and adolescents will be addressed separately in this chapter. Finally, when approaching this literature, the reader has to keep in mind a few limitations. Obviously, scarce information from the physical examination of asymptomatic subjects is scarce. Therefore, we rely mainly on published series of cases, which do not necessarily reflect the signs and symptoms of common subjects but the ones that required medical attention. Also in children, medical attention is sought by parents and not directly by the subjects themselves and probably reflects both the subjects' symptoms and the parents' perception of severity.

SYMPTOMS

Children

In his reviews, Hensinger stated that symptoms have reported to be "relatively uncommon in children" and also that "a significant number of children do not have pain and only seek medical evaluation because of postural deformity or abnormality of gait" (6,7). Perhaps such abnormalities are biased through signs- and symptoms-induced parental anxiety. A recent paper focused specifically on children diagnosed before the age of 5 (8). The authors identified eight cases (4.2%) diagnosed responding to this criterion among a group of 188 spondylolisthesis patients, all younger than 20 years old. At diagnosis, these patients were aged from 9 months to 5 years (average 3.5 years), and in two cases the etiology was traumatic or secondary to the treatment of an intradural tumor. These authors highlight the fact that postural deformities, abnormal gait secondary to hamstring tightness, and skin anomalies, rather than back pain, were the main reasons for seeking medical attention (8). Again, this is a good example of our tendency to apply adult definitions to assess children and low back pain. Children are in a general learning process, including expression of pain in an adequate and acceptable fashion, both socially and culturally (9). In younger children, reported symptoms are more a reflection of parents' beliefs and anxiety than complaints from the child himself or herself, but we should be careful not to deny analgesic treatment if it seems necessary.

Adolescents

On the contrary to children, spondylolysis appears to be symptomatic in adolescents. Around 90% of teenagers with moderate spondylolisthesis reported low back pain in a retrospective study of 149 patients (10). In cases of advanced spondylolisthesis, 11 treated conservatively and 27 surgically, symptoms also began between the ages of 10 and 15 years in 4 patients treated conservatively and 14 patients treated surgically (11), underlining the fact that symptoms are more common in adolescents and perhaps etiology differs with children. It is difficult to know the actual prevalence of pain among subjects with spondylolysis in the general population. However, figures from a cohort of more than 900 football players described by Iwamoto et al. demonstrated that roughly 80% of the subjects with spondylolysis reported low back pain as compared with one third of those without any radiological abnormalities (12). In a similar study carried out among 3,152 top notch Spanish athletes, Soler and Calderón reported that 46% of the subjects with spondylolysis and 23.5% of those without such a lesion reported low back pain at any time (13). The common presentation is an insidious onset lumbar pain, rather than lumbosacral or thoracolumbar. Initially, pain may be reported after strenuous physical activities and rest usually relieves the symptoms. With progression of symptoms, even daily living activities may become painful. Extension or rotation may increase symptoms, however the correlation between exacerbating factors and painful spondylolysis "has not been well assessed in the literature" (14). Radiations to the buttocks or the posterior aspect of the thigh may occur alone or in conjunction with low back pain. In Seitsalo's series with conservatively and surgically treated teenagers, radiating pain alone was reported by 8% and 43% of patients, respectively, and both low back and radiating pain by 8% and 40% (10). Finally, true radicular symptoms and bowel or bladder dysfunction are very rare (2,5,6), but cauda equina syndrome has been described to occur in cases of Grade 4 spondylolisthesis or spondyloptosis (2).

PHYSICAL EXAMINATION

Different clinical signs have been described. Again, scarce information is available in asymptomatic subjects and it is difficult to know the actual prevalence of such signs in the general population. Furthermore, the limits of the physical examination have been pointed out by Logroscino et al., who stated that the diagnosis of spondylolysis on the basis of a physical examination alone is impossible (2)

Children

In children with spondylolysis or Grades 1 or 2 spondylolisthesis, the physical examination may be entirely normal (6). If abnormal, the main findings are tenderness on palpation of the low back, pain and restriction in the lateral bending, severe lumbar lordosis, tight hamstrings, pelvic tilt, scoliosis, palpable lumbar step-off, and skin defects (8). In his reviews, Hensinger listed several clinical signs described in the literature and associated the particular gait (stiff-legged and short gait), previously described as a distinct syndrome by Phalen and Dickson to tightness of the hamstrings (6,7). Finally, children seldom have signs of nerve root compression (6) and even though neurologic findings have been reported to be "very rare," Beguiristain et al. recommend ruling out sacral anesthesia and bladder dysfunction by physical examination (8).

Adolescents

In adolescents, the physical examination is principally determined by muscles tightness and spasm; in advanced cases, biomechanically induced changes have been reported. Hamstring tightness defined by the popliteal angle >30 degrees to 45 degrees may be associated with the awkward gait with decreased stance phase on the affected side (5). According to the description of this gait by Logroscino et al., patients take "small steps, holding their legs rigid and rotating their pelvis" and to maintain the knees flexed, they often walk on their toes (2). In Seitsalo's paper previously mentioned (10), the prevalence of tight hamstrings defined as a straight leg raising (SLR) <60° was 3% in the group treated conservatively and 14% among those selected for surgery. However, according to Hensinger, as much as 80% of symptomatic cases may have hamstring tightness or spasm (6). A clear explanation for this finding is lacking, but hamstring tightness is seldom accompanied by neurologic signs (6) and the SLR is rarely painful (5) In cases with severe contracture of the ischiocrural muscles, patients may present with flexion of the hips and knees, retroversion of the pelvis, and flattening of the lumbar lordosis both in standing and supine positions. This posture is usually more or less fixed, and attempts to extend the hips passively are painful (2). Paraspinal muscle tenderness and spasm are also reported (5). A lumbar "sag" or scoliosis is commonly associated with secondary lumbar muscle spasm (23% to 48% of the cases) (6,7). Three patterns of scoliosis, namely sciatic, olisthetic, and idiopathic, have been described, with the first two types directly related to spondylolisthesis, while the relationship of the third type is less clear (7). In advanced cases with Grades 4 and 5, a progressive shortening of the trunk and postural changes to compensate for the anterior displacement of the center of gravity may appear with a transverse cutaneous fold forming at the level of the umbilicus. The pelvic rotation is responsible for the observed flattening of the buttocks, while active extension becomes impossible and a hyperlordosis cranial to the displaced segment may appear (2). Finally, some dynamic clinical tests have been reported with pain appearing with lumbar hyperextension or during the one-legged hyperextension test (Jackson) (5).

CONCLUSION

It is commonly accepted that the majority of children with spondylolysis or olisthesis are asymptomatic or, rather, do not seek medical attention. Children are seldom referred to medical care for pain but rather due to scoliosis, abnormal gait, or esthetic reasons. Therefore, prevalence of signs and symptoms in the general population is missing. On the contrary, low back pain alone or radiating to the buttocks is a frequent complaint of adolescents, particularly those involved in sports activities. But in either case, no symptom is pathognomonic of spondylolysis or olisthesis. Again, physical signs are scarce and unspecific in children and adolescents, and mainly related to muscle spasms and tightness. Neurologic signs are uncommon, especially in children. If almost pathognomonic signs are recognized in high grades of olisthesis, physical signs are probably totally irrelevant findings in patients with pars defects without slip or Grade I olisthesis.

REFERENCES

1. Bono CM. Low-back pain in athletes. *J Bone Joint Surg Am* 2004;86-A(2):382–396.
2. Logroscino G, Mazza O, Aulisa G, et al. Spondylolysis and spondylolisthesis in the pediatric and adolescent population. *Childs Nerv Syst* 2001;17(11):644–655.
3. Österman K, Schlenzka D, Poussa M, et al. Isthmic spondylolisthesis in symptomatic and asymptomatic subjects, epidemiology, and natural history with special reference to disk abnormalities and mode of treatment. *Clin Orthop* 1993;297:65–70.
4. Fredrickson BE, Baker D, McHolick WJ, et al. The natural history of spondylolysis and spondylolisthesis. *J Bone Joint Surg Am* 1984;66(5):699–707.
5. Lim MR, Yoon SC, Green DW. Symptomatic spondylolysis: diagnosis and treatment. *Curr Opin Pediatr* 2004; 16(1):37–46.
6. Hensinger RN. Spondylolysis and spondylolisthesis in children. *Instr Course Lect* 1983;32:132–151.
7. Hensinger RN. Spondylolysis and spondylolisthesis in children and adolescents. *J Bone Joint Surg Am* 1989;71(7):1098–1107.
8. Beguiristain JL, Diaz-de-Rada P. Spondylolisthesis in pre-school children. *J Pediatr Orthop* B 2004; 13:225–230.
9. Balague F, Dudler J, Nordin M. Low-back pain in children. *Lancet* 2003;361(9367):1403–1404. 10.
10. Seitsalo S. Operative and conservative treatment of moderate spondylolisthesis in young patients. *J Bone Joint Surg Br* 1990;72-B:908–913.
11. Harris IE, Weinstein SL. Long-term follow-up of patients with grade-iii and iv spondylolisthesis. *J Bone Joint Surg Am* 1987;69-A(7):960–969.
12. Iwamoto J, Abe H, Tsukimura Y, et al. Relationship between radiographic abnormalities of lumbar spine and incidence of low back pain in high school and college football players. *Am J Sports Med* 2004;32(3):781–786.
13. Soler T, Calderón C. The prevalence of spondylolysis in the Spanish elite athlete. *Am J Sports Med* 2000;28(1):57–62.
14. Standaert CJ, Herring SA, Halpern B, et al. Spondylolysis. *Phys Med Rehabil Clin N Am* 2000;11(4):785–803.

11

Sport, Spondylolysis, and Spondylolisthesis

E. Munting

Which attitude must be adopted toward the young athlete or the occasional sportsman or woman presenting with low back pain? No clear guidelines regarding the diagnostic work-up in these patients is agreed upon. A specific low back pain (LBP) is a very common condition in young athletes as well as in the overall population (1,2). But spondylolysis and spondylolisthesis are also common conditions arising during childhood, the symptoms of which range from none in the vast majority of the cases to incapacitating pain and neurological deficit (3).

Once isthmic spondylolysis with or without spondylolisthesis is demonstrated, what therapeutic proposal should be given? To answer this question, one needs to know the prevalence of the asymptomatic and symptomatic condition as well as its natural history in this group of patients. Micheli and Wood found that 47% of adolescent athletes presenting to a sports medicine clinic with LBP had spondylolysis as compared to a control group of adults with LBP, in whom the condition was found in only 5% of the cases (4). This significant difference in prevalence of symptomatic spondylolysis among athletes suggests that the physiopathology of the condition may be different in athletes than in nonathletic persons. Precise knowledge about all these aspects of the condition is still lacking.

EPIDEMIOLOGY AND PHYSIOPATHOLOGY OF SPONDYLOLYSIS

Isthmic spondylolysis is considered to be a fatigue fracture of the pars interarticularis (5).

Definitions

Fatigue fracture is the failure of a structure as a result of *cyclic stresses* whose intensity is within the elastic domain and far less than the ultimate tensile or compressive strength of that structure.

Pathologic fracture is a break in a bone as a result of a local or generalized weakness of the bone related to some disease affecting the material properties of the bone (osteoporosis, osteomalacia) or the structural integrity of the bone (osteolytic metastasis destroying part of the bone, screw hole after removal of an osteosynthesis plate, inadequate anatomy of part of the bone).

The fracture resistance of a structure exposed to bending and torsion stresses depends not only on the mechanical properties of its constituting material but also on its shape and design. The mathematical expression of this property is the polar moment of inertia. The polar area moment of inertia of a beam's cross-sectional area measures the beam's ability to resist torsion. The larger the polar moment of inertia, the less the beam will twist.

This is applicable to the pars interarticularis of a vertebra. The influence of the shape of the pars on its mechanical resistance is yet to be defined. There must be an optimal anatomical shape and dimension of the pars to provide adequate mechanical resistance to the stresses that are transferred through the pars. Patients with a less appropriate pars anatomy will be more prone to present spondylolisthesis. Only an anatomical study on a wide sample of vertebrae of normal and spondylolytic vertebrae can confirm this hypothesis. The importance of this factor is clearly suggested by the biomechanical studies of Cyron and Hutton (6).

Sports involving repetitive flexion, extension, or rotation of the spine are known to be associated with a high incidence of spondylolysis. These are the throwing sports (26.7%), gymnastics (11% to 17%), rowing (17%), and football, weight lifting, wrestling, diving, tennis, and volleyball (7,8). In a large radiographic study in an adolescent, athletic population, Rossi found a 15% incidence of spondylolysis (9).

Common sense leads us to suspect that the physiopathology of a spondylolysis occurring in a sedentary patient with no history of uncommon demands on his spine is not the same as that observed in the competitive weight lifter or gymnast. In the former group, a predominant "pathological fracture" mechanism is much likelier (material deficiency or/and structural deficiency: inadequate shape of the pars). In the athletic population, the tentative physiopathology of the constitution of pars defect is that of a true fatigue fracture. The repetitive, mechanical stresses on one or both pars of a vertebra imposed by the regular practice of the considered sport leads to a stress-induced reaction according to Wolff's law. The bone in the pars region reinforces itself in reaction to an increase of the local stresses and strains. This is the stage where a pathological condition may begin, influenced in some patients by some kind of genetically transmitted sensitivity. If the stresses are excessive in *intensity and frequency*, the bone remodeling and reinforcing capacity may be overrun and unable to compensate for fatigue failure of the bone, and microfractures start to occur. In this early pathological stage, the increased bone metabolism will be demonstrated with single photon emission computed tomography (SPECT) scintigraphy and may be demonstrated with magnetic resonance imaging (MRI) (10). It must be emphasized that the normal increase of metabolism related to Wolff's law, which occurs before fatigue failure, may also be picked up, although that situation is *not* pathological. On standard radiographs, the unilateral reinforcement of the pars corresponds to vertebral anisocoria. In this early stage, it seems logical that simply refraining from the causative activity may allow healing as long as there is no underlying pathological condition of the bone (material or structural).

The next stage, occurring after an accumulation of unrepaired microfractures, is overt fracture—acute spondylolysis—which is readily visible on oblique radiographs or computed tomography (CT) scans and characterized by a hot spot on scintigraphy. If the causative stresses continue to be applied, the healing process of the fracture will be compromised, leading to delayed union and finally pseudarthrosis. The scintigraphy becomes normal with time while on radiographs and CT scan the margins of the pars defect appear sclerotic. Repair of the pars at this stage can probably be obtained only by means of a surgical procedure.

The following stage, influenced by vertebral morphology, persisting mechanical strains and stresses and disc degeneration, will be spondylolisthesis, rarely progressive (3).

The questions that remain to be answered are, among others:

- Is spondylolysis in the athlete more often symptomatic than in the nonathletic population?
- When spondylolysis is symptomatic in the athlete, is it more often in the early stages?

- Is the clinical and radiographic outcome of symptomatic spondylolysis in the nonathletic population as good as in the athletic population?
- Is there a difference in the anatomy of the pars in the normal population and those people presenting with spondylolysis, and to what extent is this parameter influential in the athlete with spondylolysis?

Whatever the answer to these questions, if the physiopathology of spondylolisthesis is different in young athletes as compared to the sedentary population, the outcome of the condition may be different as well.

DIAGNOSIS

The difficulty of diagnosis is mostly related to the great variation in symptoms associated to the previously described stages. Knowing that the incidence of spondylolysis is about 3% to 6% in the Caucasian population (3,11), it is obvious that most cases go silently through the whole pathological sequence. The condition may remain undetected forever or may become symptomatic only at a late stage, following some minor or significant trauma. This is a subject of endless debate regarding compensation in work-related injuries or incidents revealing an unknown spondylolysis, presenting all radiographic characteristics of an old, ununited fracture of the pars. Obviously, any given patient may or may not become symptomatic at any stage of the condition. Adding to this fact the high frequency of nonspecific low back pain among children and adolescents, one understands that the early diagnosis of spondylolysis is not possible in all cases.

The diagnosis of pars defect cannot be made based on the history and physical examination. Sys at al. found an average delay between onset of symptoms and diagnosis of 11.3 weeks in a group of young athletes (8). Only imaging can provide the diagnosis. There is no consensus about *when* and *what type* of primary imaging modality should be used when suspecting the diagnosis of spondylolysis in an athlete. Knowing the high incidence of spondylolisthesis in the young athlete with LBP (in his or her early teens or even before), careful and detailed history about the course and the intensity of the symptoms will help in decision making about the necessity of further investigations. Athletes with LBP and practicing one of the sports known to be associated with spondylolysis will be screened earlier than the occasional athlete complaining of mild, nonspecific symptoms. In the athletic population, the prevalence of completely asymptomatic spondylolysis is not known.

The combination of bone scan, SPECT in particular, and computed tomography is the gold standard for diagnosis of spondylolysis. Plain radiography has limited sensitivity for detecting spondylolysis because of the variety of orientations of the plane of the defect: if not tangential to the radiological beam, it can be missed. MRI, though very specific for other diagnosis, has not yet been demonstrated as being equal or superior to SPECT and CT scan for the early diagnosis of spondylolysis. This modality is promising, however, and avoids exposing the patient to radiation (10).

TREATMENT AND OUTCOME

Treating and healing athletes depends on the type of stress fracture and thus the timing of diagnosis and intervention. The development of a stress fracture is a continuum that ranges from normal bone to old, ununited, inactive pars fracture and separation with spondylolisthesis. In between these two extremes, one finds stress-related hypermetabolism, changes in the marrow, microfractures, and cortical disruption with local hypermetabolism, involving one or both pars interarticularis.

Early diagnosis, at the stage of hypermetabolism associated to microfatigue fractures or just at the time of acute spondylolysis is of importance in the athlete. Indeed, in this specific population, conservative treatment is remarkably effective in the early stage of the disease, with a high rate of healing, allowing resumption of sports activity to initial levels within a mean 5.5 months after the onset of treatment in about 90% of the patients with either uni- or bilateral lesions (8).

Conservative treatment of the early forms with active metabolism around the pars, includes abstention from sports or activity modification and bracing for about 4 months. It must be noticed that the effectiveness of bracing is not demonstrated. While unilateral, early lesions are most likely to heal, nonunion is not correlated to poor clinical outcome. When the fracture is obvious but without sclerotic borders, healing is obtained in 38% to 73% of cases (12). "Old," separated fractures with sclerotic borders will not heal but may become asymptomatic under conservative treatment.

Surgical treatment is to be considered in those athletes that remain symptomatic despite 6 months of conservative treatment. Spondylolysis without listhesis and with a healthy disc are good indications for pars repair. If significant disc degeneration is present, posterolateral or interbody fusion with instrumentation (in case of associated listhesis) should be discussed.

CONCLUSION

Spondylolysis in the athlete is in most cases a benign condition with an excellent outcome under conservative management. The outcome is not affected by the bony healing of the pars. The conservative treatment is mostly abstention from the causative activity for a mean period of about 4 months. The utility of bracing has not been demonstrated.

The exact physiopathology underlying the condition probably involves a true fatigue fracture mechanism in the athlete, whereas an intrinsic fragility of the pars related to anatomy is more likely involved in the sedentary person presenting with a spondylolysis.

REFERENCES

1. Balague F, Troussier B, Salminene JJ. Non-specific low back pain in children and adolescents: risk factors. *Eur Spine J* 1999;8(6):429–438; review.
2. Szpalski M, Gunzburg R, Balague F, et al. A 2-year prospective longitudinal study on low back pain in primary school children. *Eur Spine J* 2002;11(5):459–464.
3. Fredrickson BE, Baker D, McHolick WJ, et al. The natural history of spondylolysis and spondylolisthesis. *J Bone Joint Surg Am* 1984;66:699–707.
4. Micheli LJ, Wood R. Back pain in young athletes: significant differences from adults in causes and patterns. *Arch Pediatr Adolesc Med* 1995;149:15–18.
5. Wiltse LL, Widell, Jackson DW. Fatigue fracture: the basic lesion in isthmic spondylolisthesis. *J Bone Joint Surg Am* 1975;57:17–22.
6. Cyron BM, Hutton WC. Variations in the amount and distribution of cortical bone across the partes interarticulares of L5: a predisposing factor in spondylolysis? *Spine* 1979;4:163–167.
7. Soler T, Calderón C. The prevalence of spondylolysis in the Spanish elite athlete. *Am J Sports Med* 2000;28:57–62.
8. Sys J, Michielsen J, Bracke P, et al. Nonoperative treatment of active spondylolysis in elite athletes with normal X-ray findings: literature review and results of conservative treatment. Eur Spine J 2001;10(6):498–504.
9. Rossi F. Spondylolysis, spondylolisthesis and sports. *J Sports Med Phys Fitness* 1978;18:317–340.
10. Hollenberg GM, Beattie PF, Meyers SP, et al. Stress reactions of the lumbar pars interarticularis: the development of a new MRI classification system. *Spine* 2002;15;27(2):181–186.
11. Roche MA, Rowe GG. The incidence of separate neural arch and coincident bone variations: a survey of 4,200 skeletons. *Anat Rec* 1951;109:233–252.
12. Morita T, Ikata T, Katoh S, et al. Lumbar spondylolysis in children and adolescents. *J Bone Joint Surg Br* 1995;77:620–625.

12

Conservative Treatment: Children

J. Dudler and F. Balagué

Before analyzing any treatment's modality and outcome, it seems important to define the target population. It is believed that the majority of spondylolysis and olisthesis cases in children are asymptomatic (1,2). By definition, an asymptomatic case is unlikely to receive treatment because neither the child nor the parents of the child who is asymptomatic will seek medical attention for the child, who therefore will not be treated. However, such a case could be identified by chance during a radiologic exam, and the question of a treatment may be raised. As pointed out by Fredrickson et al. in their prospective radiographic study (3), knowledge of the natural history of the disease should always enlighten our therapeutic decisions. The information available on the natural history of spondylolysis and spondylolisthesis is rather scarce, but Beutler et al. recently published a longitudinal study with an unusually long, 45-year follow-up suggesting that the natural history of asymptomatic cases is benign (4). To summarize, this study shows that a unilateral lyses is not associated with vertebral slip or disability and that subjects with bilateral L5 defects follow a clinical course similar to that of general population. Moreover, slip progression rate slows with age, at least during their follow-up (4). The most prevalent view, shared by Beutler and other authors (2,4,5), is that cases of spondylolysis or spondylolisthesis identified by chance should not and do not require treatment in the absence of symptoms. However, this opinion is not endorsed by all authors. Österman et al. recommended fusion, even in asymptomatic cases, for patients with a slip in excess of 40% (6).

CASE REPORT

A teenager initially consulted a physician at the age of 14 years for low back pain attributed to a trauma. He had progressively been involved in competitive sport (ice hockey) since the age of 6 without any major concern. The physical evaluation showed a step-off, a painful limitation of the active extension of the lumbar spine and some hamstring tightness. Standard radiographs demonstrated an L5 bilateral spondylolysis with Grade I spondylolisthesis (Fig. 12.1A), while functional radiographs in hyperflexion and hyperextension demonstrated minor translation of L5. A conservative management option was chosen after discussion with a pediatric orthopaedic surgeon, with a good functional outcome and return to the patient's previous level of sports activity. Lumbar radiographs taken 3 years later did not show any progression of the vertebral slip (Fig. 12.1B). The subject is currently aged 23 and still playing ice hockey in a team, without any specific medical attention since the last radiographs.

CONSERVATIVE TREATMENT MODALITIES

The treatment of spondylolysis and spondylolisthesis can be conservative or surgical, but the therapeutic objectives remain similar. The three main treatment objectives recognized

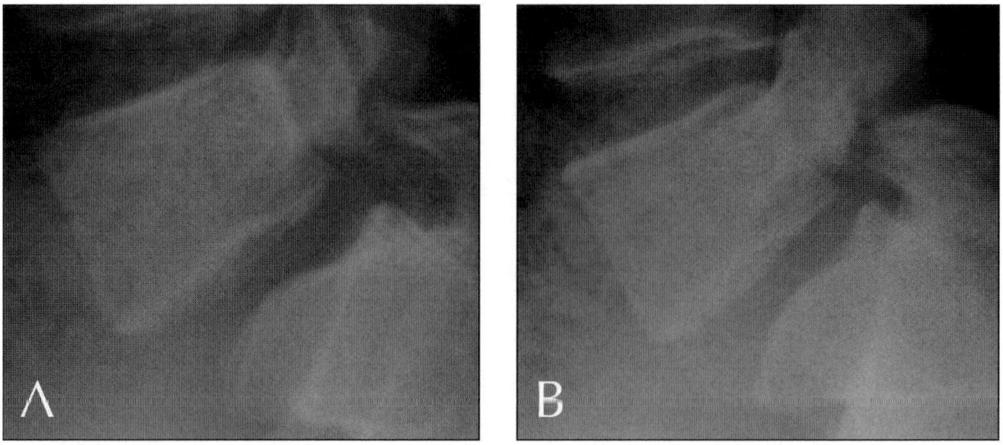

FIG. 12.1. Standard radiographs (**A** and **B**) taken 3 years apart and demonstrating bilateral spondylolysis with Grade 1 spondylolisthesis. Note the absence of either bone healing or evolution of the slip.

are bone healing, pain relief, and optimization of physical function (7). However, in their review, Herman et al. emphasize that bracing a young patient with spondylolysis is not directed at healing the defect, but that the real goal of immobilization is just alleviating symptoms (8). A similar point of view can be found in Wimberly and Lauerman's review of the topic (9). Various modalities of conservative management can be identified in the literature, from no treatment and observation, to activity modification, physical therapy, bracing, casting (5,10) or electrical stimulation (11). In all cases, information relies mainly on case reports, series of cases or cohort studies, and we failed to identified any single randomized controlled trial in these age groups. As stated before, most authors do not recommend active therapy in the case of an asymptomatic patient. According to Logroscino et al., physical activity should not be restricted in asymptomatic patients with spondylolysis, while patients with Grade 1 olisthesis should be advised to restrict sports and activities that place an increased strain on the unstable vertebra (2). However, based on their impressive longitudinal study's data, Fredrickson et al. allow full participation in sports (3). They do recommend, however, that the asymptomatic patient be informed of the existence of the lesion and told to seek medical attention if symptoms develop. Most authors agree on the beneficial effects of physical therapy, treatment that remains widely prescribed even if the demonstration of its efficiency is still lacking. A systematic review of physiotherapy for spondylolysis and olisthesis has recently been published (12). The fact that only 2 of 52 studies could finally be included in the analysis indicates the poor methodologic quality of this literature, and unfortunately neither included children or teenagers in their population. Therefore, there is an obvious lack of evidence to advise for or against physiotherapy as treatment, even if it appears reasonable (12). As a physical therapy modality, external electrical stimulation deserves a special note. Stasinopoulos has carefully reviewed the literature (11) and found that only two articles, which may be considered case reports, described the effects of such treatment in adolescents. One of these articles, describing two adolescent athletes, seems particularly promising. However, in terms of evidence, these findings are again too limited to advise for or against a generalized utilization of external electrical stimulation in this indication (11). Similarly, if external immobilization may seem an obvious mode of treatment, the timing, the role, and the best type of device continue to be a matter of debate and unresolved. In one of the original papers by Wiltse et al. (13), healing of the defects under conservative management was described in 12 cases. However, bracing ranged from no immobilization at all to a knees-to-nipples cast for 2 months. Even in the recent literature, the role and best type of external immobilization continue to be debated (1). In their review article, Herman et al. recommend for the treatment of spondylolysis immobilization in a thoracolumbosacral orthosis (TLSO) with a single-leg thigh extension or an antilordotic TLSO for a period of 6 to 12 weeks, casting being reserved for the noncompliant athlete. The period of immobilization should be adapted to bone healing, with bracing for longer than 6 months not indicated. Also, they do recommend the prescription of a rehabilitation program and a progressive return to sports activities over a 6- to 8-week period after the immobilization (8). Finally, the use of immobilization in a lightweight plaster or plastic jacket has been advocated by Hensinger for the preoperative evaluation (14).

At last, radiologists have reported in patients with either spondylolisthesis or just pars defect without vertebral slip, communication between isthmic defects and the adjacent zygapophyseal joints (15,16), and it is conceivable that a localized intervention could be beneficial. However, we did not find any studies evaluating the potential value of zygapophyseal injections in the treatment of low back pain associated with spondylolysis or olisthesis.

CONSERVATIVE TREATMENT OUTCOME

From a clinical and pathophysiologic standpoint, it appears reasonable to estimate that spondylolysis could behave differently in the presence or absence of a slip. We have separated our treatment outcome analysis accordingly. Furthermore, it is important to realize that if as doctors we tend to put a lot of emphasis on bone healing, for the patient, relief of pain and optimization of physical function are really the relevant treatment outcomes.

Spondylolysis

As already stated, treatment and outcome measures must be interpreted in the light of the natural history of the disease. One main objective of treatment is bone healing. Merbs, in a study of Canadian Inuit skeletons from a population that is known to have lived in a period when neither diagnosis or treatment of spondylolysis existed, reported evidence of spontaneous bone healing in cases of unilateral spondylolysis, but found that unilateral healing of bilateral lesions was a rare phenomenon (17). Thus, it appears that bone healing can occur to a certain extent in the absence of any treatment in unilateral case, a notion important to remember when interpreting the results on bone healing for the various treatment modalities. Fuji et al. recently evaluated retrospectively their results in 134 patients, 29 with a unilateral spondylolytic lesion and 105 with bilateral defects, for a total of 239 defects of the pars. The mean age at presentation was 13.8 years with a range from 7 to 17 years, and 109 of the patients were boys. All patients were treated conservatively with various interventions; the mean duration of follow-up was 3.4 years (range 1 to 9.8 years). Patients were initially asked to discontinue their sports activities, wear a Damen corset and undertake isometric exercises for the trunk muscles during the first 3 months of treatment. Once pain subsided, they were progressively mobilized and isotonic exercises of the trunk muscles started. If the follow-up radiographs taken at

3 months demonstrated signs of union of the defect, patients were advised against any sport for an additional 3 months; otherwise (if there was no union or if there was worsening of the defect), they were allowed to go back to their sports activities providing they reported lessening of the pain and demonstrated stronger trunk muscles. Forty of 239 defects actually healed. In those cases, once the union was demonstrated on radiographs or computed tomography (CT) scan, subjects were advised to resume sports activities with a lumbosacral support to restrict lumbar extension. The statistical analysis shows that several local, regional, and systemic variables were significantly associated with the result on bone healing (18). As might be expected, the initial aspect of the pars defects predicts bone healing. Morita et al. retrospectively reported on 185 adolescents with lumbar spondylolysis totalling 346 pars defects overall after a follow-up of 1 year with a range from 3 to 48 months (19). Initial treatment consisted of discontinuation of sports activities and the use of a conventional lumbar corset for 3 to 6 months. Follow-up radiographs were taken at 4-week intervals. Once the defects had united, patients followed a rehabilitation protocol while wearing a lumbosacral support that allows full flexion but restricts lumbar extension. Bony lesions were assessed by oblique views and CT scan and classified into early, progressive, and terminal stages. Overall, 37.9% of the pars defects had apparent radiologic healing; the actual figures were 73% for early-stage lesions, 39% for the progressive-stage, and 0 for the terminal-stage lesions (19).

A study by Miller et al. reports on 40 athletes aged 12 to 20 years suffering from spondylolysis with negative radiographs but a positive bone scintigram or single-photon emission computed tomography (SPECT) (20). The patients were followed for 7 to 11 years after conservative management, treatment consisting of a nonrigid lumbar bracing 23 hours a day and a flexion-only trunk-strengthening program started after 2 to 4 weeks of relative rest. Subjects still reporting pain at the 4-week follow-up were placed in a rigid lumbar brace. Interestingly, in terms of outcome, this represented only 5% of the cases, which means that 95% of the patients were asymptomatic or at least paucisymptomatic at 1 month. At 6 to 8 weeks, a functional progression program was then prescribed, with resumption of sports activities by week 8 to 12 wearing a nonrigid brace in pain-free subjects at rest, in unprotected hyperextension and during the subject's specific sport activity with a brace. Braces were progressively discarded over several weeks. At final follow-up, 32 patients were surveyed by phone, the low back outcome score calculated, and CT scan and lateral radiographs obtained in 11 subjects. In terms of outcomes, all subjects went back to their prior levels of sports activity. The functional outcomes were excellent with a mean score of 67.5 $\pm$ 9 out of a maximum score of 75. There were no significant differences between subgroups according to their initial anatomical grading of the defect, and the radiographic studies obtained failed to demonstrate healing of bilateral lesions regardless of the anatomical appearance on initial CT scans in this limited group (20). Thus, an important lesson from this study is that it appears that a relatively simple and short-term conservative treatment can be highly efficient in terms of both pain relief and physical function, and not too much emphasis should be put on bone healing or the appearance and grading of the initial lesion. Confirming these impressions, subjects' self-rated outcome was excellent in 82.2% of cases regardless of the lesion's group in a study by Sys et al. on 28 athletes (average age 17.2 years) with isthmic spondylolysis treated conservatively and followed for 13.2 months (3–51 months) (21). All cases were evaluated by means of radiographs, CT scan, and bone scans, including SPECT, and classified as unilateral, bilateral or pseudobilateral according to the uptake pattern. Patients were braced 23 hours/day with Boston Overlap Brace with a hinged extension to the thigh. Hamstring stretching, abdominal muscle strengthening exercises, and pelvic tilts were started when the subject was pain free during daily activities. Bracing time was individually tailored according to the scintigraphic evolution (range 12–32 weeks; average 15.9 weeks). Again, bone healing was observed in all cases with unilateral lesion, in 5 of 9 cases with bilateral lesion, and in none of those with pseudobilateral lesion, differences that were statistically significant ($P < 0.05$). Nevertheless, patients' outcome was excellent and independent of the lesion groups, emphasizing the lack of association between radiographic and clinical outcomes.

Spondylolisthesis

The same remarks concerning the relevance of the various outcomes made for spondylolysis are probably true for spondylolisthesis. In his recent review including four published series, Lonstein showed that overall two thirds or more of patients with spondylolisthesis have good results when treated by a simple combination of bracing and exercises (5). Seitsalo retrospectively reported on 149 children and adolescents with moderate spondylolisthesis (slip ≤30%) treated surgically ($n = 77$) or conservatively ($n = 72$) with a follow-up of 13.3 years. Conservative treatment consisted of rest while pain persisted, restriction of activities and stabilizing exercises for the spinal and abdominal muscles. Only five patients were treated by brace. Spontaneous bone healing, estimated in radiographs, occurred in two of the conservatively treated patients. The author concluded that a moderate grade of spondylolisthesis in adolescents usually has a benign course and suggested that spontaneous segmental stabilization may occur as a result of disc degeneration (22). If significantly more surgically treated patient were asymptomatic at long-term follow-up, 75% of the conservatively treated were pain free. Furthermore, 18 patients who were treated conservatively, despite being initially offered surgery for more severe pain and progression of the slip, fared as well as the other nonoperative patients in term of pain index and clinical results. Despite those favorable results for conservative treatment, a clinician may feel more prone to operate on a patient presenting at a very young age as opposed to an adolescent athlete. A small recent series of eight cases diagnosed in children under the age of 5 years seems to support the notion that the same conservative attitude can be applied in this age group, half of them having been managed conservatively with good results at a mean follow-up of 11.5 years (range 9 to 14 years) (23). Finally, Harris and Weinstein described the evolution of 11 cases with severe spondylolisthesis, with spondyloptosis in 6 of them. All cases were treated conservatively from a mean age of 17.8 years, with a follow-up of 18 years (range 3 to 42 years). The conservative treatment consisted of a short trial period of back brace for half of the patients only. None of them consistently used a brace, took medication, or exercised regularly. At follow-up, despite the apparent severity of the lesions, four patients were asymptomatic, six reported mild symptoms, and only one had more significant morning stiffness, which required adjustments in her work schedule. Five of these patients had some neurologic findings. Of note, almost two thirds of these patients stated that spondylolisthesis had not influenced their choice of occupation (24).

CONCLUSIONS

In conclusion and according to the literature, it seems important for clinicians to restrain themselves from being too eager to establish a causal relationship between a child's or adolescent's symptoms and the demonstration of a spondylolysis or minor spondylolisthesis. Consequently, when prescribing a treatment, our therapeutic attitude has to be cautious, as it should be for any other condition with a relatively benign natural history. Regular clinical evaluations of children with such spinal disorders without any intervention are probably all that is needed, at least for the asymptomatic patient whose spinal defect has been discovered on routine radiographs. For most symptomatic patients, a graded conservative approach with restriction of activities, some physical therapy, eventual bracing, and progressive resumption of sports activities is all that is needed in terms of pain relief and physical function. Spondylolisthesis appearing after high-energy trauma may be an exception, according to Hilibrand et al., being much more unstable and probably requiring surgical stabilization at least in adolescents and young adults (25). Some recent studies have demonstrated that initial bony lesions, particularly unilateral ones, might heal with immobilization. It may appear a priori an interesting goal. However, demonstration of an association of bone healing and the return to a pain-free previous functional level is lacking in children. Not too much emphasis should be put on bone healing at the present time, until the impact on the very long-term outcomes into adulthood is demonstrated. Finally, strong evidence is certainly missing to implement a standardized program of conservative management. From the literature, most conservative treatments seem apparently efficient, but more research is necessary to define a general attitude based on evidence and not on personal experiences or limited series of cases.

REFERENCES

1. Bono CM. Low-back pain in athletes. *J Bone Joint Surg Am* 2004;86(2):382–396.
2. Logroscino G, Mazza O, Aulisa G, et al. Spondylolysis and spondylolisthesis in the pediatric and adolescent population. *Childs Nerv Syst* 2001;17(11):644–655.
3. Fredrickson BE, Baker D, McHolick WJ, et al. The natural history of spondylolysis and spondylolisthesis. *J Bone Joint Surg Am* 1984;66(5):699–707.
4. Beutler WJ, Fredrickson BE, Murtland A, et al. The natural history of spondylolysis and spondylolisthesis: 45-year follow-up evaluation. *Spine* 2003;28(10):1027–1035.
5. Lonstein JE. Spondylolisthesis in children: cause, natural history, and management. *Spine* 1999;24(24): 2640–2648.
6. Österman K, Schlenzka D, Poussa M, et al. Isthmic spondylolisthesis in symptomatic and asymptomatic subjects, epidemiology, and natural history with special reference to disk abnormalities and mode of treatment. *Clin Orthop* 1993;297:65–70.
7. Standaert CJ. Spondylolysis in the adolescent athlete. *Clin J Sport Med* 2002;12(2):119–122.
8. Herman MJ, Pizzutillo PD, Cavalier R. Spondylolysis and spondylolisthesis in the child and adolescent athlete. *Orthop Clin North Am* 2003;34(3):461–467, vii.
9. Wimberly RL, Lauerman WC. Spondylolisthesis in the athlete. *Clin Sports Med* 2002;21(1):133–145, vii–viii.
10. Lim MR, Yoon SC, Green DW. Symptomatic spondylolysis: diagnosis and treatment. *Curr Opin Pediatr* 2004; 16(1):37–46.
11. Stasinopoulos D. Treatment of spondylolysis with external electrical stimulation in young athletes: a critical literature review. *Br J Sports Med* 2004;38:352–354.
12. McNeely ML, Torrance G, Magee DJ. A systematic review of physiotherapy for spondylolysis and spondylolisthesis. *Man Ther* 2003;8(2):80–91.
13. Wiltse LL, Widell EH Jr., Jackson DW. Fatigue fracture: the basic lesion in isthmic spondylolisthesis. *J Bone Joint Surg Am* 1975;57(1):17–22.
14. Hensinger RN. Spondylolysis and spondylolisthesis in children. *Instr Course Lect* 1983;32:132–151.
15. Sarazin L, Chevrot A, Pessis E, et al. *RadioGraphics*. 1999;19:93–104.
16. Shipley JA, Beukes CA. The nature of the spondylolytic defect: demonstration of a communicating synovial pseudarthrosis in the pars interarticularis. *J Bone Joint Surg Br* 1998;80(4):662–664.
17. Merbs CF. Asymmetrical spondylolysis. *Am J Phys Anthropol* 2002;119(2):156–174.
18. Fujii K, Katoh S, Sairyo K, et al. Union of defects in the pars interarticularis of the lumbar spine in children and adolescents: the radiological outcome after conservative treatment. *J Bone Joint Surg Br* 2004;86(2): 225–231.
19. Morita T, Ikata T, Katoh S, et al. Lumbar spondylolysis in children and adolescents. *J Bone Joint Surg Br* 1995;77(4):620–625.
20. Miller SF, Congeni J, Swanson K. Long-term functional and anatomical follow-up of early detected spondylolysis in young athletes. *Am J Sports Med* 2004;32(4):928–933.

21. Sys J, Michielsen J, Bracke P, et al. Nonoperative treatment of active spondylolysis in elite athletes with normal x-ray findings: literature review and results of conservative treatment. *Eur J Spine* 2001;10(6):498–504.
22. Seitsalo S. Operative and conservative treatment of moderate spondylolisthesis in young patients. *J Bone Joint Surg Br* 1990;72-B:908–913.
23. Beguiristain JL, Diaz-de-Rada P. Spondylolisthesis in pre-school children. *J Pediatr Orthop* B 2004;13: 225– 230.
24. Harris IE, Weinstein SL. Long-term follow-up of patients with grade-III and IV spondylolisthesis. *J Bone Joint Surg Am*1987;69(7):960–969.
25. Hilibrand AS, Urquhart AG, Graziano GP, et al. Acute spondylolytic spondylolisthesis. Risk of progression and neurological complications. *J Bone Joint Surg Am* 1995;77(2):190–196.

13

Natural Evolution and Conservative Treatment of Adult Spondylolisthesis

Michel Benoist and Raphael Vialle

Isthmic spondylolisthesis results from separation of the pars after a stress fracture or from elongation of the pars without separation. These lesions leave the posterior elements in normal position and allow forward slippage of the lumbar spine. Most cases of isthmic spondylolisthesis develop in schoolchildren. New cases may appear in adolescents or adults engaged in strenuous athletics or heavy work. Meyerding's classification is generally used to describe the degree of slippage: Grade 1 = 0–25% of slip; Grade 2 = 25%–50% of slip; Grade 3 = 50%–75% of slip; Grade 4 = over 75% of slip and spondyloptosis.

Most cases treated in adulthood are predominantly low or moderate (Grade 1 or 2) painful spondylolisthesis. High-grade listhesis is usually detected in childhood or adolescence. However high-grade lesions may have to be treated in adulthood if no major significant symptoms have necessitated surgery in adolescence. The purpose of this chapter is to discuss the natural evolution of lytic spondylolisthesis in adults, including progression of the slip and correlation of the clinical symptoms with the grading and progression of the slip. An overview of conservative treatment is also presented.

EVOLUTION OF SPONDYLOLYSIS INTO SPONDYLOLISTHESIS

Newly developed slippage in adults with spondylolysis is rare but may occur with no evidence of trauma. Such cases have been reported by some authors (1–4), as listed in Table 13.1.

PROGRESSION OF SLIPPAGE IN ADULT ISTHMIC SPONDYLOLISTHESIS

Adult progression of slippage is unusual, and many cases of spondylolisthesis remain stable for the entire adulthood. Studies on progression of the slip in adults are few, often combining adolescents and adults. Progression is even doubted by some investigators. Wiltse and Rothman (5), summarizing the natural history of isthmic spondylolisthesis, state that "significant increases in olisthesis after adulthood are sufficiently uncommon that they are not considered a substantial problem." However, there are a few reports in the literature indicating that progression of the slip does happen and may generate clinical symptoms.

In the majority of these studies, progression of slippage is described in pain-selected populations. There is, however, one study describing the natural history in subjects

TABLE 13.1. *Evolution of spondylolysis into spondylolysis in adulthood*

Authors	Number of Cases
Postacchini (1)	5
Heggeness et al. (2)	2
Virta et al. (3)	1
Ohmori et al. (4)	6

unselected for pain (6). This study by Beutler et al. was started in the early 1950s. Radiographs were obtained in 500 six-year-old schoolchildren. Twenty-two subjects (4.4%) had a spondylolysis. By adulthood, a lytic defect of the pars developed in eight more individuals. These 30 subjects were followed up for 45 years. At the last follow-up, assessment included radiographs, magnetic resonance imaging, a questionnaire on back pain, and 36-Item Short Form Health Survey (SF-36) survey. No subject was lost to follow-up evaluation once a lesion was identified. Conclusions of that report provide valuable information. First, healing of a unilateral pars defect was observed in three subjects. Second, a marked slowing of slip progression was observed in the adult decades to the age of 50 years, and in no subject did the slippage reach 40%. Most patients with bilateral pars defect and slippage followed a clinical course similar to the general population. However, the small number of subjects studied prohibits any generalization of the results.

Progression of slippage has also been reported in studies of patients selected for pain. Recently, Floman (7) has reported a clinical and radiographic review of adult patients with progressive olisthesis. Eighteen patients with low back pain and sciatica were followed during a period of 2 to 20 years (mean: 6–8 years). Slip progression started after the third decade of life, ranging from 9% to 30% (mean: 14.6%).

Marked progression of the slip (>10%) in an adult population with spondylolisthesis and back pain was documented by Virta and Osterman (8). A group of 40 nonoperated patients with Grade 1 or Grade 2 L5 spondylolisthesis was followed up for an average of 17 years. Mean progression of the slip during the observation time was 6.1%.

A clinical and radiologic follow-up study with at least 20 years of observation was published by Saraste (9) in 1987. Vertebral slippage was calculated as the distance in millimeters from the posteroinferior limit of the spondylolytic vertebra to a line through the posterior border of the vertebra below. The mean progression of slippage in 144 adults was 5 mm. Ohmori et al. (4) have followed a group of 22 patients with spondylolysis for an average of 10 years. Four patients with L5 spondylolisthesis at the first visit (mean degree of slip: 15.5 + 13.6) showed progression of the slip. The degree of slip at the second visit was 21.5+/–5).

Danielson et al. (10) have studied the radiologic progression of the slip in a group of 311 patients younger than 30 years at admission. The mean observation time was 3.8 years. A true progression (i.e., an increase >20% from admission) was found in only 3% of the patients. When progression of the slip was related to the different ages, a peak of increase of slippage was observed at age 20–25 years. Similarly, Seitsalo et al. (11), in a long-term evaluation of 272 patients, found that slippage increased in only 4% of adult patients during an observation time of 10 years. Progression of slippage in pain-selected populations is summarized in Table 13.2.

TABLE 13.2. *Progression of vertebral slippage in pain-selected populations (adults)*

Authors	Mean Progression	Observation Time in Years
Saraste H. (9)	5 mm	20
Danielson et al. (10)	3%	3,8
Seitsalo et al. Spine 1992	4%	10
Virta and Osterman (8)	6%	17
Ohmori et al. (4)	5%	10
Floman (7)	14,6	6,8

RADIOLOGIC VARIABLES ASSOCIATED WITH FURTHER SLIPPAGE

Predictive factors have been searched and discussed in studies dealing with radiologic progression of the listhesis. However, as emphasized by Beutler et al. (12), radiographic parameters vary from study to study. Radiographic positioning is not standardized and different measurements are used. For these reasons, predictive radiologic variables are difficult to identify.

The degree of slip, as well as other parameters, among them slip angle, lumbar index, cranial convexity of S1, and disc height, are often difficult to evaluate especially in Grade 3 or 4. Moreover, studies are retrospective, often mixing children, adolescents, and adults. They also lack inter- and intraobserver rating. In spite of these shortcomings and conflicting results, a few common predictive or etiologic factors of progression have been formulated by investigators.

Disc degeneration is correlated with slip progression in most studies. In this regard, the study by Floman (7) is strongly documented as disc degeneration was assessed at the slip level not only by plain radiographs but also by computed tomography or by magnetic resonance imaging. Disc narrowing was also graded according to the presence of osteophytes and of vacuum phenomenon. In all 18 cases described in Floman's study, slip increase was associated with marked disc degeneration at the slip level.

Relation between slip progression and disc degeneration is reported in other studies, including that of Beutler et al. (6). Natural history of the same group of patients had been assessed in 1990. Disc degeneration had already been disclosed as facilitating progression of the slip (13). In Saraste's study, progression of the listhesis was also correlated with disc degeneration, especially in the group with L4 spondylolisthesis. Starting in adult life, disc degeneration appears to be the key factor of slip progression. As stated by Farfan et al. (14), "Disc degeneration occurs below the pars because of rotatory and anteriorly shear forces acting on the disc." An intact disc is the only resistant structure to slip progression. However, as mentioned by Floman (7), progression of slippage and disc degeneration may be concomitant and not related.

Other etiologic factors for progression of the listhesis have been incriminated. They include the percentage of slip observed at presentation (8,11), a low lumbar index (9), or the physiologic strength of the posterior bands of the iliolumbar ligament (4). These factors are not noted by every investigator. For example, no prognostic factors were found in the study by Danielson et al. (10), who consider that the importance of the trapezoidal shape of the spondylolytic vertebrae and of the rounded endplate of the vertebra below are the consequence of the accentuated slip rather than a prognostic factor. In summary, progression in adulthood is not common, affects approximately 20% of painful spondylolisthésis (7), usually remains moderate ranging from 3% (10) to 30% (7), and is principally related to disc degeneration.

ASSOCIATION OF CLINICAL SYMPTOMS WITH DEGREE OF THE SLIP AND ITS PROGRESSION

Spondylolisthesis may remain asymptomatic. In adults, low back pain and leg pain are the most common symptoms of this condition. Pain is usually restricted to the lumbar area, with occasional referred radiation to buttocks and thighs. In the study by Beutler et al. (6) based on a population unselected for pain, there was no statistically significant difference in the pain or physical functioning scores between the spondylolytic group as a whole and those with a slip and the SF 36 norms. Similarly there was no difference in pain or function with the progression of the slip. In studies dealing with pain-selected subjects, symptoms appear to be correlated with the degree of slip. Virta and Ronnemaa (15) have reported on a cohortlike study of 20 women and 26 men with mild spondylolisthesis (Grade 1) compared with sex-matched control subjects derived from the same source. No significant difference was found in back symptoms between the two groups of men. However, women had mild back symptoms more often than the control group. In contrast, Virta and Osterman (8) conducted a follow-up study on correlations of radiographic measurements to indexes of low back pain and functional and working capacity. They followed up 148 patients (age 20–50) for 17 years. The mean degree of slip was 34.4 +1 − 19.7 (Grade 2). The degree of slip correlated positively with the pain index and the activities of daily living. Saraste's study of 255 patients followed up for 20 years found that patients had increased risk for symptoms compared to the normal population when the slip was greater than 25%. In the same study, symptoms and abnormal clinical signs were also strongly correlated with disc degeneration and a low lumbar index in L5 spondylolisthesis (9).

Listhesis at L4 level was also found in Saraste's study as a risk factor for symptoms. This is in agreement with Grober and associates (16), who conducted a retrospective multicenter study of progressive L4–L5 isthmic spondylolisthesis. Those authors concluded that L4 spondylolisthesis usually becomes symptomatic in adults and is more unstable than the L5 type and that surgery is required in a higher percentage of patients. In that multicenter study, L4 spondylolisthesis represented 9% of the entire series.

High-grade spondylolisthesis (Grades 3 and 4) is more rarely encountered in adulthood than low or moderate grades. Most instances have been detected in childhood or adolescence. Some have already been operated. Very little has been written, however, about the natural evolution of spondylolisthesis in nonoperated patients with slippage exceeding 50%, and their condition at the adult age. In this regard, interesting information is found in the paper by Harris and Weinstein (17). The clinical and radiologic course of 11 patients with high-grade slippage was studied. The average age when they were initially seen was 17 years. The average age at the time of follow-up was 37 years. At follow-up, 4 patients were asymptomatic, 6 had mild low back symptoms, and only 1 had more significant symptoms necessitating work adjustment. Surprisingly, 6 of these 11 patients had spondyloptosis: 3 were asymptomatic, 2 had mild symptoms, and 1 had more significant symptoms. Five of the 11 patients had one or more neurologic symptoms (depressed tendon reflex, mild motor weakness). Overall, patients remained active and required minor adjustment in their work and recreational activities but did not have disabling pain, neurologic symptoms, or bowel or bladder incontinence. Nine uncomplicated pregnancies occurred among the female patients. In the same paper, Harris and

TABLE 13.3. *Conservative modalities for treatment of spondylolisthesis*

Rest
Activity modification
Drugs
– Analgesics
– Nonsteroidal anti-inflammatory drugs
– Systemic steroids
– Antidepressants
Injection techniques
– Epidural steroid
– Foraminal steroid
Physical therapy
– Exercises
– Education
– Cognitive intervention
– Corsets and braces
– Transcutaneous electrical nerve stimulation
– Acupuncture

Weinstein also evaluated a group of 21 operated patients with high-grade spondylolisthesis in the same manner. Patients were operated in their teens (mean: 17 years) because of increasing pain. They all had an in situ posterior laminar arthrodesis. At the time of follow-up (mean age: 37.5 years), the 21 operated patients were less symptomatic and less restricted in their activities than the nonoperatively treated patients. It can be concluded from this study that patients with high-grade spondylolisthesis do not invariably develop disabling pain or severe neurologic symptoms later in adulthood.

CONSERVATIVE TREATMENT

Nonoperative therapy is unable to change the anatomic conditions and natural history. Its goals are relief of pain, prevention of recurrent painful episodes, restoration of function, and improvement of the patient's quality of life. The therapeutic program must be adapted to each patient according to a few parameters, including clinical symptoms, duration of symptoms, clinical pattern of evaluation, and patient's age, activities, working status, physical and intellectual level, and motivation, as well as psychosocial factors. Pathologic process (pure lysis, grade of slippage) also must be considered. Conservative modalities of treatment of adult spondylolisthesis are listed in Table 13.3. In other chapters of this book, orthoses and exercises are discussed with pertinent references. This chapter is devoted principally to drugs and injection techniques, with allusion to the other modalities. At this point it should be noted that the validity of treatment methods discussed below has not been scientifically evaluated for spondylolisthesis per se. Only a few randomized controlled trials (RCTs) exist; no Cochrane collaboration study on comprehensive nonoperative care of lytic spondylolisthesis could be found. Accordingly, and as recommended by the Quebec Task Force on Spinal Disorders, efficacy of treatments will be discussed according to their objectives and to the clinical symptoms and stage (18).

Analgesics

Medications such as aspirin or acetaminophen are the most commonly prescribed treatment to reduce symptomatic pain. Their usefulness has been considered to be scientifically proved. Randomized controlled trials of analgesics for back pain are rare and concern principally acute back pain. There is moderate evidence that analgesics are not more effective than nonsteroidal anti-inflammatory drugs (NSAIDs) (19), but they have fewer side effects. The mechanism of action of acetaminophen is still mysterious (20). Time-limited prescription of narcotic analgesics is justified and efficacious in patients with acute back pain and radicular pain. Because of potential addiction and side effects, use of narcotic analgesics for treatment of chronic low back pain is not recommended, but this question is still a matter of debate.

Nonsteroidal Anti-inflammatory Drugs

Numerous RCTs of NSAIDs in nonspecific low back pain have been performed comparing their action to a placebo or to analgesics. A systematic review of these trials reached the conclusions that evidence of efficacy is strong in acute low back pain, moderate in chronic low back pain, and less effective in acute sciatica (19). The efficacy of the various NSAIDs is similar. Moreover, their potential side effects, including gastrointestinal irritation and renal and hepatic toxicity, are similar. There is an increased risk of bleeding, perforation, and renal effects in the elderly population. Careful prescription and close observation are mandatory in this group of individuals. Cox 2 inhibitors were able to decrease dramatically the frequency of gastric ulcers with a similar efficacy. Concerns have been raised regarding unfortunate potential cardiovascular toxicities, including myocardial infarction and stroke.

Corticosteroid Therapy

Systemic steroids are currently used for acute sciatica. A high loading dose is necessary to obtain pain relief. However, the efficacy of systemic steroids has not been proven by valid clinical trials, and they carry significant risk of side effects, including osteonecrosis and steroid psychosis. To avoid these complications and enhance the anti-inflammatory effect, steroids are commonly injected by the epidural or foraminal route. No scientific test of effectiveness over the long term has been carried out in the treatment of radiculopathies caused by discal herniation or stenosis (21,22). Moreover, no specific trial of epidural or foraminal steroid injections has been carried out in the treatment of sciatica in spondylolisthesis patients. However, it should be pointed out that short-term results (23) of epidural or periradicular steroid injections are not correctly addressed in most papers. It is the authors' opinion that short-term relief may be provided, justifying their use in patients with sciatica.

Tricylic Antidepressants

Deyo (24) has carefully reviewed the trials of antidepressants for low back pain and has concluded that because of conflicting results and high dropout rates, the advantage of antidepressants over a placebo could not be demonstrated. Similar conclusions have been formulated by Van Tulder et al. (19). However, in patients with spondylolisthesis with chronic low back pain and overt or subclinical depression, the use of tricyclic antidepressants is justified in spite of the absence of specific trials in this indication. In addition to their antidepressant effect, tricyclics have analgesic properties and improve sleep.

ROLE OF PHYSICAL THERAPY

Classification of physical treatments is shown in Table 13.3. The active modalities consist of exercises and education, including "back school" and ergonomics. There is strong evidence that exercise therapy is effective for chronic nonspecific back pain (19). One study (25) has evaluated the effect of strengthening of abdominal muscles with coactivation of the lumbar multifidus in 44 adult patients with Grade 1 or 2 spondylolisthesis compared with a control group undergoing treatment directed by their respective treating practitioners. This RCT demonstrated that after intervention the specific exercise group showed a statistically significant reduction in pain intensity and functional disability levels maintained at 30-month follow-up. More studies are clearly needed to clarify the kind of exercises that would be the most effective in this category of patients. Moreover and by similarity with chronic nonspecific low back pain associated with disc degeneration, the importance of cognitive intervention to be associated with physical exercises must be stressed (26).

The rationale for lumbar corsets and braces is to impose a mechanical constraint on movement in the hope of reducing nociceptive stimulation. Corsets or braces are commonly prescribed in patients with chronic low back pain with or without spondylolisthesis. A systematic review (19) has concluded that there is no evidence for the effectiveness of orthosis in chronic nonspecific low back pain.

In spite of nonscientific evidence, it is the present author's opinion that lumbar supports used in acute or subacute episodes are better than no treatment at all, especially if they are associated with drugs or injection techniques. Additional Cochrane reviews on bracing are clearly needed.

The pain-reducing mechanism of transcutaneous electrical nerve stimulation (TENS) is based on the gate control theory at the spinal level. No scientific evidence of effectiveness of TENS for acute or chronic low back pain has been found in systematic reviews (19). No controlled trial could be identified in adult spondylolisthesis. The same can be said of acupuncture. However, as stated by Spitzer et al. (18), it seems that acupuncture can lessen pain during a series of treatments for acute or subacute episodes. This action is probably related to a placebo effect.

Currently, evaluation of treatment efficacy is based on randomized clinical trials. In the case of spondylolisthesis there is obviously a lack of studies, and especially a lack of quality studies evaluating conservative therapy, which prevents presenting a treatment program based on sound scientific evidence. However and notwithstanding the necessary effort in evidence-based medicine the personal and empirical experience of the physician is still needed. Moreover, a good physician–patient relationship and an appropriate psychological approach by the physical therapist are important factors of success. Figure 13.1 summarizes the role of conservative treatment in the management of adult spondylolisthesis as seen by the present authors.

CONCLUSIONS AND REFERRAL TO SURGERY

Low-grade spondylolisthesis in adulthood is a rather benign condition. Many adults are unaware of their spondylolisthesis, which can be detected by chance on examinations unconnected with back pain, or by symptoms appearing during the third or fourth decade of life. Progression of the slip and association with clinical symptoms in adults are closely related to degeneration of the disc at the slip level. High-grade spondylolisthesis

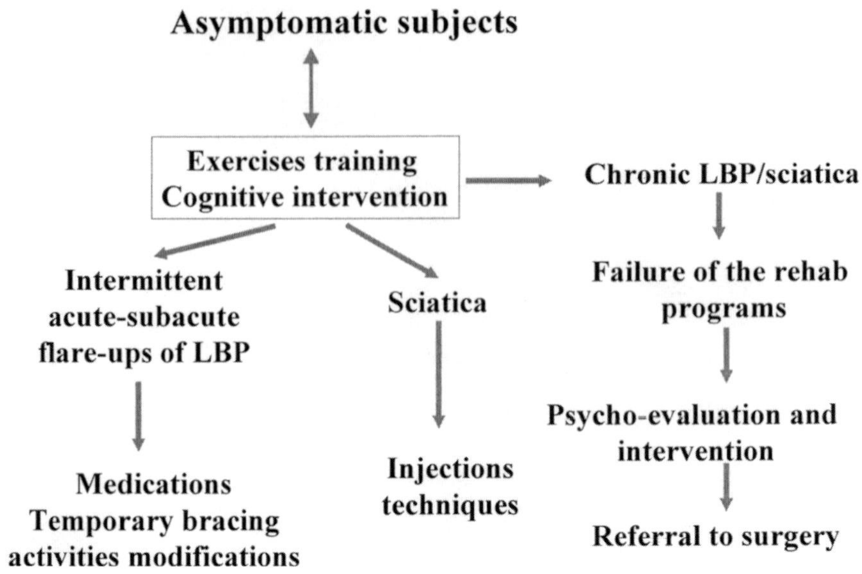

FIG. 13.1. Algorithm of conservative treatment in adult spondylolisthesis.

is less frequently encountered in adults; rather, it is usually symptomatic and discovered during adolescence or childhood.

Asymptomatic mild-moderate spondylolisthesis does not need occupational restrictions. In symptomatic adults, conservative therapy, including modification of activity and lifestyle as well as administration of the therapeutic modalities described above are usually able to control the symptoms. The rehabilitation program must be carefully structured and necessitates a multidisciplinary approach. However, a certain proportion of patients has a continued disabling low back pain or radiculopathy, sometimes with a radicular motor deficit in spite of an appropriate conservative therapy. These patients are candidates for surgery. Before deciding on surgical referral, the physician must make sure that the exercise regimen has been correctly applied, monitored, and followed and that the educational program has been performed appropriately. The risk/benefit ratio of surgical treatment must also be precisely explained to the patient. Careful selection of patients that includes psychosocial evaluation and intervention is the key to success of surgery.

REFERENCES

1. Postacchini F. The evolution of spondylolysis into spondylolisthesis during adult age. *Ital J Orthop Traumatol* 1989;15:210–216.
2. Heggeness MH, Esses SI, Kostuik JP. Acquisition of lytic spondylolisthesis in the adult. *J Spinal Disord* 1991;4:486–489.
3. Virta L. The development of isthmic spondylolisthesis in an adult. *J Bone Joint Surg Am* 1994;76:1997–1998.
4. Ohmori K, Ishida Y, Takatsu T, et al. Vertebral slip in lumbar spondylolysis and spondylolisthesis; long term follow-up in 22 adult patients. *J Bone Joint Surg Br* 1995;77:771–773.
5. Wiltse L, Rothman SL. Lumbar and lumbosacral spondylolisthesis. Classification, diagnosis, and natural history. In: Wiesel S, et al., ed. *The Lumbar Spine.* The International Society for the Study of the Lumbar Spine. 2nd edition. Philadelphia: Saunders; 1996:521–654.
6. Beutler WJ, Fredrikson BE, Murtland A, et al. The natural history of spondylolisthesis. *Spine* 2003;28:1027–1035.
7. Floman Y. Progression of lumbosacral isthmic spondylolisthesis in adults. *Spine* 2000;25:342–347.

8. Virta L, Osterman K. Radiographic correlations in adult symptomatic spondylolisthesis: a long term follow-up study. *J Spinal Disord* 1994;7:41–48.
9. Saraste H. Long term clinical and radiological follow-up of spondylolysis and spondylolisthesis. *J Pediatr Orthop* 1987;7:631–638.
10. Danielson B, Frennered K, Lass K, et al. Radiologic progression of isthmic spondylolisthesis in young patients. *Spine* 1996;16:422–425.
11. Seitsalo S, Ostermarck, Hyvarinen H, et al. Progression of spondylolisthesis in children and adolescents: a long term follow-up of 272 patients. *Spine* 1991;16:417–421.
12. Beutler WJ, Weinstein L, et al. Point of view on: natural history of spondylosis and spondylolisthesis. *Spine* 2003;28:1035.
13. Fredrikson BE. Spondylolisthesis: the natural history age 5–40. Proceedings of the North American Spine Society, 5th Annual Meeting 1990;5:105–106.
14. Farfan HF, Osteria V, Lamy C. The mechanical etiology of spondylolysis and spondylolisthesis. *Clin Orthop* 1976;117:40–55.
15. Virta L, Ronnemaa T. The association of mild-moderate isthmic lumbar spondylolisthesis and low-back pain in middle aged patients is weak and it only occurs in women. *Spine* 1993;18:1496–1503.
16. Grober U, Haugh L, Wiltse LL, et al. L4-L5 isthmic spondylolisthesis clinical and radiological review in 52 cases. Presented at the annual meeting of the American Orthopaedic Association, Coronado CA, June 1993.
17. Harris IE, Weinstein SL. Long term follow-up of patients with grade III and IV spondylolisthesis. *J Bone Joint Surg Am* 1987;69:960–969.
18. Spitzer WO, et al. Report of the Quebec Task Force on Spinal Disorders: scientific approach to the assessment and management of activity related spinal disorders: a monography for clinicians. *Spine* 1987;12 (suppl):16–21: 22–30.
19. Van Tulder MW, Koes BW, Bouter LM. Conservative treatment of acute and chronic nonspecific low-back pain: a systematic review of randomized controlled trials of the most common interventions. *Spine* 1997;22:2128–2156.
20. Bohing RM. Mechanism of action of acetaminophen: is there a cyclooxygenase 3? *Clin Infect Dis* 2003; 31(suppl 5) S:202–210.
21. Carette 5, Leclair R, Marcoux S, et al. Epidural corticosteroid injections for sciatica due to herniated nucleus pulposus. *N Engl J Med* 1991;235:1002–1007.
22. Koes BW, Schollen R, Mens J, et al. Efficacy of epidural steroid injections for low back pain and sciatica: a systematic review of randomized clinical trials. *Pain* 1995;279–288.
23. Ng LCL, Sell P. Outcomes of a prospective cohort study on peri-radicular infiltration for radicular pain in patients with lumbar disc herniation and spinal stenosis. *Eur Spine J* 2004;13:325–329.
24. Deyo RA. Drug therapy for back pain: which drugs help which patients? *Spine* 1996;21(2):841–849.
25. O'Sullivan P, Twoney LT, Allison GT. Evaluation of specific stabilizing exercise in the treatment of chronic low-back pain with radiologic diagnosis of spondylolysis or spondylolisthesis. *Spine* 1997;22:2959–2967.
26. Brox JI, Sonensen R, Friis A, et al. Randomized clinical trial of lumbar instrumented fusion and cognitive intervention and exercises in patients with chronic low back pain and disc degeneration. *Spine* 2003;28:1913–1921.

14

Spondylolisthesis and Bracing: A Critical Literature Review

Tom Bendix

Spondylolisthesis means sliding (-olisthesis) of the spine. There are mainly three types: spondylolytic, degenerative, and congenital (1,2). This chapter describes the types with regard to the possible effect of corseting or bracing and reviews the literature review on evidence found with bracing.

A brace is a stiff, body-conforming device intended to prevent or reduce movement. A corset is a fabric-based device that can be made more or less stiff by means of metal or plastic inserts. It is not as stiff as a brace.

Spondylolisthesis is seen in children above the age of 6 in whom spondylolysis at the fifth lumbar (L5) vertebra has resulted in forward sliding of the anterior aspect of L5 vertebra and the spine above (Fig. 14.1A). L4–L5 degeneration may lead to spondylolisthesis, usually above the age of 60 if, additionally, the facet joints are malformed prior to or during the period of instability (Fig. 14.1B). Furthermore, it is seen (albeit rarely) in early childhood as a result of a congenital, dysplastic dome-shaped deformation of the base of the sacral bone in combination with insufficient facet joints.

The dysplastic type virtually always progresses to the extent that surgery is the treatment of choice and a brace for primary treatment is out of the question. This type is very seldom seen and will not be considered further in this review. Other chapters in this book provide further details on classification.

SPONDYLOLYTIC SPONDYLOLISTHESIS

Spondylolysis virtually always appears in the early teen years and is most often caused by a fatigue fracture in the isthmic area (2,3). The pure spondylolytic type without spondylolisthesis is apparently rarely symptomatic, since it is often clinically evidenced later in life without the patient having any memory of pain.

There seem to be several different clinical courses:

- Symptoms occur at the time the fracture appears. Probably this is the type that is treatable with a brace (see later discussion).
- Back pain occurs around the age of 20.
- Back pain occurs later in life, most often in the 30s,when spondylolisthesis is noticed for the first time.
- The condition is never symptomatic.

Fracture pain as seen in any other fractures in the body is most likely the cause of the first mentioned, early type. Spinal instability is considered to be the cause of pain for the

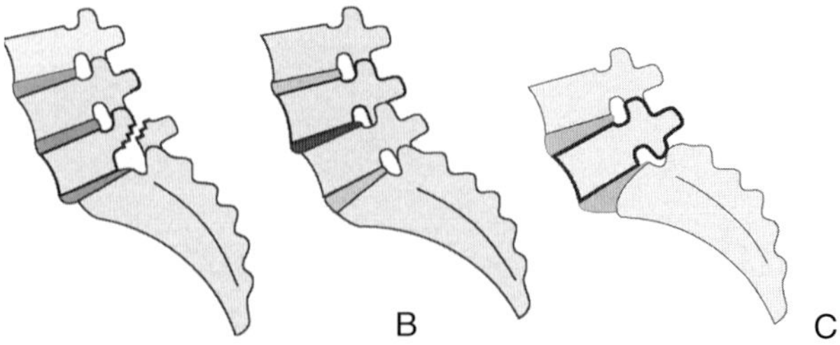

FIG. 14.1. Spondylolytic (A), degenerative (B), and congenital spondylolisthesis (C). The first two clinically present with an anterior displacement of the L4 spinal process, while the congenital type has L5 positioned forwardly.

type at age 20. The more spondylolisthesis, the more likely the appearance of symptoms during the young years.

When spondylolytic spondylolisthesis becomes a part of the clinical picture later in life, it seems related to discogenic pain, more often in L4–L5 than L5-S1.

The reason for the absence of pain despite large deformation could be the following: L5-S1 disc becomes highly deformed at an early stage and consequently severely degenerated. In most cases, the degeneration is so intensive that the nucleus degenerates quickly, changing from a jelly consistence to fibrotic tissue. One result is that the phase in the degenerative process when annular tears can be penetrated by jelly nuclear material does not occur (4). Therefore, the altered anatomy may instead influence the L4–L5 level, because that joint will receive increased demand during lumbosacral movements. Probably, this L4–L5 pathology does not differ from any other discogenic pain.

Pain and spondylolisthesis are more often associated in girls than in boys (5).

Degenerative Spondylolisthesis

The degenerative type of spondylolisthesis in later age seems highly related to spinal instability, but because this is based on discogenic components in terms of annular tears, it is difficult to distinguish what is actually the cause of a back pain. Also facet-joint pain, secondary to the reduced segmental stability, may contribute to the back pain (6). Due to anterior displacement of one part of the vertebral canal—the neural ring of L4—in relation to that of L5, the canal may be narrowed at that level, resulting in usual leg-pain claudication symptoms of spinal stenosis. Also facet-joint arthrosis and soft tissue components secondary to the reduced disc height usually contributes to this stenosis.

To make forward sliding possible, modification of the L4–L5 facet joint as illustrated in Fig. 14.2 must take place. Females seem to get symptoms from these changes more often than men (5), as in the spondylolytic version of spondylolisthesis in children.

RATIONALE FOR AND AGAINST BRACE IN SPONDYLOLYSIS/SPONDYLOLISTHESIS

The theoretical biological effect of a brace is an ability to avoid painful movements. Such movements can be either:

1. Instability
   a. Abnormal joint-mobility within the normal range of movement (ROM), or
   b. Abnormal large trunk movements

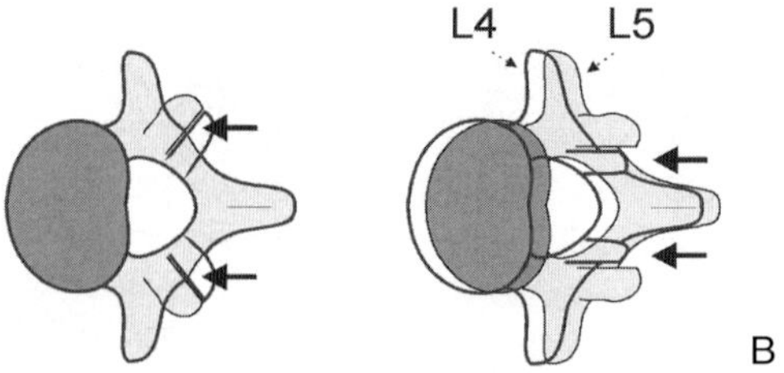

FIG. 14.2. A: Normal facet-joint orientation would not allow L4 to slide forward. **B:** A modification of the joint is mandatory and possible (although not exactly as shown in this schematic drawing).

In these cases, unexpected positioning in the course of a movement implies abnormal, uncontrolled tensions of various tissues. Instability has been studied for years, but despite a theoretical definition, no clear, clinically usable test for demonstrating instability has yet been stated. However, it seems as if lack of smoothness in the course from one end-point to another (described in list item 1a above) is a key issue, dominated by rather erratic movements.

2. Movements can also be painful in a normal movement pattern due to irritation of local receptors in deteriorated tissues, as in osteoarthritis.

The theoretical effect of a brace would be that it might be able to avoid some of these painful movements. However, at least small midrange movements do not seem to be prevented by bracing (7) and corseting offers even less prevention of movement. It could be that larger movements could be relieved to some extent. In a study (8), Spratt et al. demonstrated that bracing gave a better clinical result for a lordotic posture than for flexion/kyphosis. They hypothesized that the (slight although seemingly present) effect did not relate to possible instability but rather to the component of discogenic pain based on annular tears. Spratt et al. did look into degenerative spondylolisthesis versus retrodisplacement, but the sample was too small for subgrouping. In the present author's conception, their result may correspond well with the later demonstrated effect of extension exercises, improving those initially centralizing their pain (9).

Among other theoretical effects of braces are some new types (Orthofix) that are claimed to perform a slight traction. The first, yet unpublished, report says that these braces may have a certain pain-relieving influence, but as is the case with other such devices it is difficult to distinguish between a possible placebo effect and their biomechanical influence.

Arguing against fixation in a brace or corset is the theory of Indahl that discogenic pain is most often elicited by static muscle tension that may follow an irritated disc-surface and/or the facet-joint capsule (10,11). It is based on trials with electrical stimulation of the disc surface, which appears to facilitate contraction of the multifidus muscles. This mechanism is believed to be a normal physiological aspect of continuous stabilization; for example, during walking, contracting the right side and then the left, creating a *rhythmic* stabilization (Fig. 14.3A). In spinal pathology (e.g., discogenic pain), such stimulation of outer-annulus sensors may lead to *static* contraction (Fig. 14.3B), which may cause muscular pain as the eliciting mechanism in discogenic pain in probably a great number of patients.

The significance of such mechanisms is as yet unknown, but Indahl's theory is behind a treatment model that has been very successful in getting people with chronic low back pain to return to work (12).

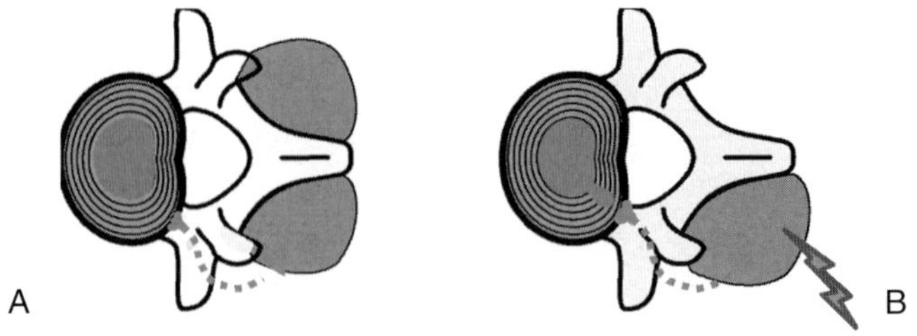

FIG. 14.3. A: During normal movements such as walking, rhythmic movements are initiated by stimulators in outer annulus. **B:** In disc pathology, such stimulation tends to cause static muscle contraction.

Such a pain mechanism might logically be worsened by a brace, facilitating a static muscle function, and conversely might be relieved by more natural, daily, rhythmic movements without a brace.

EVIDENCE FOR BRACING: WHAT DOES THE LITERATURE SAY?

A systematic literature search has been performed, having as input the keywords:

[spondylolysis OR spondylolisthesis] AND [corset OR brace].

A search of four medical literature databases (PubMed, SilverPlatter MEDLINE, EMBACE, and Cochrane) yielded 68 articles. Adding the search term "controlled trials" identified only 4 of the 68 articles.

For an assessment of possible effects of bracing in the literature, the search was disappointing. The type of information in most of the articles can be characterized as follows:

- Scoliosis was treated with a brace. Some of the patients with scoliosis had spondylolisthesis.
- Different types of surgeries were compared or evaluated. Bracing was used postoperatively and some or all patients had spondylolisthesis (as in 13,14).
- Bracing has been tested in randomized clinical trials in nonspecific low back pain (LBP), though not particularly in spondylolisthesis.

There exists only one Cochrane review on bracing, but it does not look separately at spondylolisthesis (15). In that review, VanTulder et al. investigated primarily studies on bracing and *nonspecific* LBP. Their conclusion was that in primary or secondary prevention, no effect could be demonstrated. For treatment during an episode, however, they found limited evidence that lumbar support was better than no treatment, but it remained unclear whether it was better than other treatments.

There are no controlled studies looking specifically into bracing as treatment in spondylolisthesis. There are, however, several studies documenting a beneficial prognosis after acute isthmic fracture treated with a brace, although none of them were controlled or comparative. This condition is not infrequent. In one sample by Steiner and Micheli, it was seen in 47 out of 100 consecutive adolescent athletes in a sports medicine clinic with low back pain (16). However, at the seminar in Brussels in November 2004 that was the genesis of the present book, participating back specialists had seldom seen it.

One study differentiates thoroughly between factors influencing healing during roughly 3 months in a brace for a sample of 134 children, mostly being boys in their teen years (17). The vertebra level of the acute fracture was L4 in 20 of 134. Among those 20, thirteen (65%) healed, in contrast to only 9% of the 114 with fracture at L5. The following were findings regarding prognostic signs for healing:

- Healing was better at L4 than L5 (as just mentioned).
- Pure fissures healed much better (62%) than their next "progressive" stage (9%), with rounded corners at the fissure site; the "terminal" stage, characterized by a free cleft and sclerosis, never healed. Spondylolisthesis of >5% seldom healed, and only if the whole vertebra had slipped, and not separated at the isthmic lesion.
- Whether the contralateral isthmus is intact (i.e., "unilateral spondylolisthesis") or present as a fissure did not influence healing.
- The large opportunity for sliding at the lower lumbar level—great lordosis/steep base of the sacral bone—diminishes optimal healing.
- Young bony age (i.e., the apophyseal stage) improves the healing capability, whereas chronological age within the relevant age group didn't matter.
- There was no influence from the fissure's location on the neural arch.

Also Morita et al. related the classification pure, progressive, terminal to likelihood of healing (18). They had respectively 40%, 30%, and 30% distribution in their sample of 185 children and adolescents. Healing frequencies were 73%, 39%, and 0, respectively.

Regarding contralateral involvement, another study of Sys et al., did show a trend to reduced healing if the opposite isthmus was involved (19) (see also his chapter in this book).

Another study with 73 athletes showed a favorable outcome of bracing among 80% (20). They all had isthmic lesions that were detectable by means of single-photon emission computed tomography (SPECT). Poor prognoses were associated with sudden onset, continued high-risk sports, and tight hamstrings. Most of the athletes studied returned to their sports 4 to 6 months after wearing the brace. Those with fast pain relief after few days in the brace were allowed to do light sport while wearing their brace, provided they remained pain free and avoided hyperextension. This regimen did not seem to increase the risk of nonunion or having recurrent symptoms.

Regarding SPECT scan versus computed tomography (CT) scan, it has been concluded that every single procedure overlooked some lesions, which suggests that both should be undertaken because they can supplement each other if the first type of scan does not reveal a diagnosis (21,22).

Steiner and Micheli reported 67 with symptomatic Grade 1 spondylolisthesis, treated with antilordotic brace for 6 months. Clinically 52 recovered, and 12 had radiographic evidence of healing (16).

Further consideration of the role of supplementary electrical stimulation during intended healing in a brace is suggested based on a few casuistic successes in otherwise difficult healing situations (23).

CONCLUSION

Overall, bracing does not seem to be indicated in spondylolisthesis, except probably in early isthmic fractures in teenage athletes. In that group the effect seems convincing, although controlled trials have not been carried out.

For indication of bracing such cases, SPECT scan is suggested, and being positive, it seems in itself to be a good predictor for healing. This is also the case if the cleft is narrow and if the bony age is young. A steep position of L5 reduces the chances of success. Age within the frame of the teen years, uni- or bilateral, as well as position on the neural arch did not influence the chance of healing (4).

The lack of general effect of bracing in spondylolisthesis should be seen in light of the fact that analysis of subgroups is almost nonexistent, except those with acute isthmic fracture. Therefore, specific indications may still appear.

REFERENCES

1. Wiltse LL. Spondylolisthesis. *West J Med* 1975;122:152–153.
2. Wiltse LL, Newman PH, MacNab I. Classification of spondylolisis and spondylolisthesis. *Clin Orthop* 1976; 23–29.
3. Wiltse LL. Spondylolisthesis in children. *Clin Orthop* 1961;21:156–163.
4. Krämer J. Presidential address: natural course and prognosis of intervertebral disc diseases. *Spine* 1995;20:635–639.
5. Kjaer P, Leboeuf-Yde, Korsholm L, Sorensen JS, Bendix T. Magnetic resonance imaging and low back pain in adults—a diagnostic imaging study of 40-year old men and women. *Spine* 1990;15:111–113.
6. Butler D, Trafimow J, Andersson GBJ, et al. Discs degenerates before facets. *Spine* 1990;15:111–113.
7. Miller RA, Hardcastle P, Renwick SE. Lower spinal mobility and external immobilization in the normal and pathologic condition. *Orthop Rev* 1992;21:753–757.
8. Spratt KF, Weinstein JN, Lehmann TR, et al. Efficacy of flexion and extension treatments incorporating braces for low-back pain patients with retrodisplacement, spondylolisthesis, or normal sagittal translation. *Spine* 1993;18:1839–1849.
9. Long A, Donelson R, Fung T. Does it matter which exercise?: a randomized control trial of exercise for low back pain. *Spine* 2004;29:2593–2602.
10. Indahl A, Kaigle A, Reikeras O, et al. Electromyographic response of the porcine multifidus musculature after nerve stimulation. *Spine* 1995;20:2652–2658.
11. Indahl A, Kaigle AM, Reikeras O, et al. Interaction between the porcine lumbar intervertebral disc, zygapophysial joints, and paraspinal muscles. *Spine* 1997;22:2834–2840.
12. Indahl A, Velund L, Reikeraas O. Good prognosis for low back pain when left untampered: a randomized clinical trial. *Spine* 1995;20:473–477.
13. Christensen FB, Karlsmose B, Hansen ES, et al. Radiological and functional outcome after anterior lumbar interbody spinal fusion. *Eur Spine J* 1996;5:293–298.
14. Johnsson R, Stromqvist B, Aspenberg P. Randomized radiostereometric study comparing osteogenic protein-1 (BMP-7) and autograft bone in human noninstrumented posterolateral lumbar fusion: 2002 Volvo Award in clinical studies. *Spine* 2002;27:2654–2661.
15. van Tulder MW, Jellema P, van Poppel MN, et al. Lumbar supports for prevention and treatment of low back pain. *Cochrane Database Syst Rev* 2004;CD001823.
16. Steiner ME, Micheli LJ. Treatment of symptomatic spondylolysis and spondylolisthesis with the modified Boston brace. *Spine* 1985;10:937–943.
17. Fujii K, Katoh S, Sairyo K, et al. Union of defects in the pars interarticularis of the lumbar spine in children and adolescents: the radiological outcome after conservative treatment. *J Bone Joint Surg Br* 2004;86:225–231.
18. Morita T, Ikata T, Katoh S, et al. Lumbar spondylolysis in children and adolescents. *J Bone Joint Surg Br* 1995;77:620–625.
19. Sys J, Michielsen J, Bracke P, et al. Nonoperative treatment of active spondylolysis in elite athletes with normal x-ray findings: literature review and results of conservative treatment. *Eur Spine J* 2001;10:498–504.
20. d'Hemecourt PA, Zurakowski D, Kriemler S, et al. Spondylolysis: returning the athlete to sports participation with brace treatment. *Orthopedics* 2002;25:653–657.
21. Congeni J, McCulloch J, Swanson K. Lumbar spondylolysis: a study of natural progression in athletes. *Am J Sports Med* 1997;25:248–253.
22. Standaert CJ, Herring SA. Spondylolysis: a critical review. *Br J Sports Med* 2000;34:415–422.
23. Fellander-Tsai L, Micheli LJ. Treatment of spondylolysis with external electrical stimulation and bracing in adolescent athletes: a report of two cases. *Clin J Sport Med* 1998;8:232–234.

15
Rehabilitation

Margareta Nordin

Herbiniaux, a Belgian obstetrician, noted a bone prominence of the sacrum that was obstructing labor in 1782. The term *spondylolisthesis* was first used by Dr. Kilian in 1854 and is derived from the Greek *spondylos* (vertebrae) and *olisthy* (to slip or slide). Spondylolysis occurs with a prevalence of 4% to 6% in the general population. Although the etiology of this lesion is unclear, it has been shown to have both hereditary and acquired risk factors. Prevalence is twice as high in females as in males, and prevalence increases in athletes participating in certain high-risk sports (1,2). Spondylolisthesis occurs in persons with bilateral spondylolysis; slip progression is greatest early in the life span (1). Predicting risk factors for progression of the slip has proven difficult, and slippage is uncommon in adults (3). The rehabilitation literature for nonsurgical treatment of the condition is sparse, and only a few randomized controlled trials exist (3,4). Rehabilitation involves bracing or exercises or both, in combination with education to the patient about the condition. The purpose of these treatments is to stabilize the spine, prohibit further slippage, decrease pain, and increase function. Most patients do well with conservative treatment regimen; however, it is estimated that 9% to 15% of patients with spondylolysis or low-grade spondylolisthesis need surgery (3). The purpose of this brief chapter is to comment on the natural history in patients with spondylolysis and spondylolisthesis and to summarize the evidence of prescribed brace and exercise regimens.

THE NATURAL HISTORY OF THE DISORDERS

The natural history in young adults (n = 47) with isthmic spondylolisthesis who sought medical care was studied by Frennered et al. (5). The mean age at diagnoses was 12.2 years (range: 1.6–16.9 years) and follow-up was 7 years. These patients presented with low-grade spondylolisthesis (≤50% slip), and progression of slip was rare during follow-up. Eighty-three percent of the individuals seeking care had no pain or occasional pain that did not interfere with their daily activities. No significant prognostic indicators were found for either progression of slip or subsequent surgery. Thirty percent underwent surgery because of pain or progression of slip, and the authors' conclusion is that, based on the findings of this relatively small prospective cohort over 7 years, the natural history of low-grade spondylolisthesis is benign.

In 1994, a follow-up study in Finland was conducted on correlations of radiographic measurements of isthmic spondylolisthesis to indexes of low back pain and functional and working capacity. One hundred forty-eight middle-aged patients treated for low back pain an average of 17 years earlier participated as a patient population (6). Fifty percent of the patients had undergone posterior or posterolateral fusion, decompression had been performed in 23% of patients, and 27% of the patients had been treated conservatively.

The level of progression of the slip, instability of the olisthetic segment, or radiologic nonunion of spinal fusion did not correlate with either the pain index or function measured as the activities of daily living (ADL) index (6).

A prospective study of spondylolysis and spondylolisthesis was initiated in the United States in Buffalo, New York, in 1955 with a radiographic and clinical study of 500 first-grade children (1). The purpose of the study was to determine the natural history of spondylolysis and spondylolisthesis. In this population studied from the age of 6 years to adulthood, 30 individuals were identified to have pars lesions. Data collection at a 45-year follow-up assessment included magnetic resonance imaging, a back pain questionnaire, and the 36-Item Short Form Health Survey (SF-36) survey. No subject with a pars defect was lost to follow-up evaluation once a lesion was identified. Subjects with unilateral defects never experienced slippage over the course of the study. Progression of spondylolisthesis slowed with each decade. There was no association of slip progression and low back pain. There was no statistically significant difference between the study population SF-36 scores and those of the general population the same age. Subjects with pars defects follow a clinical course similar to that of the general population. There appears to be a marked slowing of slip progression with each decade, and no subject has reached a 40% slip (1).

In summary from these three prospective studies on the natural history of mild to moderate spondylolysis/spondylolisthesis (Grades 1 and 2), it could be concluded that the condition has a relatively benign natural history from childhood and no clear indicators or predictors for progression of a slip of ≤50% in long-term follow-up of 7 to 45 years. One study suggests that the progression of slippage decreases for each decade.

The findings are supported by a study using stereophotogrammetry (7). Eight patients with mostly Grade 1 spondylolisthesis and long-term back pain (no sciatica) were matched with healthy controls for gender, afflicted segment and grade of disc degeneration. Patients and matched controls underwent external fixation test and stereophotogrammetry. The conclusion of the study was that the spondylolytic defect in the pars does not cause permanent instability or hypermobility detectable in the adult population with low back pain and low-grade spondylolisthesis. The lumbosacral intervertebral translations were measured from recumbent to erect position. The mean sagittal translation was 1.8 mm (range 1.1–3.1 mm) for the spondylolytic group and 1.8 mm (range 0.3–2.5 mm) for the matched healthy control group. Similar results were found for the vertical translations with no difference between the groups (7). Although few patients were included, the study is noteworthy; however, the results from the study may change when further studies with improved technology such as open magnetic resonance imaging and simultaneous motion can be studied.

REHABILITATION

Rehabilitation for spondylolysis or spondylolisthesis often includes bracing, activity modification, and special exercises. Overall, little evidence for or against these treatments is available.

Bracing

Bracing is used to stabilize the spine while the patient maintains activity. The brace is worn for 2 to 6 months. Gradual increased activity and progressing exercises are performed until bony healing is achieved if a fracture has occurred, such as a fracture of pars intra-articularis (8) Three theories are predominant for the bracing: one is to maintain the spine in lordosis, the second is to maintain the spine in an antilordotic position, and the third theory to use a "nonspecified" brace to limit extension. In uncontrolled studies, the results leading to bony healing were similar (8).

One study from Japan studied the efficacy of conservative treatment in athletes with severe low back pain and spondylolysis with the focus on returning the athlete to the original sports activities (9). One hundred four athletes (96 males and 8 females, mean age 20.7 years), who consulted in a sports medicine clinic during the 11-year period because of low back pain with an apparent defect of the pars interarticularis on plain radiographs, were subjected to conservative treatment. Forty percent of the patients discontinued sports activities due to severe low back pain. They were conservatively treated with activity restriction and antilordotic lumbosacral bracing, which was aimed at relieving low back pain by achieving stability of the fracture partly associated with fibrous union. After their low back pain was markedly reduced, the brace was removed, and then individual training to return to the original sports activities was started. Thirty-five patients (87.5%) could return to their original sports activities in an average of 5.4 months (range: 1.0–11.5 months) after the onset of treatment, and could continue the activities for at least 6 months despite nonbony union. These results suggest that the outcome of conservative treatment with activity restriction and bracing appears to be satisfactory in controlling symptoms and returning to original sporting activities. Randomized controlled trials are needed to confirm the results.

In summary, virtually no evidence exists for efficacy of brace treatment in patients with spondylolysis or low-grade spondylolisthesis; the field is wide open for research.

Exercises

McNeeley et al. (4) performed a systematic review on physiotherapy for spondylolysis and spondylolisthesis including 71 articles published in peer review journals. Only two randomized controlled studies showed acceptable quality and were included in the systematic review. Both studies indicate that an exercise regimen is superior to control groups. O'Sullivan et al. (10) evaluated the effect of strengthening of abdominal muscles with co-activation of the lumbar multifidus for 10 weeks compared to a treatment recommended by medical practitioners. Forty-four patients (Slippage Grade 0–2) participated; they were randomly allocated to two groups. The results for stabilizing exercises were effective up to 30 months and clinically and statistically significant for pain reduction and disability perception. The authors and systematic reviewers concluded that the proposed exercise regimen lends itself to reproducibility in clinical settings.

Spratt et al. (11) randomized patients (n = 65) to one group with flexion exercise and a flexion brace; a second group with extension exercise and an extension brace; and a third group as control group with sham exercise. The study group with extension exercise and an extension brace showed significantly better results than the two other groups. The authors suggest that these results may indicate advanced disc diseases as the underlying pathology. There was a larger dropout rate in the flexion group, and the results suffered consequently. Both studies provide some evidence to suggest that specific exercise interventions alone or in combination with other treatments may have a positive effect on pain and function in patients with spondylolysis or spondylolisthesis. Summarizing these two studies and the systematic literature review, there is weak to moderate evidence that an exercise regimen will reduce pain and perceived disability in patients with low-grade spondylolisthesis. Exercises including those to stabilize the trunk and extension exercises are possibly superior; however, more research is needed to confirm these statements.

Moller and Hedlund (12) performed a prospective randomized study with the purpose of determining whether posterolateral fusion in patients with adult isthmic spondylolisthesis results in an improved outcome compared with an exercise program. One hundred eleven patients were randomly allocated to an exercise program (n = 34) or posterolateral fusion with or without transpedicular fixation (n = 77). The inclusion criteria were lumbar isthmic spondylolisthesis of any grade, at least 1 year of low back pain or sciatica, and a severely restricted functional ability in individuals 18 to 55 years of age. The patients were followed up for 2 years; the follow-up rate was 93%. The functional outcome, as assessed by the Disability Rating Index and pain reduction, was better in the surgically treated group than in the exercise group at both the 1-year and 2-year follow-up assessments (P <0.01). In the exercise group, the Disability Rating Index did not change at all, whereas the pain decreased slightly (P <0.02). This study showed that careful patient selection and surgical management of adult isthmic spondylolisthesis improves function and relieves pain more efficiently than an exercise program over 2 years. In a follow-up 9 years later of the same patients, the same authors conclude:

> Posterolateral fusion in adult lumbar isthmic spondylolisthesis results in a modestly improved long-term outcome compared with a 1-year exercise program. Although the results show that some of the previously reported short-term improvement is lost at long term, patients with fusion still classify their global outcome as clearly better than conservatively treated patients. Furthermore, because the long-term outcome of the patients conservatively treated most likely reflects the natural course, one can also conclude that no considerable spontaneous improvement should be expected over time in adult patients with symptomatic isthmic spondylolisthesis (13).

This statement stands until further longitudinal studies are performed.

CONCLUSIONS

Young patients with spondylolysis/olisthesis (low grade) seem to do well with activity modification and possibly a brace regimen. However, no randomized studies exist to support these regimens although they are common clinical practice.

Adult patients with spondylolysis or low-grade spondylolisthesis may improve with an exercise program; however, the evidence is still weak and the studies related to exercise are few. Bracing is less well understood in adult patients presenting with spondylolysis or low-grade spondylolisthesis, and evidence of efficacy is lacking. The questions of what kind of brace or exercise or the contribution of each modality cannot be answered because studies are lacking, especially quality studies. Comparing exercise to surgery, the short-term effect of selective adult patients with 1 year of low back pain for surgery, the efficacy of surgery seems to be superior to exercise for decreasing pain and increasing function. However, the long-term effect over a decade seems to be rather similar for surgery or exercise. This is important information to patients and their choice of treatment.

REFERENCES

1. Beutler WJ, Fredrickson BE, Murtland A, et al. The natural history of spondylolysis and spondylolisthesis: 45-year follow-up evaluation. *Spine* 2003;28(10):1027–1035.
2. McTimoney CA, Micheli LJ. Current evaluation and management of spondylolysis and spondylolisthesis. *Curr Sports Med Reports* 2003;2(1):41–46.

3. Standaert CJ, Herring SA. Spondylolysis: a critical review. *Br J Sports Med* 2003;34:415–422.
4. McNeely ML, Torrance G, Magee MJ. A systematic review of physiotherapy for spondylolysis and spondylolisthesis. *Man Ther* 2003;8(2):80–91.
5. Frennered AK, Danielson B, Nachemson AL. Natural history of symptomatic isthmic low-grade spondylolisthesis in children and adolescents: a seven-year follow-up study. *J Ped Orthop* 1991;11(2):209–213.
6. Virta L, Osterman K. Radiographic correlations in adult symptomatic spondylolisthesis: a long-term follow-up study. *J Spinal Disord* 1994;7(1):41–48.
7. Axelsson P, Johnsson R, Stromqvist B. Is there increased intervertebral mobility in isthmic adult spondylolisthesis? A matched comparative study using roentgen stereophotogrammetry. *Spine* 2000;25(13):1701–1703.
8. Grobler LJ, Wiltse LL. Classification, and non-operative and operative treatment of spondylolisthesis. In: Frymoyer JW, ed. *The Adult Spine: Principles and Practice.* 2nd edition. Philadelphia: Lippincott-Raven; 1997: 1865–1884.
9. Iwamoto J, Takeda T, Wakano K. Returning athletes with severe low back pain and spondylolysis to original sporting activities with conservative treatment. *Scand J Med Sci Sports* 2004;14(6):346–351.
10. O'Sullivan PB, Twomey LT, Allison GT. Evaluation of specific stabilizing exercises in the treatment of chronic low back pain with radiologic diagnosis of spondylolysis or spondylolisthesis. *Spine* 1997;22(24):2959–2967.
11. Spratt KF, Weinstein JN, Lehmann TR, et al. Efficacy of flexion and extension treatments incorporating braces for low-back pain patients with retrodisplacements, spondylolisthesis, or normal sagittal translation. *Spine* 1993;18(13):1839–1849.
12. Moller H, Hedlund R. Surgery versus conservative management in adult isthmic spondylolisthesis-a prospective randomized study: part 1. *Spine* 2000;25(13):1711–1715.
13. Ekman P, Moller H, Hedlund R. The long-term effect of posterolateral fusion in adult isthmic spondylolisthesis: a randomized controlled study. *Spine J* 2005;5(1):36–44.

16

Surgical Treatment of High-Grade Spondylolisthesis: An Analysis of 18 Patients

Maryline Mousny and André Kaelin

Spondylolisthesis was first described in 1782 by Herbiniaux, a Belgian obstetrician (1). Taillard precisely defined this condition only in 1957 (2). Nowadays spondylolisthesis is a well-known condition and remains the commonest identifiable cause of low back pain in children and adolescents (3). The exact incidence of dysplastic spondylolisthesis is unknown, but this type makes up 14% to 24% of treated cases in large series, with a 2:1 female:male ratio (4). Today, most of the authors agree on the treatment of mild to moderate spondylolisthesis, but controversy still exists over the most appropriate method for managing high-grade spondylolisthesis (5). A lot of treatment options are proposed in the current literature (6–10).

In our institution, we perform a posterior interbody and posterolateral fusion with segmental pedicle fixation when the slip is greater than 50% with a lumbosacral kyphosis. No forceful intraoperative reduction maneuver is performed, but a partial reduction is usually obtained by positioning the patient. In cases of spondylolisthesis with radiographic progression or greater than 50% slip but without lumbosacral kyphosis, we perform an in situ posterolateral instrumented fusion. The purpose of the present report is to evaluate retrospectively the radiographic and functional outcome of patients operated on for moderate to high-grade dysplastic spondylolisthesis.

MATERIALS AND METHODS

Eighteen patients who were operated on for moderate to severe dysplastic-type spondylolisthesis from 1988 to 2000 at Hôpital des Enfants in Geneva were reviewed retrospectively. Clinical records and serial radiographs were evaluated.

The surgical indications included severe L5-S1 spondylolisthesis (Meyerding (11) Grades 3 or 4), radiographic progression (six patients), and severe pain. All patients complained of unremitting pain. All the cases presented radiographic features of severe dysplasia and were therefore classified as dysplastic-type spondylolisthesis according to the Wiltse classification (12,13).

We recorded the relevant points in the personal and familial previous history of each patient. The practice of any sports activity was noted. Pre- and postoperative clinical measurements included activity level, symptoms, posture (presence or absence of a lumbosacral kyphotic deformity and lumbar hyperlordosis, a lumbar step-off, an associated scoliosis), lumbar forward flexion, neurologic findings, straight leg raising, and gait pattern.

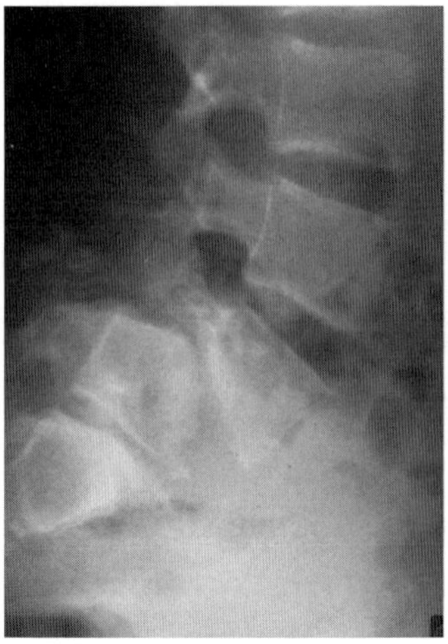

FIG. 16.1. High-grade spondylolisthesis, with slipping of L5, L5–S1 kyphosis, and dysplastic change of vertebrae.

Mean clinical and radiologic follow-up was 6.5 years (range 3 to 14.5 years). At latest follow-up, all patients but two had reached skeletal maturity.

Patients

The 18 patients who underwent operative stabilization had symptomatic dysplastic-type spondylolisthesis (Fig. 16.1). Nine were female, and nine were male. The average age at the initial symptom was 14 years (range 11 to 17 years). The average age at diagnosis was 15.2 years (range 6 to 18 years). The average age at diagnosis is less than the average age at initial symptom because the diagnosis was fortuitously made in two patients and they became symptomatic later. Regarding the other patients, the average interval from first complaints to time of diagnosis was 11 months (range 0 to 36 months).

All patients had conservative treatment prior to surgery: physiotherapy and medication for 15 patients, physiotherapy and bracing for 8 patients. All patients were improved with the bracing, but the pain reappeared when they tried to wean.

The average age at surgery was 16 years (range 11.7 years 10 months to 20.1 years). The interval from time of diagnosis to time of operation averaged 11 months (range 1 to 60 months). Nine patients hadn't reached skeletal maturity at surgery. All the patients but one had no history of trauma. Four patients participated in repetitive lower risk sports, and one patient in high-risk sports (gymnastics). Three patients had a familial history of spondylolisthesis (direct relatives). Regarding the associated conditions, one patient suffered from anorexia nervosa, one patient had been treated for hip dysplasia, one patient for bilateral Legg-Calvé-Perthes disease, and one patient for clubfoot.

Back pain was the most common complaint at the first visit. All patients described lumbar pain. Eight patients had concomitant radicular pain about one or their two lower extremities. One of these patients had typical cruralgia, while the other patients complained of sciatic-type pain. Seven patients were concerned by their postural deformity and abnormal gait. All patients complained of tight hamstrings, and 12 had a significant step-off deformity in the lumbosacral area. All patients had lumbosacral kyphosis. Four patients had scoliotic deformity.

Eight patients had a neurologic finding on preoperative evaluation. Two patients had a one-grade decrease on motor testing of L5 innervated muscles (one in both legs and two in the left leg). Three patients had positive Lasegue test without motor deficit at clinical examination. One patient had mild sensory disturbance (dysesthesia) in L5-S1 distribution and decreased ankle jerk test in the right leg. One patient had decreased quadriceps jerk test on the right side. Four patients had an abnormal, waddling-type gait.

Radiographic Evaluation

Standing lateral and anteroposterior radiographs were measured at the following intervals: at diagnosis, preoperatively; at 3 months, 6 months, and 1 year postoperatively; and at last follow-up. These radiographs were taken with the patient standing because the slip angle can change more than 11 degrees between standing and supine radiographs (14). Hyperextension and hyperflexion radiographs were taken preoperatively.

Radiographic measurements included: (a) percentage of slip (i.e., anterior displacement of L5 /or L4 on S1 /or L5) (2) and (b) slip angle of L5 on the sacrum, using the inferior endplate of L5 and the perpendicular to the posterior body of S1 (14). We used the percentage of slip and the displacement index to determine preoperatively the presence or absence of instability on the dynamic radiographs. We also measured the lordosis angle L1–L5. The radiologic criteria for fusion was the presence of a fusion mass on plain radiographs, posteriorly when only a posterolateral fusion was performed, or posteriorly and between the two vertebral bodies when a posterolateral and interbody fusion were performed.

The disc spaces were preoperatively assessed by magnetic resonance imaging. If the L4–L5 disc was intact, a single-level L5-S1 fusion was performed; if it showed signs of degeneration, a L4-S1 fusion was performed.

Surgical Technique

The patient was placed prone, on a four-poster soft frame, with the hips and the knees in a 90-degree flexed position (genupectoral position). Nerves roots monitoring for sensitory and motor pathways were installed. A longitudinal midline posterior incision was made and subperiosteal dissection from the spinous process of L3 to S2 was performed. The L5 lamina was removed. The nerve roots (L5, S1) were decompressed and the cauda equina was freed gently from the posterosuperior zone of the first sacral vertebral body. Transpedicular screws (CD Instrumentation or CD Horizon) were inserted at L5 (or L4) and S1 level under the control of image intensifier, for the last cases under CAOS (Medivision). A lateral roentgenogram was obtained to confirm the proper position of the screws. The screws were intentionally inserted in a lateral and convergent fashion. The goal was to obtain a "triangulation effect" and therefore good stability. A slight distraction was performed to open L5-S1 disk space. The L5-S1 intervertebral disk was removed and a 0.5-cm sacral dome osteotomy was performed. Corticocancellous graft was placed in the interbody space. A cage (posterior lumbar interbody fusion, or PLIF) was also used when the foraminal space was not enough open. Then the position of the patient was changed, and the hips were extended to permit the movement of the pelvis under L5. During this maneuver, a direct visualization of the nerve roots was possible, allowing detection of any nerve impingement.

Changing the position of the patient allowed partial correction of the lumbosacral kyphosis (Fig. 16.2). The rods (CDI) were first inserted proximally and then progressively

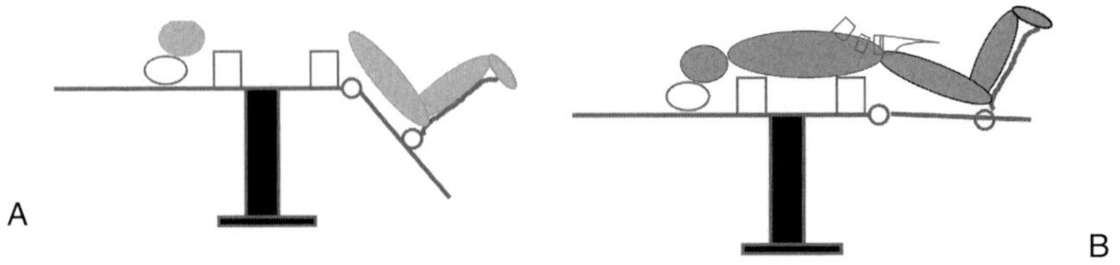

FIG. 16.2. **A:** Installation prereduction. **B:** Installation postreduction.

fixed to the sacrum. A satisfactory correction of the kyphosis was obtained when the L5 transpedicular screws were parallel to the S1 screws. Usually the discectomy allowed good mobilization of the L5 vertebra. The sacral dome osteotomy prevented any tension on the nerve roots. Segmental compression was applied between the two vertebrae. The compressive forces applied on the construct helped to maintain the achieved reduction (the restored lumbar lordosis). Local autogenous and allogenous bone graft was placed posteriorly and posterolaterally on all available surfaces after decortication. Postoperatively, under brace protection, ambulation was permitted as soon as possible. The patient was discharged at 6 to 8 days after surgery; the removable orthosis was worn 4 months. Activity was restricted until solid fusion occurred. Twelve patients had L5-S1 fusion, and 6 patients had L4-S1 fusion. All patients with high-grade spondylolisthesis (≥50°) had posterior interbody and posterolateral fusion.

RESULTS

Clinical

All patients operated on described improvement of their back pain. At latest follow-up, 13 patients had complete resolution of their back and lower leg pain. One patient still described some discomfort at the lumbar spine; four had occasional pain during sports activities. Regarding their sports ability, all patients were at the activity level they desired and returned to their former activities. No patient had hamstring tightness postoperatively. The patients with scoliosis showed no progression of their curves at the latest follow-up. All patients had improvement in their cosmetic appearance as well as in their gait. Two patients still clinically demonstrated a lumbar hyperlordosis. Two patients had L5 mild paresis, one with full recovery at 2 weeks postsurgery, one with partial recovery (patient needed a second surgery).

Radiographic

As previously mentioned, all patients had dysplastic-type spondylolisthesis. Seventeen patients had an obviously rounded upper sacrum. Regarding associated vertebral malformations, six patients had spina bifida (one at L5, three at S1, one at L5-S1, and one at L4-L5-S1). A hypoplasia of the posterior arch of L5 and S1 was noted during the surgical procedure in one patient.

The mean percentage of slip was 73.1% (range 56.7% to 100%). The mean L5 slip angle was 38 degrees (range 21° to 51°). The mean sacral inclination was 44.3 degrees (range 13° to 62°). The lumbar lordosis measured an average of 58.1 degrees (range 40°

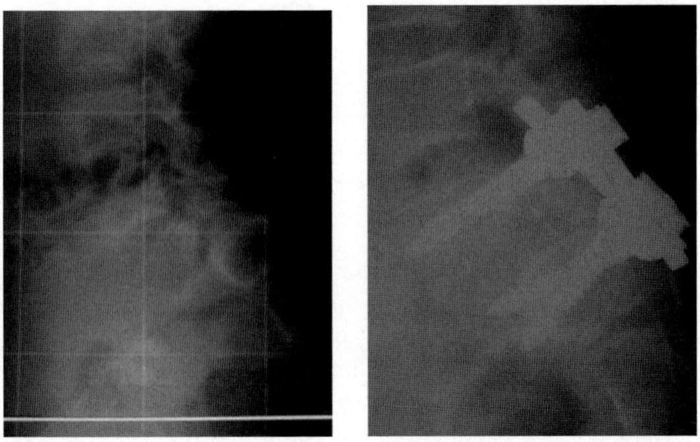

A B

FIG. 16.3. X-ray pre- and postreduction done by posterior approach, sacral osteotomy, PLIF, and posterior instrumentation in compression.

to 80°). Four patients had an associated scoliosis. Two patients had a thoracic curve, convex to the right, and two a lumbar curve.

Postoperatively, the mean percentage of slip was 42% (range 5% to 70%). All patients showed an improvement of the slippage with a mean improvement of 31%. Using Meyerding classification, six patients improved by one grade, five patients by two grades, and four patients showed no improvement. At latest follow-up, the mean percentage of slippage was 44% (range 16% to 73%). Three patients nevertheless showed a small loss of reduction.

The mean postoperative L5 slip angle was 5 degrees (range −3° to 10°). At latest follow- up, the L5 slip angle worsened in one of the three patients, showing a postoperative progression. The final result was nevertheless an improvement of the slip angle, with a mean angle of 6 degrees (range 3° to 11°).

The mean postoperative lumbar lordosis averaged 45.1 degrees (range 18° to 66°). No statistically significant difference was noted at the last follow-up (Fig. 16.3).

The three patients with associated scoliosis showed no worsening of the curves. Regarding the hardware, one sacral pedicular screw was found broken in two patients, one patient after 6 months and one patient after 3 years, without consequence. Among the three patients with postoperative worsening, both sacral pedicular screws were found broken in one patient at 1 year.

The quality of the fusion at 6 months was difficult to assess in four patients. One of these patients (patient 1) has been followed up for 6 months, and two others presented a postoperative progression. All patients but one (patient 1, with a 6-month follow-up) had a radiographically mature fusion 1 year postoperatively.

Complications

Postoperatively, two patients had mild paresis of the anterior tibialis. The recovery was spontaneous and complete for one patient. One patient operated on for a high-grade spondylolisthesis (L5-S1 fusion) showed a recurrence of the slippage with appearance of neurologic signs in the lower extremities and had secondary surgery 1 week after the first procedure. No other complications were noted.

DISCUSSION

Although most authors agree on the treatment of low-grade spondylolisthesis, there is still a lot of controversy about the treatment of high-grade spondylolisthesis. Harris and Weinstein (5) have found that 57% of patients (21 patients, age ranging from 11 to 25 years) treated with in situ posterolateral fusion were asymptomatic compared with 36% of patients (11 patients, age ranging from 10 to 24 years) treated conservatively. The operative group were less symptomatic and more active than the nonoperative group. It seems thus that the outcome is better for the operated patients. But controversy remains over what procedure must be performed and a lot of surgical techniques have been described in the literature, including for example in situ posterolateral fusion (7,13,15–21), reduction and fusion through a posterior approach (10,22–30), reduction and posterolateral fusion followed by anterior interbody fusion L5-S1 (31), reduction and anterior interbody fusion (32), reduction and combined fusion (3,33–36), L5 corporectomy (8,37). The main arguments against fusion in situ have been a higher rate of pseudarthrosis (5,14,18,20), a higher risk of postoperative slip progression (14), and the persistence of the cosmetic deformity (14,15,18). Among the surgeons performing reduction, it's usually accepted that correction of the kyphosis is of primary importance, while correction of the anterior shift is of only secondary importance (14,26,29,38–41). The improvement of the lumbosacral kyphosis offers some advantages as compared with fusion in situ. It improves spine mechanics above the fusion, and it creates a spinal balance that is favorable for the achievement of a good fusion (42). It also improves the global sagittal contour and cosmetic appearance. But it's noteworthy that very few patients complain about their cosmetic deformity (15,17,18,20). In their comparative study, Harris and Weinstein (5) noticed that no patients were dissatisfied with their cosmetic appearance. Whatever surgical option chosen, the goal must be to obtain stable fusion (39,40,43,44). It has been observed that once bony union or stability has been achieved, resolution of pain occurs, even in the presence of minor neural deficits, and hamstring spasm as well as the associated gait abnormalities resolve (14,15,45–47). Haraldsson et al. (48) compared spondylolisthesis in adolescents and children and showed that the most important cause of the preoperative symptoms observed in young people were instability at the level of the defect. Therefore, they suggested that the goal of treatment was to obtain stabilization. In our study, only four patients were concerned by their cosmetic appearance. Back pain was the most common complaint. At latest follow-up, 13 patients had complete resolution of their back pain, and two patients still complained of some lumbar discomfort but without consequence on their activity level. All patients but one had a radiographically mature fusion mass at latest follow-up. We have tried to assess as precisely as possible the radiographic results by taking different measurements, but it must be noted that the regional landmarks are often obscure, making inherent error in measurement possible. This problem of inaccuracy of landmarks during roentgenographic measurements has also been pointed out by other authors (5,29,49,50).

Some authors use a one-stage posterior procedure to perform posterolateral and interbody fusion in high-grade spondylolisthesis (26,27,30,33,38,51,52,54). In 1982, Bohlman and Cook (51) described a one-stage procedure using a posterior approach to realize decompression and in situ posterolateral and interbody fusion by placing a fibula from S1 to the displaced body of L5 in high-grade spondylolisthesis. Roca et al. (53) used the same technique to treat 14 patients with severe spondylolisthesis. No reduction was attempted, but the sacral prominence was osteotomized to remove all pressure on the dura. They used a fibular strut graft placed between S1 and L5 without instrumentation.

Twelve patients demonstrated incorporation of the graft with solid fusion. Two patients showed pseudarthrosis of the graft with increased slippage in one of these cases. The authors concluded that the use of instrumentation could improve the results and proposed to use a transvertebral screw. In these studies, the authors performed a fusion in situ, and the goal of the sacroplasty was to prevent any acute cauda equina syndrome. It must be noted that these studies didn't distinguish between adults and children. Among authors performing a reduction through a posterior approach, most of them used an instrumented reduction (24,25,39). Fabris and Costantini (49) performed the same posterior interbody fusion after sacral osteotomy and reduction and used segmental pedicle fixation to treat 11 young patients (age 13–18 years) with severe L5-S1 spondylolisthesis. The method of reduction was nevertheless different than the "positional method" performed in our study. They used a temporary device placed bilaterally between L1 and the sacral wings to achieve reduction by distraction. The mean correction of slipping was 79.5 ± 7%. The follow-up period ranged from 6 to 36 months. No neurologic complications were described. The hardware had to be removed from one patient 2 years after surgery because the patient experienced regional discomfort. The authors concluded that the posterior interbody fusion (and eventual sacral dome osteotomy) associated with posterior segmental pedicle instrumentation allowed both root decompression and achievement of solid fusion. Shufflebarger (55) reported on a prospective study of 18 adolescents operated on for severe spondylolisthesis. The surgical procedure included a L5 nerve decompression, temporary distraction for reduction, excision of the sacral dome, posterior lumbar interbody structural graft placement, and compression pedicle screw construct. All arthrodesis were performed at the lumbosacral level. The average preoperative slippage was 77% (70% to 90%) and improved to 13% (5% to 25%). The average slippage angle improved from 35 degrees to 4 degrees. Forty percent had preoperative neurologic deficits, but all deficits resolved after surgery. There were no neurologic complications, infections, or instrumentation complications. Boachie-Adjei et al. (38) used a technique of partial lumbosacral kyphosis reduction, posterior decompression, posterior interbody fusion, and pedicle screw transfixation of the lumbosacral junction to treat six patients with high-grade spondylolisthesis. The partial reduction was obtained by positioning the patient with the hips in maximum extension and by performing a reduction maneuver with an interbody spreader placed between L5 and S1. A sacral dome resection was performed to make the reduction easier. The mean slip angle was improved from 62 degrees to 28 degrees and there was no significant improvement in the percentage of slip. The mean follow-up was 42.6 months, and no progression of the slip angle or percentage of slip was noted. All patients had good results regarding pain control, function, and overall satisfaction with the procedure. The authors concluded that this posterior approach was safe and effective in obtaining a solid arthrodesis and restoring sagittal balance, and that the goal of surgery in treating high-grade spondylolisthesis was to obtain partial correction of the slip angle and not to correct the percentage of slip. In our study, we didn't use forceful instrumented reduction, but rather a "positional reduction" (i.e., reduction obtained by the preoperative or intraoperative positioning of the patient). The mean preoperative percentage of slip for the patients with severe L5-S1 spondylolisthesis was 73.1%. Postoperatively, the percentage of slip averaged 44.2% for these patients. The mean correction was 40.3%. Regarding patients with severe spondylolisthesis, the mean L5 slip angle was 38 degrees preoperatively and 9.9 degrees postoperatively. Two patients (one with L4–L5 spondylolisthesis and one with L5-S1 spondylolisthesis) were still skeletally immature at latest follow-up (1 year), but in one patient (L5-S1 spondylolisthesis), the last x-rays demonstrated a solid fusion without any progression. All patients but two described no pain at latest follow-up. The two other patients described only some lumbar discomfort. All patients could resume their previous activities. Like many authors (14,29,38,40,41), we think that the purpose of surgery is to obtain a correction of the lumbosacral kyphosis rather than the percentage of slip, in order to improve the sagittal alignment and therefore the spine mechanics.

The reduction carries risks of neurologic compromise. The commonest complication associated with reduction of L5 spondylolisthesis is paresis of the L5 nerve roots; paresis of the L4 and S1 roots as well as cauda equina syndrome have also been reported (14,56–58). Permanent motor deficits have been reported in as high as 25% of patients with reduction by instrumentation, and a higher incidence of transient deficits has been observed by others (6,25). Dubousset (6) described that the greatest danger to the L5 nerve root during the reduction maneuver occurred during the last 25% of the reduction of the slippage. These complications can be prevented to a great extent by using intraoperative spinal cord monitoring in the form of the wake-up test or somatosensory evoked potentials (SEP).

To determine the extent of fusion, each patient had preoperative magnetic resonance imaging to assess the quality of the intervertebral disc above and below the spondylolisthesis level. Six patients with L5-S1 spondylolisthesis showed deterioration of the L4–L5 disc and had L4–L5–S1 fusion. It seems that the quality of the intervertebral disc above the spondylolisthesis level cannot be predicted with the grade of slipping. Fusion to L4 theoretically reduces the number of motion segments but it seems that the long-term follow-up of these patients is good, with no reduction in their functional abilities (5,18,20).

The reported incidence of pseudarthrosis after posterior in situ arthrodesis varies from 0% to 60% in the literature (14,16–18,44,59).

The quality of the fusion mass is an important factor affecting the outcome. Newton and Johnston (60) studied adolescent patients with poor outcome following in situ arthrodesis for severe spondylolisthesis. They found that the incidence of poor result was higher in patients demonstrating a bad-grade fusion and concluded that the quality of fusion mass correlated with outcome.

Postoperative slippage progression after in situ posterolateral fusion has been described even though a solid arthrodesis was obtained because of bending and shear forces on the fusion mass (4,14,17,18,61,62). Nowadays a lot of authors use modern transpedicular fixation systems, which offer more stable fixation and should therefore enhance the rate of fusion and decrease the rate of secondary displacement (33,42,49,57,58). But some studies also describe progressive postoperative recurrence of the slippage despite use of fixation systems and bone grafts (25,33,58,59,63,64). Boos et al. (33) treated 10 patients (mean age 23.6 years, range 9 to 50 years) with severe spondylolisthesis with reduction and pedicular fixation. Six patients had a single posterolateral fusion. All four patients with a spondyloptosis had an additional interbody fusion, via a transperitoneal approach in three cases and by a posterior approach in one case. These four patients had solid fusion without loss of reduction. Five of the six patients treated by a single posterolateral fusion demonstrated loss of reduction, nonunion, and implant failure. Four of these patients were reoperated. The authors concluded that the pedicular fixation systems might only allow permanent reduction and fusion of severe spondylolisthesis if a combined interbody and posterolateral fusion was performed. The same observation was made by Steffee and Sitkowski (58). In the study of Molari et al. (44), the frequency of instrumentation failure and partial loss of reduction was higher in group 2 (i.e., patients treated by reduction and posterior L4-sacrum fusion). All instrumentation complications occurred in sacral-pelvic fixation. As a conclusion, the authors recommended anterior column bone grafting and the use of four-point sacral-pelvic fixation using bicortical S1 screws and bilateral iliac screws. The main disadvantage of these iliac screws is the need for removal. In our study, we used the Cotrel-Dubousset instrumentation. Screw breakage was found in three patients. Only one (with initial Grade 4 spondylolisthesis) of them showed a loss of reduction. The main advantage of this instrumentation is to allow early ambulation without need of cast immobilization. Some authors (6) think that instrumentation at the lumbosacral junction may be excessively bulky and prominent, necessitating removal later. In our series, no patient complained of prominent hardware.

CONCLUSION

At the present time there is no consensus regarding treatment of high-grade spondylolisthesis. In this chapter, the authors explain their philosophy regarding treatment of spondylolisthesis and describe their technique of reduction and segmental fusion of high-grade spondylolisthesis associated with a lumbosacral kyphosis using a posterior approach. This technique has the advantage to provide good reduction of the lumbosacral kyphosis through a unique posterior approach, nerve decompression, solid fixation and fusion while allowing early ambulation, without the need of a prolonged postoperative cast immobilization. As with any spondylolisthesis reduction technique, neurologic risk should limit this procedure to well-selected patients. This is a technically demanding procedure and the surgeon must have substantial hands-on experience in this demanding technique. The number of patients is too small to draw statistical conclusions. It's likely that a lot of techniques are good for the treatment of high-grade spondylolisthesis, but the goal must be to achieve a solid bone union allowing resolution of the pain and the hamstring tightness and if possible improvement of the neurologic complaints. Whatever the technique chosen by the surgeon, the goal must be the same, and the surgeon must perform the procedure he or she is the most used to.

REFERENCES

1. Herbiniaux G. *Traité sur divers accouchements laborieux, et sur polypes de la matrice.* Brussels: JL DeBroubers; 1782.
2. Taillard W. *Les spondylolisthesis*. Paris: Masson; 1957.
3. Hensinger RN. Spondylolysis and spondylolisthesis in children and adolescents: current concept review. *J Bone Joint Surg Am* 1989;71:1098–1107.
4. Lonstein JE. Spondylolisthesis in children: cause, natural history and management. *Spine* 1999;24:2640–2648.
5. Harris IE, Weinstein SL. Long-term follow-up of patients with Grade-III and IV spondylolisthesis: treatment with and without posterior fusion. *J Bone Joint Surg Am* 1987;69:960–969.
6. Dubousset J. Treatment of spondylolysis and spondylolisthesis in children and adolescents. *Clin Orthop* 1997; 337:77–85.
7. Ishikawa S, Kumar SJ, Tores BC. Surgical treatment of dysplastic spondylolisthesis: results after in situ fusion. *Spine* 1994;19:1691–1696.
8. Lehmer SH, Steffee AD, Gaines RW Jr. Treatment of L5-S1 spondyloptosis by staged L5 resection with reduction and fusion of L4 onto S1. *Spine* 1994;19:1916–1925.
9. O'Brien J, Mehdian H, Jaffray D. Reduction of severe lumbosacral spondylolisthesis: a report of 22 cases with a ten-year follow-up period. *Clin Orthop* 1994;300:64–69.
10. Poussa M, Schlenzka D, Seitsalo S, et al. Surgical treatment of severe isthmic spondylolisthesis in adolescents. *Spine* 1993;18:894–901.
11. Meyerding HW. Spondylolisthesis. *Surg Gynecol Obstet* 1932;54:371–377.
12. Wiltse LL, Newman PH, MacNab W. Classification of spondylolysis and spondylolisthesis. *Clin Orthop* 1976;117:23–29.
13. Wiltse LL, Rothman LG. Spondylolisthesis: classification, diagnosis and natural history. *Semin Spine Surg* 1989;1:78–94.
14. Boxall D, Bradford DS, Winter RB, et al. Management of severe spondylolisthesis in children and adolescents. *J Bone Joint Surg Am* 1979;61:479–495.

15. Freeman BL, Donati NL. Spinal arthrodesis for severe spondylolisthesis in children and adolescents: a long-term follow-up study. *J Bone Joint Surg Am* 1989;71:594–598.
16. Frennered AK, Danielson BI, Nachemson AL, et al. Midterm follow-up of young patients fused in situ for spondylolisthesis. *Spine* 1991;16:409–416.
17. Grzegorzewski A, Kumar SJ. In situ posterolateral spine arthrodesis for grades III, IV and V spondylolisthesis in children and adolescents. *J Pediatr Orthop* 2000;20:506–511.
18. Johnson JR, Kirwan EO. The long-term results of fusion in situ for severe spondylolisthesis. *J Bone Joint Surg Br* 1983;65:43–46.
19. Pizzutillo PD, Mirenda W, MacEwen GD. Posterolateral fusion for spondylolisthesis in adolescence. *J Pediatr Orthop* 1986;6:311–316.
20. Seitsalo S, Osterman K, Hyvarinen H, et al. Severe spondylolisthesis in children and adolescents: a long-term review of fusion in situ. *J Bone Joint Surg Br* 1990;72:259–265.
21. Stanton RP, Meehan P, Lovell WW. Surgical fusion in childhood spondylolisthesis. *J Pediatr Orthop* 1985; 5:411–415.
22. Balderston RA, Bradford DS. Techniques for achievement and maintenance of reduction for severe spondylolisthesis using spinous process traction wiring and external fixation of the pelvis. *Spine* 1985;10:376–382.
23. Harrington PR, Dickson JH. Spinal instrumentation in the treatment of severe progressive spondylolisthesis. *Clin Orthop* 1976;117:157–163.
24. Herman S, Pouliquen JC. Spondylolisthésis à grand déplacement chez l'enfant et l'adolescent: résultats de 12 cas de réduction-fixation postérieure. *Rev Chir Orthop* 1988;74:614–621.
25. Hu SS, Bradford DS, Transfeldt EE, et al. Reduction of high-grade spondylolisthesis using Edwards instrumentation. *Spine* 1996;21:367–371.
26. Louis R, Tropiano P, Nazarian S. Traitement chirurgical des spondylolisthesis à grand déplacement par la technique de la réduction-fusion par double abord. *Rachis* 1990;2:449–460.
27. Roy-Camille R. Spondylolisthesis. In: *Conferences d'enseignement 1986* (Cahiers d'enseignement de la SOFCOT, n° 26). Paris: Elsevier; 1986:89–101.
28. Schöllner D. One stage reduction and fusion for spondylolisthesis. *Int Orthop* 1990;14:145–150.
29. Schwend RM, Waters PM, Hey LA, et al. Treatment of severe spondylolisthesis in children by reduction and L4-S4 posterior segmental hyperextension fixation. *J Pediatr Orthop* 1992;12:703–711.
30. Vidal J, Fassio B, Buscayret C, et al. Surgical reduction of spondylolisthesis using a posterior approach. *Clin Orthop* 1981;154:156–165.
31. Laursen MB, Thomsen K, Eiskjaer SP, et al. Functional outcome after partial reduction and 360 degree fusion in grade III-V spondylolisthesis in adolescent and adult patients. *J Spinal Disord* 1999;12:300–306.
32. Bitan F, Padovani JP, Glorion C, et al. Les spondylolisthésis à grand déplacement de l'enfant et de l'adolescent: résultats de la réduction-arthrodèse par plaque antérieure. *Rev Chir Orthop* 1990;76:425–436.
33. Boos N, Marchesi D, Zuber K, et al. Treatment of severe spondylolisthesis by reduction and pedicular fixation: a 4-6-year follow-up study. *Spine* 1993;18:1655–1661.
34. Bradford DS, Gotfried Y. Staged salvage reconstruction of grade-IV and V spondylolisthesis. *J Bone Joint Surg Am* 1987;69:191–202.
35. Dick WT, Schnebel B. Severe spondylolisthesis: reduction and internal fixation. *Clin Orthop* 1988;232:70–79.
36. Smith MD, Bohlman HH. Spondylolisthesis treated by a single-stage operation combining decompression with in situ posterolateral and anterior fusion: an analysis of eleven patients who had long-term follow-up. *J Bone Joint Surg Am* 1990;72:415–421.
37. Gaines RW, Nichols WK. Treatment of spondyloptosis by two stage L5 vertebrectomy and reduction of L4 onto S1. *Spine* 1985;10:680–686.
38. Boachie-Adjei O, Do T, Rawlins BA. Partial lumbosacral kyphosis reduction, decompression and posterior lumbosacral transfixation in high-grade isthmic spondylolisthesis: clinical and radiographic results in six patients. *Spine* 2002;27:E161–E168.
39. Edwards C, Bradford D. Controversies-Instrumented reduction of spondylolisthesis. *Spine* 1994;19:1535–1537.
40. Jouve JL. Spondylolyse et spondylolisthesis lombosacre. In: *Conferences d'enseignement 2001* (Cahier d'Enseignement de la SOFCOT). Paris: Elsevier; 2001.
41. McPhee IB, O'Brien JP. Reduction of severe spondylolisthesis: a preliminary report. *Spine* 1979;4:430–434.
42. Muschik M, Zippel H, Perka C. Surgical management of severe spondylolisthesis in children and adolescents: anterior fusion in situ versus anterior spondylodesis with posterior transpedicular instrumentation and reduction. *Spine* 1997;17:2036–2043.
43. Kaelin A. Spondylolyse et spondylolisthésis de l'enfant et de l'adolescent. In: *Progrès en médecine physique et de réadaptation*. Paris: Masson; 1998:403–419.
44. Molinari RW, Bridwell KH, Lenke LG, et al. Complications with surgical treatment of pediatric high-grade isthmic dysplastic spondylolisthesis: a comparison of 3 surgical approaches. *Spine* 1999;24:1701–1711.
45. Johnson LP, Nasca RJ, Dunham WK. Surgical management of isthmic spondylolisthesis. *Spine* 1988;13:93–97.
46. Shelokov A, Haideri N, Roach J. Residual gait abnormalities in surgically treated spondylolisthesis. *Spine* 1993;18:2201–2205.
47. Meyers LL, Dobson SR, Wiegand D, et al. Mechanical instability as a cause of gait disturbance in high-grade spondylolisthesis: a pre- and postoperative three-dimensional gait analysis. *J Pediatr Orthop* 1999;19:672– 676.
48. Haraldsson S, Willner S. A comparative study of spondylolisthesis in operations on adolescents and adults. *Arch Orthop Trauma Surg* 1983;101:101–105.

49. Fabris DA, Costantini S, Nena U. Surgical treatment of severe L5-S1 spondylolisthesis in children and adolescents: results of intraoperative reduction, posterior interbody fusion, and segmental pedicle fixation. *Spine* 1996;21:728–733.
50. Lindholm TS, Ragni P, Ylikoski M, et al. Lumbar isthmic spondylolisthesis in children and adolescents: radiologic evaluation and results of operative treatment. *Spine* 1990;15:1350–1355.
51. Bohlman HH, Cook SS. One-stage decompression and posterolateral and interbody fusion for lumbosacral spondyloptosis through a posterior approach: report of two cases. *J Bone Joint Surg Am* 1982;64:415–418.
52. Cloward RB. Spondylolisthesis: treatment by laminectomy and posterior interbody fusion. *Clin Orthop* 1981; 154:74–82.
53. Roca J, Ubierna MT, Caceres E, et al. One-stage decompression and posterolateral and interbody fusion for severe spondylolisthesis: an analysis of 14 patients. *Spine* 1999;24:709–714.
54. Wiltse LL, Jackson DW. Treatment of spondylolisthesis and spondylolysis in children. *Clin Orthop* 1976;117: 92–100.
55. Shufflebarger HL. High grade isthmic spondylolisthesis: monosegmental surgical treatment. Scoliosis Research Society Annual Meeting, New York, NY, 1998.
56. Dewald RL, Faut MM, Taddonio RF, et al. Severe lumbosacral spondylolisthesis in adolescents and children: reduction and staged circumferential fusion. *J Bone Joint Surg Am* 1981;63:619–626.
57. Matthias HH, Heine J. The surgical reduction of spondylolisthesis. *Clin Orthop* 1986;203:34–44.
58. Steffee AD, Sitkowski DJ. Reduction and stabilization of grade IV spondylolisthesis. *Clin Orthop* 1988;227: 82–89.
59. Sherman FC, Rosenthal RK, Hall JE. Spine fusion for spondylolysis and spondylolisthesis in children. *Spine* 1979;4:59–67.
60. Newton PO, Johnston CE. Analysis and treatment of poor outcomes following in situ arthrodesis in adolescent spondylolisthesis. *J Pediatr Orthop* 1997;17:754–761.
61. Ghosez JP, Himmer O, Devyver B, et al. Traitement chirurgical du spondylolisthésis isthmique: etude comparative de 3 types d'arthrodèse. *Rev Chir Orthop Reparatrice Appar Mot* 1992;78:515–528.
62. Leyvraz PF, Guigoz JP. Resultats du traitement chirurgical du spondylolisthésis par greffes postérolatérales intertransversaires: a propos of 39 cases. *Rev Chir Orthop Reparatrice Appar Mot* 1987;73:137–141.
63. Boos N, Marchesi D, Aebi M. Treatment of spondylolysis and Cotrel-Dubousset instrumentation: a preliminary report. *J Spinal Disord* 1991;4:472–479.
64. Michel CR, Caton J, Samani J, et al. Apport de la technique de E. Luque dans la chirurgie des grands spondylolisthésis de l'enfant. *Chir Pediatr* 1984;25:161–163.

17

Direct Repair of the Pars Interarticularis for Spondylolysis

F. Pellisè and A. Malik

Spondylolysis, defined as a defect of the vertebral pars interarticularis, is estimated to occur in 3% to 7% of adults and is usually clinically asymptomatic (1,2). For patients with symptomatic spondylolysis, a variety of management strategies have been advocated (3–5). Conservative management resolves the problem of pain in most patients and should be attempted prior to surgery. The alternative forms of nonsurgical treatment may include rest, adaptation of physical activity and sports, active physiotherapy, bracing, and medication. Activity restriction followed by rehabilitation and strengthening exercises are often successful in improving symptoms (3). Nonetheless, a small percentage of patients fail conservative treatment, and a surgical alternative may be considered for this subgroup (6).

Several procedures have been proposed and used over the years for the surgical management of symptomatic spondylolysis or spondylolisthesis with minimal displacement. The traditional surgical procedure to manage this condition has been spinal fusion (6); decompression by total excision of the loose lamina (7) with or without fusion has also been advocated. As an alternative to fusion techniques that eliminate a mobile segment, surgical procedures repairing only the pars defect were introduced (4,8). The aim of this surgery is to ensure consolidation of the pars interarticularis fracture without modifying the functional anatomy around the defect. With the restoration of normal anatomy, preservation of motion at the affected spinal segment is theoretically possible. Surgical success is directly related to accurate localization of the source of pain. In a patient with a pars defect, pain can potentially originate from the defect itself or from an adjacent degenerative disc (9). Most reports point out that the ideal candidates for direct repair are younger patients without degenerative findings, but identification of the actual source of pain may be more important than the consideration of age (10). Several diagnostic tools have been used to select ideal surgical candidates: Pars infiltration to confirm the pars defect as the source of pain, and magnetic resonance imaging (MRI) and discography to rule out discogenic pain.

In 1968, Kimura (8) was the first to introduce direct repair of the defect, using bone graft without any internal fixation. Patients were confined to bed-rest for 2 months and thereafter wore a brace for an additional 4 to 6 months. In 1970, Buck was the first to use internal fixation (lag screws) across the pars interarticularis to repair the fracture (4). Other authors have since reported direct repair of the pars defect using wire (11–14), hook screws (15–20), cable-screws (21), screw-rod hooks (22–25), and other internal fixation techniques (26,27).

Buck admitted that accurate placement of translaminar screws is technically difficult (28). The technique requires considerable skill, and with relatively few cases being operated, most surgeons will have limited surgical experience (14). Scott was the first to apply a simple and effective means of repairing spondylolytic defects through the use of bone grafts and wiring in 1968. However, his results were not published until 1986 (14). It was later found that segmental wiring can also be accompanied by technical difficulties when passing the wire under the transverse process of L5, because of the overlapping iliac crest (12). Furthermore, placement of the wire under the transverse process can lead to substantial bleeding and carries a risk of nerve root injury (20).

In order to avoid passing a wire around the transverse process, the use of pedicular screws to anchor the tension band wire was suggested in 1993 (27). In this modified screw-wire technique, the wire is anchored around the spinous process to hold down graft bone that bridges the pars defect. However, with this system, the compression force exerted against the graft bones is diverted away from the lamina. The strength and linkage of wires as well as the inadequate direction of the force attained through fixation are unfavorable for achieving fusion (25). The use of Buck screws across the pars defect is advantageous in that the direction of the compression force they exert is the same as that of the lamina. Nevertheless, the presence of the screw limits the size of the bone graft mass on the surface of the defect.

In 1984, Morscher introduced the screw-hook technique (29). As compared with the compression screw alone, the hook had the advantage of providing a solid grasp in dysplastic vertebral arches. The main problem with the Morscher technique was seen to be the high incidence of screw loosening, which presented as swelling and pain (18,20).

Pseudoarthrosis may develop after repair of the defect and often leads to poor clinical results (13,19,30). The most frequent cause of pseudoarthrosis has been found to be the use of internal fixation techniques that do not provide sufficient stability (31). More rigid fixation techniques lead to a lower prevalence of pseudoarthrosis and hence, better clinical results. The clawlike configuration of the screw-rod-hook construct, which incorporates elements of standard spine instrumentation, offers good mechanical stability (32). However, a potential drawback of this technique lies in the bulkiness of the instrumentation, which makes radiographic evaluation of the pars difficult (24). Although several studies have analyzed the effectiveness of the different systems, the series are small in number and no comprehensive or detailed comparisons among them have been made. These reduced bibliographic reviews do not appear to favor any one surgical technique over another (18).

Professional athletes have a higher prevalence of isthmic defects than the general population (33). It is currently believed that the most likely cause of isthmic spondylolysis in athletes is a fatigue fracture. A direct relationship has been observed between this condition and intense sports activities in athletes between the ages of 5 and 15 years (34). Most patients with symptomatic spondylolysis in general, and professional athletes in particular, have mechanical back pain related to activity and movement. This is a limitation that prevents such athletes from performing at a maximum level. If symptoms are not reduced through conservative measures, the affected athlete must either retire from sports activities or undergo some type of surgical treatment. When surgery is chosen, however, a relatively long period of activity restriction is required, which usually leads to deterioration in athletic performance. The implications of these factors cause both physicians and athletes to hesitate before considering surgery. At present, information is insufficient concerning the long-term outcome of athletes treated for symptomatic spondylolysis in terms of their return to sports activity (34).

To elucidate some of the uncertainties related to spondylolysis surgery, we compared the results of different surgical techniques used in this pathology according to their complications, fusion rates, clinical outcomes, and return to sports activities; we evaluated the effects of patient characteristics such as age on the surgical outcome. The comparison is based on a review of the literature following a Medline search using as key words "spondylolysis" and "repair."

REVIEW OF THE LITERATURE

We found 78 references for spondylolysis repair, published between June 1970 and April 2004. Thirty-five items that specifically focused on direct repair of the lysis, and reported the results of cohorts of more than four patients were selected. Case reports and technical descriptions were excluded from this review. In total we evaluated 28 full text papers and seven abstracts (11,16,17,35,37,38).

The literature review covers 668 patients. The mean number of patients per paper was 19.65 (standard deviation 22.43; range 4 to 113). The mean age at the time of surgery was 23.16 years (SD 6.17; range 12 to 35.8). The mean of the minimum age of the cohorts was 14.77 years (SD 3.48; range 7 to 21), and their mean maximum age was 38.04 years (SD 10.32; range 15 to 60). Males were predominant in the majority of papers, and represented 67.5% of the total series (range 20 to 100). Low back pain was the main preoperative symptom, being present in 99.3% of the patients. Radicular pain was associated with back pain in many cohorts of patients and was present in 27.8% of each sample (range 0% to 80%). The studies retrieved were retrospective and evaluated patients after a mean postoperative follow-up period of 59.43 months (range 8.5 to 130.8). Minimum follow-up ranged from 5 to 114 months, while maximum follow-up ranged from 17 to 204 months.

Eleven papers (4,9,18,30,31,35,36,39–42) reported the results of a total of 169 patients treated with the Buck technique. Seven papers (15–20,43) reported the results of 206 patients treated with the Morscher technique. Six papers (11–14,34,44) reported the results of 96 patients treated with the Scott-wiring technique. Four (22–25) papers reported the results of 36 patients treated with the screw-rod-hook technique. Five papers (10,21,26,45,46) included a heterogeneous group with a total of 141 patients treated by different techniques, whereas two abstracts did not specify the surgical technique used (37,38). Few papers gave detailed information on the different parameters related to this surgery. The mean operating time, reported in three papers, was 115 minutes (range 84 to 146), and mean blood loss, reported in five papers, was 271.8 cc (range: 146 to 430).

No prospective randomized studies were found, and clinical outcomes were assessed with nonstandardized scales in the vast majority of papers (94%). The Henderson scale was the most frequently used tool to evaluate clinical outcome. The Henderson criteria describe the result as *excellent* when the patient is pain-free and returns to full activity and *good* when there is only occasional pain or limitation in undertaking strenuous physical activities. Clinical outcomes as reported in the 35 papers are included in this review. The rate of excellent and good clinical outcomes varied between 40% and 100%, with a weighted mean value of 84.43% (range 78.91% to 90.35%). Although correlations are difficult to establish in this type of study, statistical analysis showed that clinical outcome correlated inversely with the existence of bilateral pseudoarthrosis ($r = -0.82, p = .00$) and with patient age ($r = -49, p = .00$). There was also a trend toward poorer clinical outcomes in papers published earlier ($r = 0.32, p = 0.06$).

The comparison between surgical techniques showed no significant statistical differences, although there was a trend toward better results with the screw-rod-hook technique (88.89% excellent and good; range 80.8% to 97.6%). The mean weighted rates of

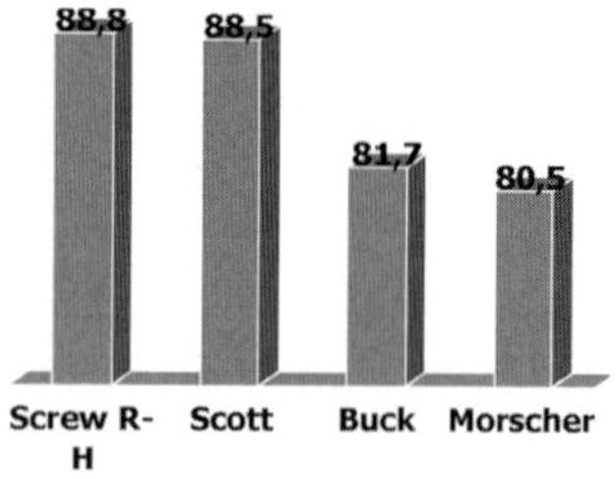

FIG. 17.1. Mean weighted rates of excellent and good results ($p > .05$).

excellent and good results for the other techniques are shown in Figure 17.1. Eleven papers reported the percentage of patients who returned to sports activities (22,39,44); the weighted mean value of success, defined as return to sports, was 79.17% (range 69.78% to 89.82%).

Patients with an unsatisfactory clinical outcome underwent revision surgery to fuse the affected spinal segment. The weighted mean rate of revision to an arthrodesis was 5.33% (range 2.48% to 11.47%). The percentage of patients who eventually achieved fusion was smaller in the cohorts treated with the screw-rod-hook technique (2.78%; range 0.40% to 19.19%), although again the differences between surgical techniques were not statistically significant (Fig. 17.2).

Among the 25 papers including information on postoperative complications, the weighted mean rate of complications was 13.48% (range 8.68% to 20.95%). The majority (7.87%; range 3.71% to 16.68%) were mechanical failures, with early failures being due to incorrect instrumentation placement and late failures associated with bilateral pseudoarthrosis. Neurologic complications due to nerve root impingement developed in 2.7% of patients (range 1.03% to 7.04%) and resolved spontaneously in half of them. Wound complications were reported in 1.92%. Comparisons between the different surgical techniques showed differences that were not significant, although there was a trend toward fewer complications in the patients treated with the screw-rod-hook technique (Fig. 17.3).

To evaluate pars reconstruction (consolidation) at follow-up, plain radiographs were used in 19 studies and a combination of radiographs plus computed tomography (CT) scanning was used in eight. Eight papers did not state the methods used to assess pars fusion. With regard to nonunion, the weighted rate of bilateral pseudoarthrosis was 13.32% (range 9.20% to 19.29%). The Scott and screw-rod-hook techniques had fusion

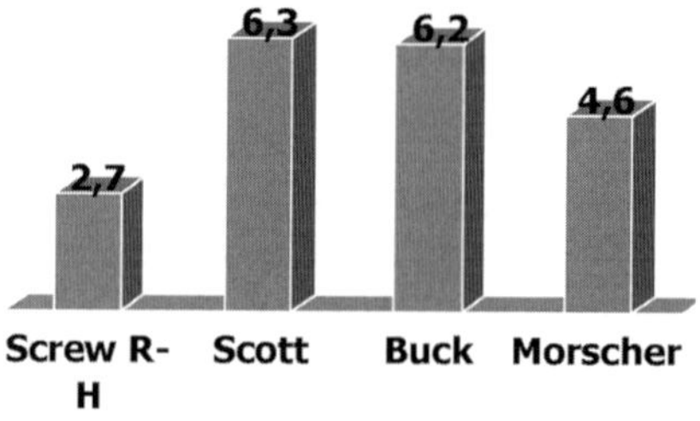

FIG. 17.2. Weighted mean rate of revision surgery to fuse ($p > .05$).

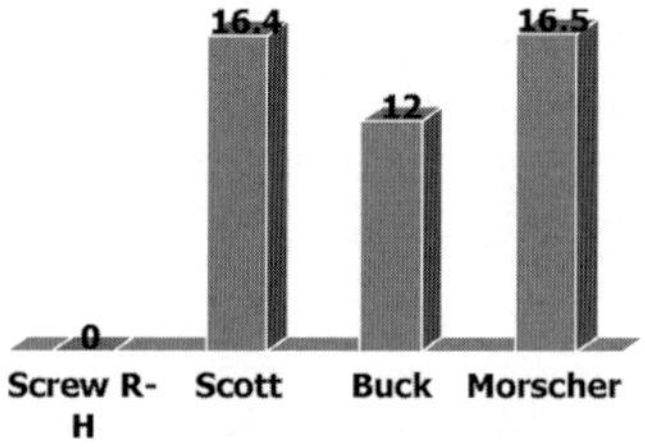

FIG. 17.3. Weighted mean rate of complications ($p > .05$).

rates higher than 90%, while the Buck and Morscher techniques had lower fusion rates. Differences were not statistically significant (Fig. 17.4).

DISCUSSION

Our review of the literature shows that direct repair of the pars interarticularis for spondylolysis in a small group of adequately selected patients will substantially improve the clinical situation in up to 85% of the cases while allowing return to presymptomatic levels of sport activity in 80%. In 5% of patients, surgery fails and revision surgery is required in the midterm to fuse the repaired segment. Presence of bilateral nonunion and older age at the time of surgery were seen to have a direct correlation with poor clinical outcomes.

Although differences were not statistically significant, the Buck and Morsher techniques tended to have a lower fusion rate than the Scott and screw-rod-hook techniques. These findings contradict the results reported by Deguchi et al. in 1999 (32). In this experimental study carried out on calf lumbar spines, the four fixation systems offered as much resistance to flexion and torsion as the normal spine throughout the loading regimen, with no significant differences among the instrumented spines. However, the screw-rod-hook and Buck techniques provided more secure fixation with less motion across the defect than the Scott and modified Scott techniques. In their experimental setting, the authors evaluated a perfectly placed Buck screw. However, Buck's technique is demanding, and there are several reports of incorrect intraoperative placement of the screw (28,31). It is likely that the amount of fixation provided by an incorrectly placed translaminar screw intraoperatively will be less than that found in experimental settings. Furthermore, in Buck's technique the screw crosses the defect and reduces the bony surface for fusion. These two parameters, incorrect screw placement and reduced bony surface, might explain the higher rate of nonunion associated with Buck screws in the present study despite better experimental fixation.

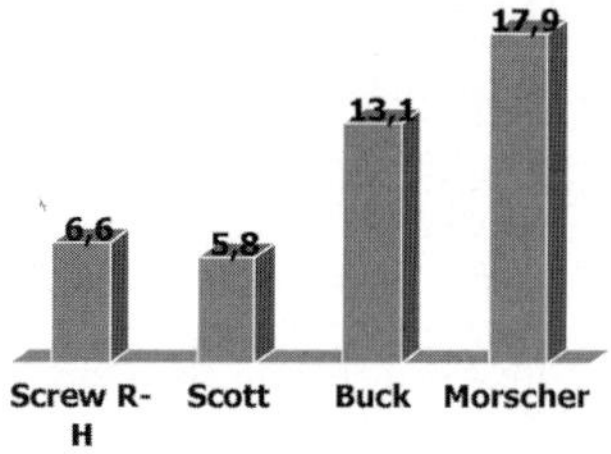

FIG. 17.4. Weighted mean rate of bilateral pseudoarthrosis ($p > .05$).

Comparatively, the screw-rod-hook technique is associated with better clinical outcome and fewer complications than the other techniques. This technique provides a good bed for the bone graft with excellent fixation and avoids the technical difficulties and complications associated with translaminar screw placement and periapophyseal wiring. In 1999, we communicated our results of direct repair using the screw-rod-hook fixation technique, with fusion being assessed by CT scanning (24). Our study, with an average postoperative follow-up of 41 months, showed that good clinical outcomes with return to sports activities could be obtained even when bilateral pseudoarthrosis was evident on CT scans.

Clinical improvement after isthmic reconstruction surgery is based on the fact that the area of lysis and the mobility of the posterior vertebral arch, which might be the origin of pain, has been restored to a more anatomical state. Several papers have supported this hypothesis. Schneiderman (47) identified free nerve endings with a nociceptive function in the area of lysis. Eisenstein (48) described neuropeptides in the isthmic defect, which have been associated with nociception within the autonomous nervous system and were thought to mediate in the sensation of pain caused by movement of the affected area. Nordström (49) isolated local inflammatory mediators within the defect that stimulate the local neural elements originating pain. The great stability conferred by pedicle screws and laminar hooks associated with surgical debridement at the site of spondylolysis may explain the favorable clinical outcome at midterm even when consolidation of the pars had not been achieved.

In conclusion, direct pars repair in spondylolysis is a safe and effective modality to treat selected patients in whom conservative measures have failed. Isthmic reconstruction appears to be a logical and less drastic surgical option than fusion, with the theoretical advantage of restoring anatomy. Factors such as the age of the patient and failure to obtain bilateral pars fusion may influence in the clinical outcome. However, it has been shown that some reconstruction techniques provide very solid fixation and can result in good clinical outcome despite unsuccessful pars reconstruction.

REFERENCES

1. Amato M, Totty WG, Gilula LA. Spondylolysis of the lumbar spine: demonstration of defects and laminal fragmentation. *Radiology* 1984;153:627–629.
2. Fredrickson BE, Baker D, McHolick WJ. The natural history of spondylolysis: spondylolisthesis. *J Bone Joint Surg Am* 1984;66:699–707.
3. Blanda J, Bethem D, Moats W. Defects of pars interarticularis in athletes: a protocol for non-operative treatment. *J Spinal Disord* 1993;6:406–411.
4. Buck JE. Direct repair of the defect in spondylolisthesis. Preliminary report. *J Bone Joint Surg Br* 1970; 52(3):432–438.
5. Moller H, Hedlund R. Instrumented and non-instrumented posterolateral fusion in adult spondylolisthesis: a prospective randomized study: Part 2. *Spine* 2000;25:1716–1721.
6. Hensinger RN. Current concepts review. Spondylolysis and spondylolisthesis in children and adolescents. *J Bone Joint Surg Am* 1989;71:1098-1107.
7. Gill GG, Manning JG, White HL. Surgical treatment of spondylolisthesis without spine fusion. *J Bone Joint Surg Am* 1955;37:493–520.
8. Kimura M. My method of filling the lesion with spongy bone in spondylolysis and spondylolysthesis. *Orthop Surg* 1968;19:285–295.
9. Suh PB, Esses SI, Kostuik JP. Repair of pars interarticularis defect. The prognostic value of pars infiltration. *Spine* 1991;16(8-S):S445–S448.
10. Wu SS, Lee CH, Chen PQ. Operative repair of symptomatic spondylolysis following a positive response to diagnostic pars injection. *J Spinal Disord* 1999;12(1):10–16.
11. Andersen L. Lumbar spondylolysis treated with cerclage using the method of the 80s. *Ugeskr Laeger* 1994;156(26):3888–3890.
12. Bradford DS, Iza J. Repair of the defect in spondylolysis or minimal degrees of spondylolisthesis by segmental wire fixation and bone grafting. *Spine* 1985;10(7):673–679.

13. Johnson GV, Thompson AG. The Scott wiring technique for direct repair of lumbar spondylolysis. *J Bone Joint Surg* 1992;74B(3):426–430.
14. Nicol RO, Scott JHS. Lytic spondylolysis. Repair by wiring. *Spine* 1986;11(10):1027–1030.
15. Albassir A, Samson I, Hendrickx L. Traitement de la spondylolyse douloureuse par le crochet de Morscher. *Acta Orthop Belg* 1990;56(2):489–495.
16. Buess E, Waldis M. Direct screwing in spondylolysis: results and observations on indications. *Schweiz Rundsch Med Prax* 1994;83(17):515–518.
17. Chen JF, Lee ST. A physiological method for the repair of young adult simple isthmic lumbar spondylolysis. *Changgeng Yi Xue Za Zhi* 2000;23(2):92–98.
18. Dreyzin V, Esses SI. A comparative analysis of spondylolysis repair. *Spine* 1994;19(17):1909–1915.
19. Hefti F, Seelig W, Morscher E. Repair of lumbar spondylolysis with a hook-screw. Inter Orthop 1992;16:81–85.
20. Sales de Gauzy J, Vadier F, Cahuzac JP. Repair of lumbar spondylolysis using Morscher material. 14 children followed for 1–5 years. *Acta Orthop Scand* 2000;71(3):292–296.
21. Songer MN, Rovin R. Repair of the pars interarticularis defect with a cable–screw construct: A preliminary report. *Spine* 1998;23(2):263–269.
22. Kakiuchi M. Repair of the defect in spondylolysis. Durable fixation with pedicle screws and laminar hooks. *J Bone Joint Surg Am* 1997;79(6):818–825.
23. Lundin DA, Wiseman D, Ellenbogen RG, et al. Direct repair of the pars interarticularis for spondylolysis and spondylolisthesis. *Pediatr Neurosurg* 2003;39:195–200.
24. Pellisè F, Toribio J, Rivas A, et al. Clinical and CT scan evaluation alter direct repair in spondylolysis using segmental pedicular screw hook fixation. *J Spinal Disord* 1999;12(5):363–367.
25. Tokuhashi Y, Matsuzaki H. Repair of defects in spondylolysis by segmental pedicular screw hook fixation. A preliminary report. *Spine* 1996;21(17):2041–2045.
26. Gillet P, Petit M. Direct repair of spondylolysis without spondylolisthesis, using a rod-screw construct and bone grafting of the pars. *Spine* 1999;24(12):1252–1256.
27. Salib RM, Pettine KA. Modified repair of a defect in spondylolysis or minimal spondylolisthesis by pedicle screw, segmental wire fixation, and bone grafting. *Spine* 1993;18(4):440–443.
28. Buck JE. Further thoughts on direct repair of the defect in spondylolysis. *J Bone Joint Surg Br* 1979;61:123.
29. Morscher E, Gerber B, Fasel J. Surgical treatment of spondylolisthesis by bone grafting: direct stabilization of spondylolysis by means of a hook screw. *Arch Orthop Trauma Surg* 1984;103:175–178.
30. Pedersen AK, Hagen R. Spondylolysis and spondylolisthesis: treatment by internal fixation and bone-grafting of the defect. *J Bone Joint Surg Am* 1988;70(1):15–24.
31. Beckers L. Buck's operation for treatment of spondylolysis and spondylolisthesis. *Acto Orthop Belg* 1986; 52(6):819–823.
32. Deguchi M, Rapoff AJ, Zdeblick TA. Biomechanical comparison of spondylolysis fixation techniques. *Spine* 1999;24(4):328–333.
33. Soler T, Calderon C. The prevalence of spondylolysis in the Spanish elite athlete. *Am J Sports Med* 2000;28(1):57–62.
34. Nozawa S, Shimizu K, Miyamoto K, et al. Repair of pars interarticularis defect by segmental wire fixation in young athletes with spondylolysis. *Am J Sports Med* 2003;31(3):359–364.
35. Bonnici AV, Koka SR, Richards DJ. Results of Buck screw fusion in grade I spondylolisthesis. *J R Soc Med* 1991;84(5):270–273.
36. Buring K, Fredensborg N. Osteosynthesis of spondylolysis. *Acta Orthop Scand* 1973; 44:91–92.
37. Prasartritha T. Surgical repair of pars defects in spondylolysis. *Thai J Med Assoc* 2001;84(9):1235–1240.
38. Reitman CA, Esses SI. Direct repair of spondylolytic defects in young competitive athletes. *Spine J* 2002;2(2):142–144.
39. Hardcastle PH. Repair of spondylolysis in young fast bowlers. *J Bone Joint Surg Br* 1993;75(3):398–402.
40. Ohmori K, Suzuki K, Ishida Y. Translamino-pedicular screw fixation with bone grafting for symptomatic isthmic lumbar spondylolysis. *Neurosurgery* 1992;30(3):379–384.
41. Roca J, Moreta D, Fuster S, et al. Direct repair of spondylolysis. *Clin Orthop* 1989; 246:86–91.
42. Tonino A, van der Werf G. Direct repair of lumbar spondylolysis: 10 year follow-up of 12 previously reported cases. *Acta Orthop Scand* 1994;65(1):91–93.
43. Ivanic GM, Pink TP, Achatz W, et al. Direct stabilization of lumbar spondylolysis with a hook screw: mean 11-year follow-up period for 113 patients. *Spine* 2003;28(3):255–259.
44. Askar Z, Wardlaw D, Koti M. Scott wiring for direct repair of lumbar spondylolysis. *Spine* 2003;28(4): 354–357.
45. Dai LY, Jia LS, Yuan W, et al. Direct repair of defect in lumbar spondylolysis and mild isthmic spondylolisthesis by bone grafting, with and without facet joint fusion. *Eur Spine J* 2001;10(1):78–83.
46. Jeanneret B. Direct repair of spondylolysis. *Acta Orthop Scand* 1993;64(suppl 251):111–115.
47. Schneiderman GA, McLain RF, Hambly MF, et al. The pars defect as a pain source. *Spine* 1995;20:1761–1764.
48. Eisenstein SM, Ashton IK, Roberts S, et al. Innervation of the spondylolysis "ligament." *Spine* 1994;19:912–916.
49. Nordström D, Santavirta S, Seitslao S, et al. Symptomatic lumbar spondylolysis: neuroinmunologic studies. *Spine* 1994;19:2752–2758.

18

Isthmic Reconstruction with Pedicle Screws and a V-Shaped Rod in Spondylolysis without Degenerative Disk Disease

Philippe Gillet

Spondylolysis is a fatigue fracture thought to be the result of repetitive microtrauma of the pars interarticularis or isthmus of the posterior arch of lower lumbar vertebrae. Although spondylolysis can lead to back pain and referred leg pain, true sciatica, or even neurologic deficit and progressive deformity of the spine in the sagittal plane, it is often well tolerated during a patient's lifetime. Surgery is needed by a very restricted number of patients. Spondylolisthesis defines an anteroposterior displacement of the pathologic vertebra in regard of the lower vertebrae. It can be the result of the pars interarticularis defect, but spondylolisthesis can also occur in degenerative disorders of the spine because of dysplasia of posterior facet joints and after severe trauma. In spondylolisthesis or spondylolysis, many patients presenting with thigh pain or even leg pain do not really suffer from root entrapment; the pain can be referred pain. Even true radicular pain does not mean that a true decompression of the nerve root must be performed. Root pain can be initiated by local inflammatory conditions due to excessive motion of the mobile segment; a stabilization procedure without decompression may lead to disappearance of radicular symptoms as well as back pain and muscle contracture. True entrapment of nerve roots can, however, exist in severe vertebral slippage and severe disk narrowing deforming the neural foramen or in the case of associated herniated disks. When spondylolisthesis is due to dysplasia of the lumbosacral facets or to degenerative conditions, multiple root compromise can occur and may be severe because the whole vertebra including the posterior arch slips forward, causing central canal stenosis in addition to foraminal stenosis.

These different pathologic conditions may lead to intractable pain and functional deficit requiring surgical treatment. The type of surgery should be tailored to each individual situation and should be as least aggressive as possible. Depending on the anatomical status, an isolated fusion, a fusion with correction of the deformity, a combined fusion, and decompression must be considered. Fusion is generally performed across a mobile segment (arthrodesis) but may also be considered at the level of the pars itself, without sacrifice of spinal mobility.

GUIDELINES FOR SURGICAL TREATMENT

The following sections summarize the author's current guidelines for surgical treatment to be considered in the various pathologic situations associated with spondylolysis or spondylolisthesis:

Spondylolysis Without Associated Disk Disease and Without Spondylolisthesis

A pars defect reconstruction is advised whenever possible to avoid loss of mobile segments and increased stress on adjacent structures. In cases where a L5 spondylolysis is present with an intact L5-S1 disk but with degenerative disk changes at the L4–L5 level, isthmic reconstruction of L5 may have been considered to avoid L4-S1 fusion. The reconstruction is performed in such cases in the hope that the L5 spondylolysis is the main cause of back pain; results have been satisfactory in our hands but inferior to those in the isolated spondylolysis cases. Such a therapeutic option should be considered with caution and only in carefully selected cases.

Spondylolysis with Associated Disk Disease and Grade 0 or 1 Spondylolisthesis

A posterolateral in situ fusion with or without posterior instrumentation is the classical procedure; reduction of a Grade 1 slip is optional. If the nerve root is entrapped, resection of the posterior arch should be performed and, if needed, removal of a herniated disk.

In heavy patients who anticipate engaging in strenuous work, if disk material has been removed or if the disk space is high, a posterior lumbar interbody fusion (PLIF) with posterior instrumentation is a recommended option to avoid secondary kyphosis due to progressive narrowing of the disk space.

Spondylolysis with Associated Disk Disease and Grade 2 or 3 Spondylolisthesis

A PLIF with partial or total reduction of the slip and moreover restoration of an adequate lumbosacral lordosis combined with posterior instrumentation is recommended. If the disk space is very narrow, if there is no significant loss of lumbosacral lordosis, and if no neurologic symptoms are present, a posterolateral in situ fusion with posterior instrumentation would be an option, especially in Grade 2 slips.

Spondylolysis with Associated Disk Disease and Grade 4 Spondylolisthesis or Spondyloptosis

A posterior reduction with a PLIF, or a combined anterior and posterior approach with anterior lumbar interbody fusion (ALIF) and posterolateral fusion and posterioror instrumentation should be considered, remembering that correction of the lumbosacral kyphosis is more important than correction of the slip. If true spondyloptosis is present, the Gaines procedure may be an option.

Lysis at the Level of the Pedicle

If a unilateral pedicle lysis associated with contralateral spondylolysis is present or if a bilateral pedicle lysis is present, the only option is an interbody fusion since a posterolateral bone graft will not stabilize the vertebral body and the motion segment; a PLIF or ALIF would be our procedure of choice.

Dysplasic Spondylolisthesis

A thorough posterior midline and lateral decompression must be performed, keeping in mind that severe narrowing of the spinal canal may be present with severe compromise of the cauda equina. Further injury of the nerve roots must be avoided during the intracanalar use of surgical instruments. Reduction and fusion are performed according to the abovementioned rules.

Degenerative Spondylolisthesis

In symptomatic degenerative spondylolisthesis, spinal stenosis is the rule, and the main or the sole indication for surgical treatment is often the neurologic deficit. In the event of primary severe instability or postlaminectomy instability, a posterolateral fusion, instrumented or not, a PLIF or a lateral retroperitoneal ALIF should be considered (since degenerative spondylolisthesis often occurs at L3–L4 or L4–L5). The aim of the fusion in this specific indication is more often to avoid iatrogenic secondary increase of the spondylolisthesis than to treat back pain.

Details on these different techniques have been described elsewhere (5).

Pars Repair or Isthmic Reconstruction

A small number of patients presenting with isolated pars interarticularis defect suffer from chronic disabling low back pain, sometimes radiating to the thighs without true sciatica. These symptoms can be accounted for by hypermobility of the loose posterior arch with stimulation of the defect tissue, which seems rich in nociceptive nerve endings, and the relative instability of the vertebral body, which induces excessive stress to the underlying disk.

Removal of the pathologic soft tissue and bone grafting of the defect to restore the stabilizing role of the posterior arch is a logical form of treatment in this small group of patients. “Isthmic reconstruction” or “direct repair of the pars interarticularis” has been proposed by different surgeons since 1968.

Kimura (8) used an isolated bone graft followed by postoperative bed rest and a cast. Most procedures include some sort of internal fixation in order to improve the fusion rate and promote more rapid return to active life, if possible without external support. Buck (2) used a screw across the pars. Nicole and Scott (12) described a technique using the passage of wires under the laminae and transverse processes. Salib and Pettine (16) and Songer and Rovin (17) similarly proposed wiring the posterior arch but fixing the cable on pedicle screws. Morsher et al. (11) designed a special screw-hook construct. Louis (10) proposed bone grafting of the pars associated with temporary fixation of the lumbosacral junction with his butterfly plate. We reported on an original technique using a V-shaped rod and pedicle screws, associated with direct bone grafting of the pars defect (4).

PATIENT SELECTION

Since the beginning of our experience with the original V rod technique starting in 1992, patients have been selected to be candidates for pars repair when they meet the following criteria. They have to suffer from chronic disabling pain, located in the low back, possibly radiating to the thighs, which has been resistant to conservative treatment for at least 1 year and incompatible with comfortable everyday life, work, or sports. The absence of degenerative disk disease has to be confirmed by a normal T2 weighted magnetic resonance imaging (MRI) scan. If there is still doubt after the MRI, a provocative discogram is performed at the suspect spinal level and there must be absence of pain during injection of the dye or saline. We did not consider patients presenting with spondylolisthesis from

Grade 1 on to be candidates for this conservative surgery. However, in slight spondylolisthesis, the disk is not necessarily pathologic and pars repair has been performed in such cases by other authors (10). Increased pain upon hyperextension of the lumbosacral spine was considered a positive provocative sign. Infiltration of the pars defect with saline or lidocaine was not used in this study but may be recommended for optimal selection. Litigation or compensation cases are considered relative contraindications as in all other surgical procedures. Smoking may favor nonunion but is not considered a specific contraindication against the choice of a pars interarticularis repair technique instead of an intervertebral fusion procedure.

SURGICAL TECHNIQUE AND POSTOPERATIVE CARE

The technique described here is for a L5 pars repair. Anatomical landmarks should be adapted accordingly for L4 and L3 levels.

The patient can be positioned on any operating table the surgeon is familiar with; however, the sagittal alignment of the lumbosacral spine is important. Access to the isthmic defect is easier with the patient in slight kyphosis, but placement of the instrumentation in this position may lead to impingement between the instrumentation and the underlying vertebra when the patient stands. We place the patient prone on a Hall frame with the hips flexed no more than 20 degrees to 30 degrees in order to avoid disturbing the lordosis of the lumbar spine. Alternatively, the surgeon may choose to put the patient on an operating table that allows moving the lower limbs during surgery in order to perform the cleaning and decortication of the defect as well as the graft placement easily in kyphosis and the instrumentation in lordosis.

The lumbosacral area is approached through a midline incision from the L3–L4 level down to the S1–S2 level. Subperiosteal dissection is performed laterally down to the origin of the transverse processes at the L5 level—far enough to properly locate the entry point of the pedicular screws, but not farther than the articular processes at the L5-S1 level. Care is taken to preserve the capsuloligamentous structures of the L4–L5 and L5-S1 facet joints. However, to prevent stress being put on the isthmus of L5 by the overlying inferior L4 facets during spine extension, which could possibly lead to recurrence of the spondylolysis, 2 or 3 mm of the distal aspect of these facets is removed with an osteotome, as described by Louis (8), taking care to remove as little capsular structure as possible. The soft tissue situated in the pars defect is removed using rongeurs; if the preoperative MRI shows no root impingement (which is most often the case in these patients), a very thin layer of soft tissue is preserved at the bottom of the defect to avoid migration of the bone graft in the foramen. The sides of the defect, the upper half of the L5 laminae and the lateral, extra-articular aspect of the upper L5 articular process joint are exposed down to bleeding bone. Lumbar pedicular screws 35 mm long and 5 mm in diameter are inserted in the L5 pedicles, avoiding violating the L4–L5 joint. An autologous iliac bone graft is harvested and trimmed to be fitted in the defects. To prevent inadvertent anterior migration of the bone graft, a posterior fin is trimmed to rest on the border of the laminae (Fig. 18.1). The fusion mass is further augmented by putting an onlay graft on top of the posterior aspect of the L5 laminae and on the lateral extra-articular aspect of the L5 upper articular processes (Fig. 18.2). The pedicle screws are placed with their grooves oriented 30 degrees to 45 degrees to the longitudinal axis of the patient. A 6-mm diameter rod, usually 8–10 cm in length, is bent in a V shape and put under the L5 spinous process after the L5-S1 interspinous ligament has been removed. The rod is firmly fixed against the spinous process and the laminae, offering the possibility of both

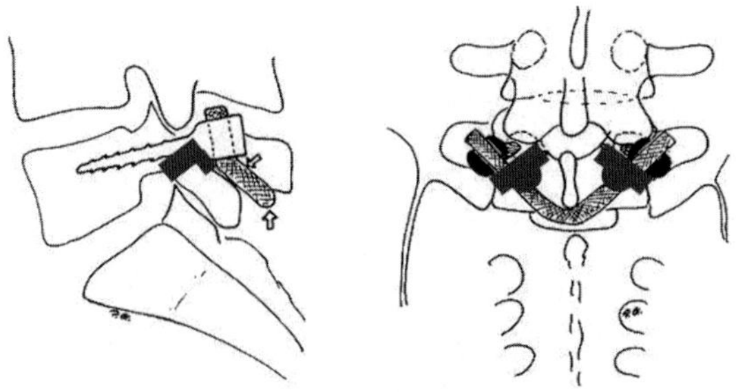

FIG. 18.1. Positioning of the grafts: bone blocks are fitted in the defects (*dark gray*), with a small posterior fin resting on the laminae to avoid inadvertent migration in the foramen.

compressing the graft in the defect and stabilizing the posterior arch. Sometimes, a slight bending of the rod is necessary in the sagittal plane to fit it properly against the posterior arch of the vertebra and in the grooves of the open pedicle screws. Finally, the locking bolts are firmly tightened against the rod to fix it to the pedicle screws while, using a compression clamp, some compression is applied between the apex of the bent rod and the screws to stabilize the graft. Care is taken to avoid any impingement between the rod and the superior aspect of the S1 spinous process during extension of the spine; sometimes, a few millimeters of bone must be removed from the base of the S1 spinous process (Fig. 18.3).

We have used either stainless steel or titanium implants over the years. It is clear that proper bending of titanium alloy rods can be difficult in this technique and that the importance of the angle of the bend poses a theoretical risk for fatigue fracture of the rod. However, we have never observed such a complication in the surgeries we have performed. It is believed that the stress imposed on this construct remains much lower than when a mobile segment is fixed; hence titanium implants are now routinely preferred for postoperative imaging purposes.

Patients can sit and walk 1 or 2 days after surgery and are usually discharged at day 4. No brace is recommended, the construct is considered solid enough to secure the posterior arch until fusion of the bone graft is obtained; this position is based on the experience the author has with the same spinal instrumentation in the stabilization of more unstable conditions of the spine (e.g., lumbar degenerative scoliosis, spondylolisthesis of Grades 2 and 3) where the absence of postoperative bracing has also been the rule without apparent unfavorable influence on the results. Patients are encouraged to walk as

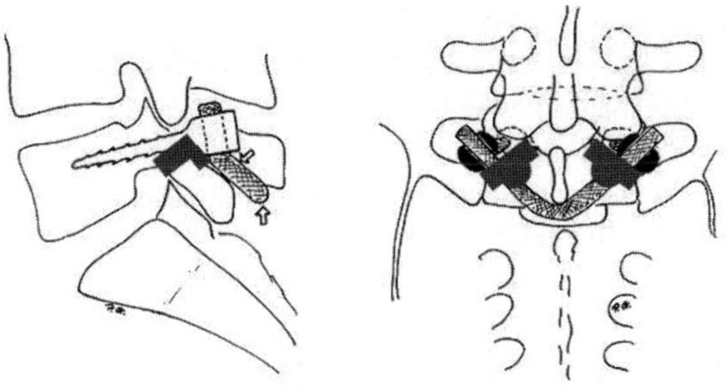

FIG. 18.2. Positioning of the grafts: a supplementary onlay graft is put on the lateral extra-articular aspect of the superior articular facets and on the laminae (*light gray*).

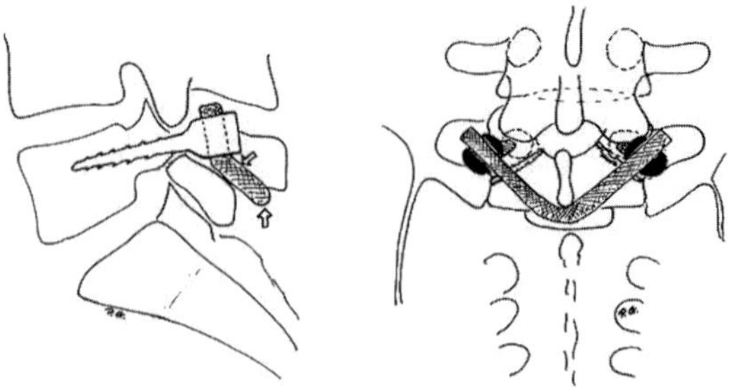

FIG. 18.3. Positioning of the instrumentation with adequate bending in AP and lateral views; note the compression points on the posterior arch (*arrows*) under the spinous process and on the laminae.

much as possible, anterior bending is discouraged but not strictly forbidden, and physiotherapy and exercises are avoided for 3 months. Return to work is possible at 1 month if there is no mechanical stress on the spine. Return to strenuous occupations or sports is delayed until the fourth or sixth postoperative month.

The existence of a spina bifida occulta is a contraindication to the use of this technique because of the impossibility to obtain adequate posterior arch stability with our construct when a midline cleft is present.

RESULTS

The early results of the first patients who underwent this procedure have been reported (4). At present time, 33 patients benefited from pars repair using the V rod technique over a 12-year period. This relatively low number illustrates the fact that few spondylolysis patients require surgical treatment when no disk degeneration or true local instability is associated. The mean age at surgery was low, about 25 to 30 years old, but older patients (up to 48 years) were considered eligible because of normal disk status. Sex distribution was in favor of male patients (75%). Return to normal everyday life and return to profitable and sometimes strenuous work and sport was obtained in the vast majority of cases.

Bone union of the pars was assessed by plain lateral and in some cases oblique radiographs or tomograms. Evaluation of the fusion is difficult on regular radiographs, even more so than in other spinal fusion procedures. Computed tomography (CT) may be used in the case of suspected nonunion and titanium implants.

One patient with residual pain sustained a secondary ALIF procedure after a positive discography, the result remained poor. Hardware removal was not performed except in one patient with residual pain while the bone fusion appeared solid; a late fair result was obtained, but the role of implant removal remained questionable in this particular case. No hardware breakage or loosening was observed. Donor site pain was not encountered in this series, possibly thanks to the small amount of bone necessary for this procedure and to a meticulous harvesting technique.

In the case of early (6- to 12-month follow-up) unsatisfactory result with residual back pain, nonunion should be ruled out if proper preoperative imaging has been performed. In late bad results, nonunion still must be considered, but also the occurrence of disk degeneration at the level of the spondylolysis or at any adjacent segment; since those patients are allowed to perform freely any activity, they are (like any other population) at risk for disk injury, both acute or chronic.

DISCUSSION

Reconstruction of the pars interarticularis, an operation referred to as "direct repair of the pars" or "isthmic reconstruction," seems a logical and less aggressive approach than lumbosacral fusion in the small group of patients presenting with painful spondylolysis without associated slip or degenerative disk disease. It is indeed the only true reconstructive surgical procedure that can be performed on the spine. Other operations usually imply fusion of one or more mobile segments or necessitate removal of some anatomical structures. For this reason, pars repair should deserve consideration.

Kimura (8), in 1968, seems to be the first to have described a technique of direct pars repair. He used isolated bone grafting of the pars, with no instrumentation. The patients operated with this technique had to remain recumbent for a number of weeks, followed by external immobilization by a cast for up to 6 months. Buck (2), in 1970, described internal fixation with direct screwing through the pars. Unfortunately, this technique decreases the area available for bone grafting, which remains the essential part of the operation. Proper placement of the screws is reported to be difficult. A number of authors reported satisfactory results with the Buck technique (1,3,9,13–15,19,20). Scott (12), beginning in 1970, used a wiring technique to stabilize the posterior arch. This technique has some drawbacks: placement of the wires under the transverse processes is difficult and can lead to significant bleeding, potential nerve root injury is a risk, wires are not very strong, and patients must wear a postoperative brace (7). Hambly and Wiltse (6), in 1994, described a modification of the Scott technique, the main difference being the use of a paraspinous instead of a midline approach. Louis (10), in the 1970s, developed a technique of temporary fixation of the lumbosacral junction with an original butterfly plate. The advantages are a large area available for the bone graft and the avoidance of possible shortening of the pars interarticularis as can happen with techniques putting compression over this area. Excellent results have been reported in a large series by the author. However, implant removal as a secondary procedure is mandatory, and postoperative bracing is advised for 3 months. Morsher (11), in 1984, presented a special hook-screw device that makes it possible to fix the posterior arch and the bone graft under compression, without the need for extensive dissection. This elegant technique is demanding, however, as regards the placement of the instrumentation; moreover, since the instrumentation is small, its relative weakness necessitates postoperative protection with a brace (3,20). Custom-made "Morsher-like" constructs have been employed by some surgeons using different "universal" rod-hook-screw instrumentations; they seem to offer greater solidity (to the author's knowledge, these techniques have been presented in meetings but are not published). All these "Morsher" techniques do not offer a link between the left and right aspects of the instrumentation; this could lead to greater instability of the posterior arch and graft then our V-rod technique. Salib and Pettine (16) and Tokuhashi and Matsuzaki (18) reported original techniques with satisfactory results in case reports, Songer and Rovin (17) published a technique using a cable passing underneath the lamina, fixed on a pair of pedicle screws; their technique requires specific instrumentation; they report good or excellent results in all seven patients operated. All authors report fusion in 3 to 6 months.

Our original V-rod technique reported here seems to offer several advantages. The whole construct is one piece, offering global stability of the posterior arch and bone graft. The strength of the hardware (rod and screws) avoids the need for postoperative immobilization, and everyday nonstrenuous activities are possible during the first weeks following surgery. The placement of pedicle screws is done in a classical way; any surgeon accustomed with pedicle screw systems should be able to use this technique very rapidly.

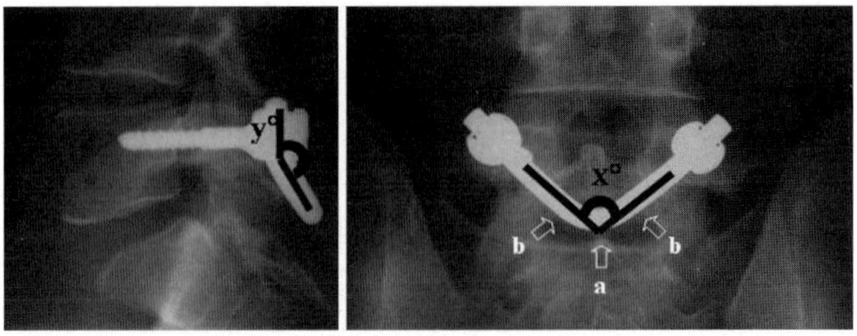

FIG. 18.4. Postoperative radiographs show the contact points between the rod and the posterior arch (*arrow a:* spinous process, *arrows b:* laminae) and the custom-made bending of the rod in the frontal (*x* angle) and sagittal (*y* angle).

In our series, different versions of the Cotrel–Dubousset instrumentation were elected according to their availability over the years (CCD, Horizon, Legacy; Medtronic, Memphis, USA), but the same construct can be made with any comparable rod and screw system and there is no need for special instrumentation.

The bone grafting procedure is not hindered by the hardware, compression of the graft fitted in the pars defect is possible, and the possibility to supplement the graft by onlay grafting of the laminae and zygapophyseal facets further enhances the chances for solid fusion. Implant removal is not to be considered as a routine procedure since all adjacent segments remain free.

The only demanding points of the procedure are proper bending of the rod and meticulous avoidance of any impingement between the rod and the posterior arch of the underlying vertebra (Fig. 18.4). Proper placement of the patient, with respect to normal lordosis, is essential in this regard; it makes the preparation of the pars defect more difficult but it avoids any misplacement of the hardware that could lead to a mechanical conflict and pain.

Proper evaluation of the underlying disk is done with MRI and only patients with normal T2 weighted images are considered candidates for surgery (Fig. 18.5). Routine use of discography in patients who are candidates for isthmic reconstruction may be excessive due to the inherent risks of the technique, but the question remains debatable. It is interesting to point out that Louis did not recommend systematic evaluation of the adjacent disk by discography or MRI; he considered that the conventional radiologic aspect

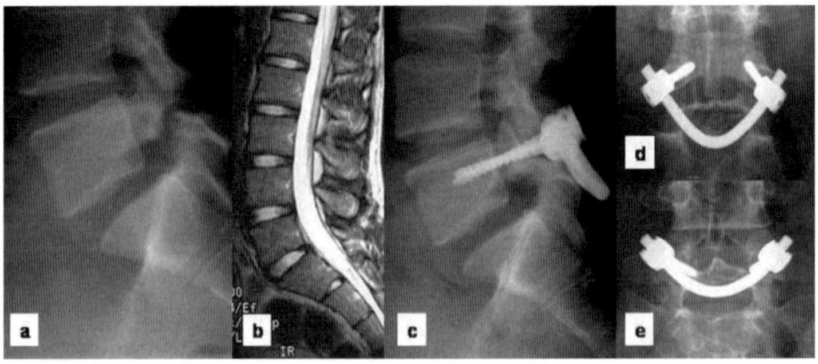

FIG. 18.5. A: Preoperative lateral radiograph showing L5 spondylolysis. **B:** T2 weighted MRI. **C, D, and E:** Postoperative lateral and anteroposterior radiographs with fused isthmus; note that the entry point of the pedicular screw must not impinge on the L4 inferior articular facet.

of the disk space was satisfactory if its height was at least two thirds of its normal height and if there was no slip of more than 10 mm (10). This could, in view of his good results, extend the number of patients in which pars interarticularis repair could be contemplated in comparison of the stricter criteria used in our series.

Overall follow-up of our patients is short, even if half of our cases have a 5- to 10-year follow-up. Two years' observation seems sufficient to evaluate the effectiveness of a technique designed to obtain fusion of the pars articularis. However, longer follow-up studies are needed to evaluate the advantages offered by a technique of direct repair of a pars defect compared to a one-level lumbosacral fusion procedure in patients presenting with isolated spondylolysis.

CONCLUSIONS

The technique described in this study seems to be a satisfying option in the treatment of patients presenting a L4 or L5 spondylolysis without any associated spondylolisthesis or degenerative disk disease. The motion segments are preserved. Solid fusion appears to have been obtained in all cases according to our radiologic results, however, proper radiologic assessment is difficult due to the instrumentation, and nonunion could be overlooked. Return to a comfortable everyday life was obtained early, in a matter of weeks; return to work or demanding sports was obtained in the majority of cases after a 4-month period. The technique is readily available to surgeons accustomed to the use of any rod and screw system and should have a short learning curve. Proper patient selection is mandatory, in the presence of a less than perfect MRI result, discography should probably be considered, but its potential complications must not be overlooked. As with all surgical procedures designed to treat patients whose main complaint is back pain, the psychological profile of the patients and a compensation background may influence the end result.

REFERENCES

1. Bonnici AV, Koka SR, Richards DJ. Results of Buck screw fusion in grade I spondylolisthesis. *J Rl Soc Med* 1991;84:270–273.
2. Buck J. Direct repair of the defect in spondylolisthesis: preliminary report. *J Bone Joint Surg Br* 1970; 52,432–437.
3. Dreyzin V, Esses SI. A comparative analysis of spondylolysis repair. *Spine* 1994;19:1909–1915.
4. Gillet P, Petit M. Direct repair of spondylolysis without spondylolosthesis, using a rod-screw construct and bone grafting of the pars defect. *Spine* 1999;24:1252–1256.
5. Gillet P. Spondylolysis with or without spondylolisthesis. In: DuParc J, ed. *Surgical Techniques in Orthopaedics and Traumatology. Vol. 2. Spine*. Paris: Elsevier; 2003 (55-130-B-10).
6. Hambly M, Wiltse L. A modification of the Scott wiring technique. *Spine* 1994;19:354–356.
7. Johnson G, Thompson A. The Scott wiring technique for direct repair of lumbar spondylolysis. *J Bone Joint Surg Br* 1992;74:426–430.
8. Kimura M. My method of filling the lesion with spongy bone in spondylolysis and spondylolisthesis. *Orthop Surg* 1968;19:285–295.
9. Kip Ph, Esses S I, Doherty B, et al. Biomechanical testing of pars defect repairs. *Spine* 1994;23:2692–2697.
10. Louis R. Reconstruction isthmique des spondylolyses par plaque vissèe et greffes sans arthrodëse (pars interarticularis reconstruction for spondylolysis by plate and screws with grafting without arthrodesis). *Rev Chir Orthop* 1988;74:549–557.
11. Morscher E, Gerber B, Fasel J. Surgical treatment of spondylolisthesis by bone grafting and direct stabilization of spondylolysis by means of a hook screw. *Arch Orthop Trauma Surg* 1984;103:175–178.
12. Nicol R, Scott J. Lytic spondylolysis, repair by wiring. *Spine* 1986;11:1027–1030.
13. Ohmori K, Suzuki K, Ishida Y. Translamino-pedicular screw fixation with bone grafting for symptomatic isthmic lumbar spondylolysis. *Neurosurgery* 1992;30:379–384.
14. Pedersen A, Hagen R. Spondylolysis and spondylolisthesis, treatment by internal fixation and bone grafting of the defect. *J Bone Joint Surg Am* 1988;70:15–24.
15. Roca J, Moretta D, Fuster S, et al. Direct repair of spondylolysis. *Clin Orthop* 1989;246:86–91.

16. Salib R, Pettine K. Modified repair of a defect in spondylolysis or minimal spondylolisthesis by pedicle screw, segmental wire fixation and bone grafting. *Spine* 1993;18:440–443.
17. Songer M., Rovin R. Repair of the pars interarticularis defect with a cable-screw construct, a preliminary report. *Spine* 1998;23:263–269.
18. Tokuhashi Y, Matsuzaki I. Repair of defects in spondylolysis by segmental pedicular screw hook fixation, a preliminary report. *Spine* 1996;21:2041–2045.
19. Van der Werf G, Tonino A, Zeegers W. Direct repair of lumbar spondylolysis. *Acta Orthop Scand* 1985; 56:378–379.
20. Winter M, Jani L. Results of screw osteosynthesis in spondylolysis and low-grade spondylolisthesis. *Arch Orthop Trauma Surg* 1989;108:96–99.

19

Treatment of Lumbar Spondylolisthesis and Related Unstable Spinal Lesions: The Usefulness of PLIF with Cages and Semirigid Interpedicular Posterior Fixation for Circumferential Arthrodesis and Prevention of Adjacent Degeneration

Gilles Perrin

Posterior lumbar interbody fusion (PLIF) with cages is optimal not only for intervertebral fusion but also in re-establishing weight bearing to the anterior structures and in restoring the disc height and foraminal opening for nerve root decompression (1–4). Posterior fixation is indicated for immediate stabilization in order to enhance osteogenesis and to allow early mobilization without external contention in order to prevent muscle atrophy and spinal balance deterioration. PLIF as a distractive technique and posterior interpedicular fixation in compression restore physiologic lordosis and indeed protect the adjacent spine. Semirigid fixation with an interpedicular damper significantly reduces the risk of screw fracture and enhances the bone fusion by maintaining constraints on the cages. Prevention of adjacent degenerative disease by using semirigid extension to the overlying vertebra of the posterior interpedicular fixation as a nonfusion method is indicated for protection of the adjacent spinal level in case preoperative imaging shows a pathologic disc adjacent to the forecasted fusion.

Delayed complications after lumbar fusion with recurrence of back pain and neurologic symptoms are now commonly reported and related to degenerative lesions at the adjacent intervertebral level above a fused spinal segment (5–8). A retrospective study reported by Gillet (9) on the fate of the adjacent motion segment pointed out that 41% of the patients with follow-up over 5 years developed transitional segment alterations such as collapsed discs, osteophyte formation with degenerative spondylolisthesis, or stenosis, and 20% needed a second surgery for extension of the fusion. This adjacent degeneration is related to reactional hypermobility and biomechanical hypersolicitation above a rigid fused segment (10–12). The reported rate of symptomatic adjacent segment disease in a meta-analysis of the literature performed by Park et al. (13) is higher in patients with transpedicular instrumentation (12.2% to 18.5%) than in patients who underwent fusion with other forms of instrumentation or with no instrumentation (5.2% to 5.6%). Logically, the risk of such adverse effects of fusion is related to the length of the fusion and the presence of preoperative degenerative discal lesions above the forecasted fusion (14,15). If monosegmental fusion is with very low adjacent reactional hypersolicitation, bisegmental fixation indicated by severely slipped spondylolisthesis requires protection of the adjacent disk through the creation of a transitional zone between the fused vertebral segments and the overlying hypermobile spine (16). This intermediate zone can be protected by using a semirigid interpedicular element as a nonfusion method that allows controlled intervertebral motion (4 mm in flexion extension and 2 mm in vertical extension and compression).

The aims of this retrospective study were not only to assess the clinical outcome and fusion rate in the group of patients treated with circumferential arthrodesis achieved in one stage with a posterior approach, but also to determine in a subgroup of patients with long-term follow-up over 8 years the clinical and anatomical benefits of protection of the adjacent level by means of posterior semirigid stabilization in order to prevent recurrent symptoms.

MATERIALS AND METHODS

Study Design

From 1978 to September 2003, PLIF was performed in a personal consecutive series of 1,500 patients with clinical presentation of nerve root compression related to unstable bone or discoligamentous lumbar lesions such as

- Isthmic spondylolisthesis, 1,095 cases (73%)
- Foraminal stenosis with collapsed disc and degenerative spondylolisthesis, 259 cases (17.2%)
- Lesions, documented by dynamic x-rays, which are either discoligamentous degenerative or iatrogenic unstable, 148 cases (9.8%)

In this series, 430 patients were operated on between 1993 and 2000 for lumbar stabilization of isthmic spondylolisthesis with circumferential arthrodesis in one stage through a posterior approach by using cages for PLIF and posterior interpedicular fixation and 290 patients were reviewed for clinical and radiologic evaluation with long-term follow-up (>4 years). Thirty-four of the 290 patients underwent surgery for isthmic spondylolisthesis between June 1993 and April 1997 with PLIF and posterior fixation and semirigid protection of the pathologic adjacent disc and were reviewed with a mean follow-up of 8.27 years to assess the evolution of adjacent spinal levels.

Surgical Procedure

The intervertebral space was approached posteriorly. The mobile posterior vertebral arch is completely removed. The lateral recesses and the foramina were widely open with total resection of the articular facets. Restoration of the intervertebral height in order to open the foramina and to achieve a total nerve root decompression was achieved by using distracting probes after discal resection. Such distraction with restoration of normal intervertebral discal height results in partial reduction of horizontal slippage. This partial reduction is sufficient for nerve root decompression. Total reduction of Grade 3 or 4 spondylolisthesis is not advisable because such reduction creates reactional excessive constraint to the overlying spine with a high risk of adjacent degeneration. It seems more logical to preserve the acquired adequate sagittal balance between the spine and the pelvic incidence (17). Cortical bone of the vertebral endplates was carefully kept intact. PLIF to distract the disc space was performed by using large intervertebral cages filled

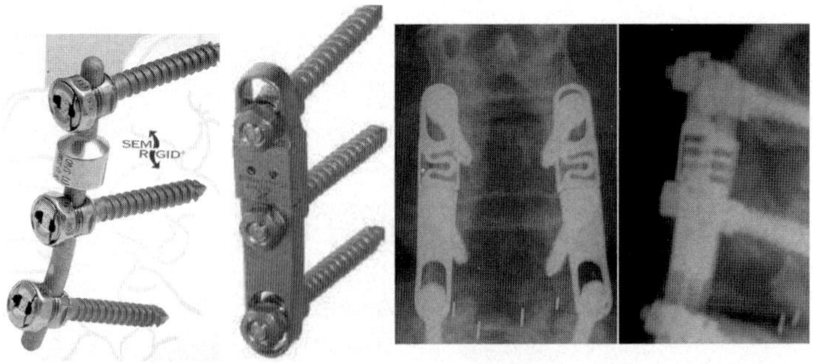

FIG. 19.1. Semirigid TTL rod and Aladyn plate-postoperative x-ray control of Aladyn plate.

with cancellous bone from laminectomy. Cylindric or threaded cages were implanted in 50 cases. Large parallelepiped titanium cages were used in 290 cases, and since 1997 PEEK polymer ADONIS cages have been inserted for PLIF in 90 patients.

Posterior interpedicular fixation in compression was performed for immediate stabilization and restoration of lordosis. Rigid plates or rods were used in 98 cases. Semirigid ISOLOCK or Aladyn plates or semirigid TTL rods with an interpedicular damper (Fig. 19.1) have been used since 1993 for posterior fixation in 332 cases. In case of low-grade spondylolisthesis (Grade 0, 1, or 2) with the adjacent disc found to be normal by preoperative found by magnetic resonance imaging (MRI), monosegmental PLIF and short posterior fixation were performed. In case of severely slipped spondylolisthesis and/or an adjacent pathologic but not compressive disc, the circumferential arthrodesis performed at the level of the severe unstable lesion was completed with adjacent semirigid interpedicular stabilization (Figs. 19.2 and 19.3). In case of adjacent compressive prolapsed or excluded disc, adjacent discectomy with second PLIF was performed. Getting up and walking without any external contention was allowed the day after the surgical procedure. Patients were discharged after 5 days, and rehabilitation was immediately begun with the main purpose of restoration of posterior muscles and well-balanced lumbar lordosis. Each patient was ergonomically trained to prevent excessive flexion and axial rotation.

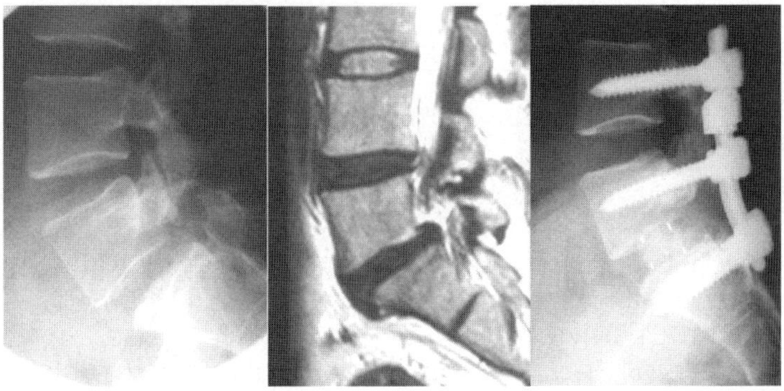

FIG. 19.2. Isthmic L5-S1 spondylolisthesis with adjacent L4–L5 pathologic disc treated with circumferential arthrodesis L5-S1 (PLIF with PEEK polymer cages and posterior fixation) and adjacent protection of the L4–L5 disc with a posterior interpedicular semirigid element.

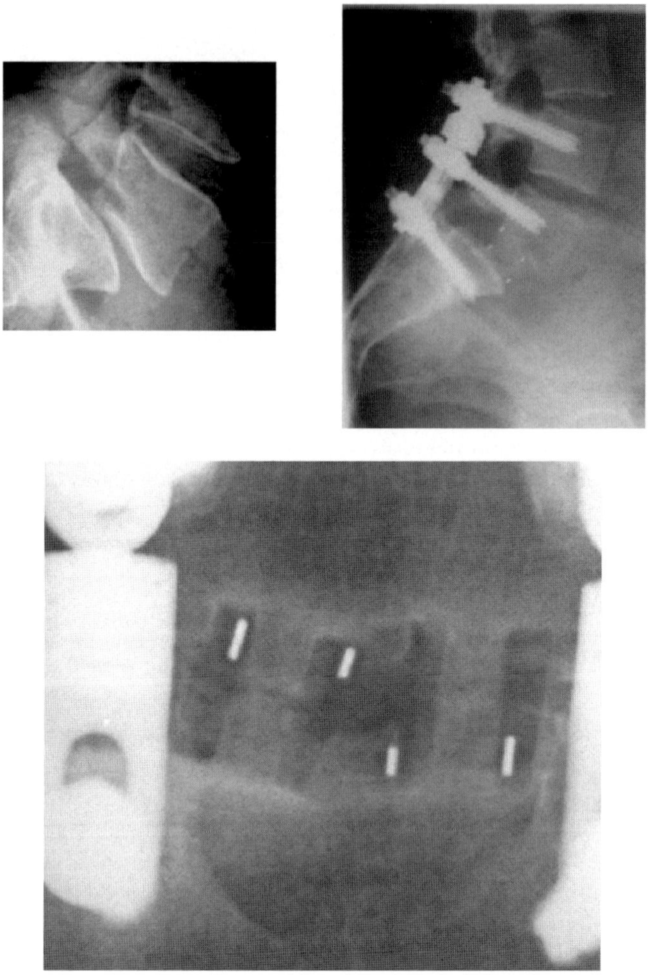

FIG. 19.3. PLIF for Grade 2 L5-S1 isthmic spondylolisthesis; note the restoration of L5-S1 intervertebral height and foraminal opening. Fusion is well documented with the intervertebral bone bridges.

RESULTS

Fusion Rate

Two hundred ninety patients who were operated on between 1993 and 2000 for lumbar stabilization of isthmic spondylolisthesis with cages for PLIF and posterior interpedicular fixation (semirigid posterior fixation in 332 cases) were reviewed for clinical and radiologic evaluation with long-term follow-up (>4 years). No local infection was observed. No patient required second surgery for clinical complications or for removal of a dismantled or broken fixation system.

In these 290 reviewed cases, 285 patients (98.3%) demonstrated bone fusion with radiologic documentation of new intervertebral bone bridges, with increased bone density within the cages, without osteolysis or bone lucencies at the interface with the implants, and without intervertebral motion on the dynamic x-rays (Figs. 19.4 and 19.5).

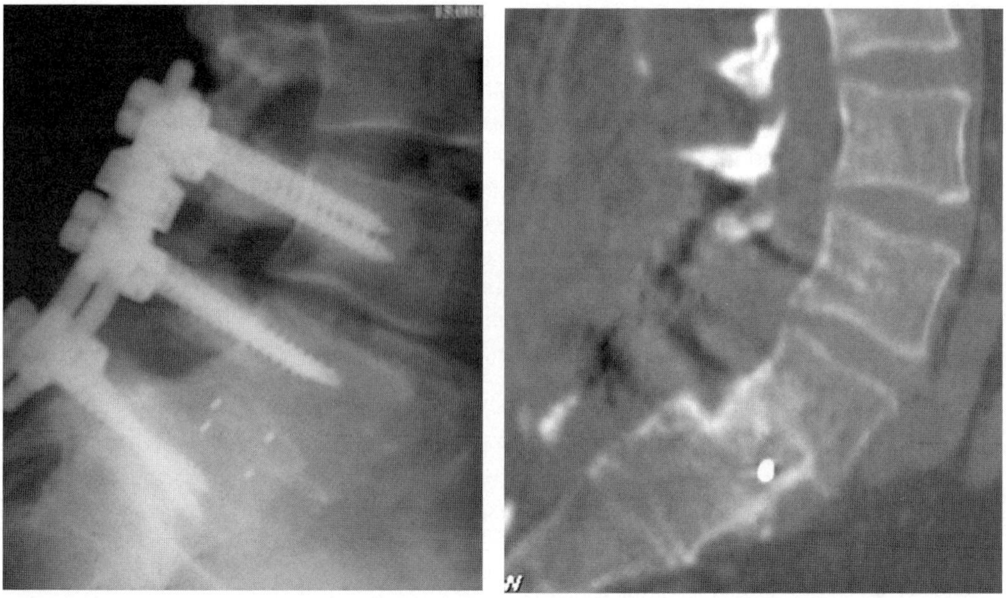

FIG. 19.4. Isthmic spondylolisthesis at L5-S1: Documentation of intervertebral fusion 7 years after surgery.

In only two cases, the postoperative x-ray control documented bone subsidence with intracorporeal penetration of the cages. This complication induces loss of the intervertebral height restoration without any incidence on the fusion. In five cases, it was not possible to document bone growth, but dynamic x-rays showed no intervertebral motion.

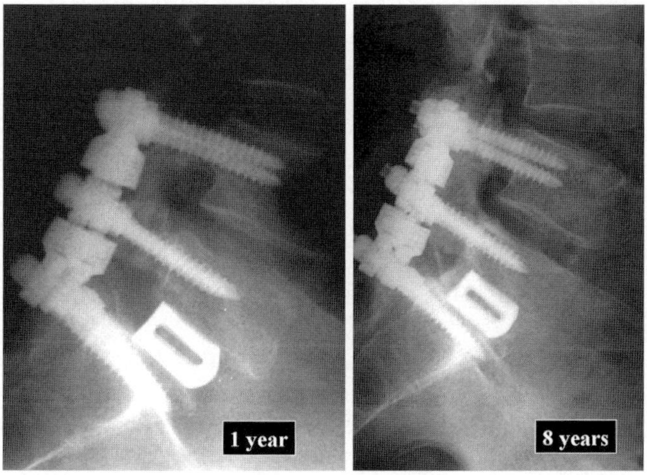

FIG. 19.5. X-rays control 8 years after surgery of a Grade 1 spondylolisthesis at L5-S1. Note evidence of fusion L5-S1 with bone bridges back to the titanium cages. The intervertebral L4–L5 discal height is well maintained, and no new degenerative lesion is documented at the "free" L3–L4 level.

Clinical Outcome

No radicular complication or any kind of iatrogenic clinical complication due to the posterior fixation or the intervertebral implants was experienced in this series. The clinical outcome assessed by the degree of persistent radicular pain, the consumption of analgesics, and the evaluation of walking distance and the working ability was excellent (i.e., improvement of the functional score >50%) in 245 patients (84.5%). The clinical outcome assessed by using the Stauffer–Coventry criteria was evaluated as excellent in 221 cases (76.2%), fair in 61 cases (21%), and poor in 8 patients (2.7%). Assessment using the modified Prolo score showed the clinical outcome to be excellent in 109 patients (37.6%), good in 121 patients (41.7%), fair in 53 patients (18.3%), and poor in 7 patients (2.4%).

Evolution of the Adjacent Disc

In order to assess the long-term benefits of the semirigid intervertebral stabilization as a protective nonfusion technique for pathologic adjacent disc, a specific retrospective study was carried out in a subgroup of 34 patients operated on between June 1993 and April 1997 for isthmic spondylolisthesis L4–L5 or L5-S1 by PLIF and posterior bisegmental fixation for radicular decompression, stabilization, and protection of the adjacent pathological disc by using a semirigid interpedicular damper without grafting. Twenty-two cases were reviewed with clinical evaluation and radiologic assessment after a mean long-term follow-up of 8.27 years. Results are as follows:

1. Radiologic evidence of fusion of disc treated by means of PLIF was documented in all the patients (22 of 22) with new intervertebral bone bridges and absence of intervertebral motion on dynamic x-rays. No vertebral endplate subsidence and fracture or dismantling of the fixation system were noted. Loss of the restored intervertebral height was observed in one case (4.5%).
2. Radiologic assessment after long-term follow-up of the adjacent pathologic disc protected by the semirigid interpedicular element documented spontaneous interarticular facets fusion in four cases (18.5%). Persistence of intervertebral motion on dynamic x-rays was evident in 15 cases (68.2%) with important motion over 4 mm in 3 cases and within the range of 4 mm in 12 cases. Conservation of the discal intervertebral height was well documented in 18 cases (82%).
3. Severe new degenerative lesions with significant discal collapsus, sagittal mobility, and horizontal slipping or new arthrotic conditions of the neohinge free disc adjacent to the instrumented bisegmental vertebral segment was observed in only one case (4.6%). No spontaneous fusion of this neohinge disk was documented. Persistence of intervertebral motion of this disk was evident in 21 cases (95.4%) with a normal range of motion over 4 mm in 10 cases and within 4 mm in 11 cases. The total balance of the overlying spine was assessed with a physiologic harmonious lordosis in 16 cases (72.7%).
4. In this subgroup of patients, the clinical outcome after long-term follow-up was evaluated by using a low back pain visual analogue scale for self-rated assessment. In 18 cases (81.5%), pain was rated under 4 on a scale of 10. The mean evaluation of low back pain was for all the patients at the preoperative period at 8.36 years (after the 1-year follow-up at 5.12 and after the 8.27-year follow-up, at 3.4. Radicular leg pain was rated as less than 1 on a scale of 10 in 15 cases (68.2%). The mean evaluation of radicular leg pain was for all the patients at the preoperative period at 6.23 (after 1-year follow-up at 3.2 and after 8.27-year follow-up at 2.1). The patient's satisfaction

index was assessed by using the 36-item Short Form Health Survey (SF-36) (scale from 1 = strongly agree to 5 = strongly disagree). In 21 patients (91%), the satisfaction index was rated at Grade 1, and the patient's comment was agreement for second similar surgery if it would be necessary.

DISCUSSION

Lumbar circumferential arthrodesis with a reconstruction of both anterior and posterior columns in one stage with posterior approach in the surgical treatment of nerve root compression related to isthmic spondylolisthesis or discoligamentous unstable lesions is an efficient technique for the nerve root decompression and for the spinal stabilization with an optimal fusion rate. Stabilization of isthmic spondylolisthesis with posterior fixation and posterolateral grafting without anterior column reconstruction is not able to decompress the nerve root ant to maintain foraminal opening. Some mechanical problems were reported to the posterior fixation elements and associated with excessive stress in spinal flexion (7). Using only PLIF without posterior fixation is not sufficiently reliable to achieve vertebral fusion. Elias et al. (18) reported a bad pseudoarthrosis rate (34%) in patients operated on with threaded cages as a stand-alone system. Twenty-one percent of patients in his series underwent secondary surgery to treat pseudoarthrosis. In our series with circumferential arthrodesis, the fusion rate was 97.2%. The posterior approach is logical for patients with clinical presentation of radicular symptoms related to bone lesions or to discal collapsus. This procedure requires a large foraminal opening completed by total resection of the facet joints to achieve a total nerve root decompression. With complete preoperative visual control of the nerve root freedom, it is possible to retract the radicular structures for the insertion of large intervertebral implants for distracting PLIF without any risk implant protrusion and neurologic complication. Such decompressive bone resection induces additional iatrogenic intervertebral instability and legitimizes vertical, horizontal, and axial stabilization achieved by PLIF and complementary posterior fixation. This protocol avoids the second surgery proposed by several authors for anterior intervertebral fusion (ALIF) after posterior decompression and fixation. This anterior approach has a high risk of vascular or neurologic morbidity. PLIF, easily performed with a totally open canal, lateral recesses, and foramina, has a very low risk of radicular complication. Nevertheless, this technique requires radicular dissection and can be difficult and dangerous for patients with previous posterior approach and epidural fibrosis. For revisional surgery, it could be necessary to perform the circumferential arthrodesis in two stages: first, posterior decompression and interpedicular fixation, and second, anterior intervertebral fusion. Intervertebral distraction with restoration of normal intervertebral discal height results in partial reduction of the horizontal slippage. This partial reduction is sufficient for nerve root decompression. Total reduction of Grade 3 or 4 spondylolisthesis is not advisable because such reduction creates reactional excessive constraint on the overlying spine and induces destabilization of the neoequilibrium between lumbar spine and pelvic incidence (19). Distractive PLIF performed by using large implants and posterior fixation in compression is efficient to restore physiologic lordosis. Such sagittal spinal balance is the best way to prevent adjacent biomechanical complications like discal degeneration, slippage, arthrotic proliferation, or kyphotic deformation. The risk of adjacent degeneration is logically very important for patients with preoperative pathologic adjacent disk above the forecasted intervertebral fusion (20). As a new neohinge disc, this pathologic disk will be unable to absorb additional mechanical hypersolicitation. To prevent worsening of this adjacent degeneration, it seems advisable to protect this disc from excessive hypermobility and constraints by using a nonfusion technology device like the intervertebral semirigid system that controls intervertebral motion. In this series, the use of the semirigid interpedicular element above the fused intervertebral segment meets all the mechanical requirements for the adjacent discal protection. In our series, no complication related to the hardware was experienced. Conservation of the discal height (82% of the patients) under the posterior semirigid stabilization, and the absence of degenerative lesions at the level above the instrumentation after long-term follow-up over 8 years in 96% of the patients, are evidence of the reliability of the semirigid system and evidence of the legitimacy and efficiency of the concept of the transitional nonfused intervertebral zone created by the semirigid interpedicular stabilization between the rigid fused segment and the hypermobile hypersolicited level above the instrumentation.

CONCLUSION

The high rate of fusion and the absence of failure of the fixation system emphasize the efficiency of using both intervertebral cages and posterior fixation for lumbar stabilization. Radiolucent polyetheretherketone (PEEK) cages are useful because they provide easy x-ray controls and they improve the bone fusion through their own resilience, which is close to the physiologic cortical bone elasticity and unlike the stiffness of titanium alloys. Semirigid fixation significantly reduces the risk of screw fracture by the absorption of the stress on the interpedicular damper and enhances the bone fusion by maintaining constraints on the cages, which remain under a compressive load (Wolff's law). This semirigid fixation system prevents the stress-shielding phenomenon. Fusion with polymer cages and semirigid fixation, avoidance of postoperative corset, and early rehabilitation for restoring lordosis and powerful posterior muscles collectively meet all the requirements not only for pain relief but also for definitive stabilization without iatrogenic spinal complication or further destabilization of spine at the adjacent level to the arthrodesis. Preventive protection of the intervertebral level adjacent to the fused segment is indicated in case of adjacent degenerative disc or adjacent arthritic conditions. Semirigid fixation, which allows controlled intervertebral motion for this adjacent level, seems to create the mechanical conditions for a transitional intervertebral zone between the rigid fused segment and the "free" adjacent hypersolicited level above the spinal instrumentation. This biomechanical intermediate zone seems to be very important before the restoration of physiologic lordosis achieved by recovery of efficient posterior muscles. Such semirigid fixation seems to be an efficient measure to prevent adjacent level degeneration and recurrence of symptoms.

Semirigid ISOLOCK or Aladyn plates, TTL rods, ADONIS PEEK cages and related spinal implants are made by Scient'X Company, Cedex, France.

REFERENCES

1. La Rosa G, Conti A, Cacciola F, et al. Pedicle screw fixation for isthmic spondylolisthesis: does posterior lumbar interbody fusion improve outcome over posterolateral fusion? *Spine* 2003;99(2):143–150.
2. Perrin G. Surgical treatment of severe lateral and foraminal spine degenerative stenosis. Gunzburg R, Szpalski M, ed. *Lumbar Spinal Stenosis*. Philadelphia: Lippincott Williams & Wilkins; 2000:313–320.
3. Perrin G. Usefulness of intervertebral titanium CH cages for PLIF and posterior fixation with semi-rigid Isolock plates. Szpalski M, Gunzburg R, Spengler DM, et al., ed. *Instrumented Fusion of the Degenerative Lumbar Spine: State of the Art, Questions, and Controversies*. Philadelphia: Lippincott-Raven; 1996:271–279.

4. Szpalski M., Gunzburg R. Lumbar spinal stenosis in the elderly: an overview. *Eur Spine J* 2003;12(suppl 2): 170–175.
5. Brunet JA, Wiley JJ. Acquired spondylosis after spinal fusion. *J Bone Joint Surg Br* 1984;66(5):720–724.
6. Eck JC, Humphreys SC, Hodges SD. Adjacent-segment degeneration after lumbar fusion: a review of clinical, biomechanical, and radiological studies. *Am J Orthop*1999;28(6):336–340.
7. Harris RI, Wiley JJ. Acquired spondylolysis as a sequel to spine fusion. *J Bone Joint Surg Am* 1963;45(6):1159–1170.
8. Whitecloud T, Davis J, Olive P. Operative treatment of the degenerated segment adjacent to a lumbar fusion spine. *Spine* 1994;19:532–536.
9. Gillet P. The fate of the adjacent motion segments after lumbar fusion. *J Spinal Disord* 2003;16(4):338–345.
10. Axelsson P, Johnsson R, Stromqvist B. The spondylolytic vertebra and its adjacent segment: mobility measured before and after posterolateral fusion. *Spine* 1997;22(4):414–417.
11. Dekutoski MB, Schendel MJ, Ogilvie JW, et al. Comparison of in vivo and in vitro adjacent motion after lumbar fusion. *Spine* 1994;19(15):1745–1751.
12. Ha KY, Schendel MJ, Lewis JL, et al. Effects of immobilization and configuration on lumbar adjacent segment biomechanics. *J Spinal Disord* 1993;6(2):99–105.
13. Park P, Garton HJ, Gala V, et al. Adjacent segment disease after lumbar or lumbosacral fusion: review of the literature. *Spine* 2004;29(17):1938–1944.
14. Nagata H, Schendel MJ, Transfeldt EE, et al. The effects of immobilization of long segments of the spine on the adjacent and distal facet force and lumbosacral motion. *Spine* 1993;18(16):2471–2479.
15. Okuda S, Iwasaki M, Miyauchi A, et al. Risk factors for adjacent segment degeneration after PLIF. *Spine* 2004;29(14):1535–1540.
16. Wimmer C, Gluch H, Krismer M, et al. AP-Translation in the proximal disc adjacent to spine fusion: a retrospective comparison of mono- and polysegmental fusion in 120 patients. *Acta Orthop Scand* 1997; 68(3):269–272.
17. Perrin G, Cristini A. Prevention of adjacent level degeneration above a fused vertebral segment: long-term effects, after a mean follow-up of 8.27 years, of the semi-rigid intervertebral fixation as a protective technique for pathological adjacent disc. IMAST 2003 Meeting, Rome.
18. Elias WJ, Simmons NE, Kaptain GJ, et al. Complications of posterior lumbar interbody fusion when using a titanium threaded cage device. *Spine* 2000;93(1):45–52.
19. Rajnics P, Templier A, Skalli W, et al. The association of sagittal spinal and pelvic parameters in asymptomatic persons and patients with isthmic spondylolisthesis. *J Spinal Disord* 2002;15:24–30.
20. Etebar S, Cahill DW. Risk factors for adjacent-segment failure following lumbar fixation with rigid instrumentation for degenerative instability. *Spine* 1999;90(2):163–169.

20

A New Spondylolisthesis Reduction Technique

Abraham Rogozinski and Chaim Rogozinski

Open reduction of high-grade spondylolisthesis in combination with posterior instrumentation and fusion is intended to restore sagittal balance, reduce the slip angle, and provide anatomical restoration of the spine. This allows reduced tension of the lumbar nerves (1–4). Clinical benefits to the patient include decreased postoperative pain, immediate mobilization of the patient without bracing, a halt to the progression of the deformity, the ability for the surgeon to perform complete neural decompression, the promotion of successful arthrodesis, and the restoration of body posturing mechanisms with corresponding improvement in appearance and self-image (2–6).

Decompression of spondylolisthesis alone has been associated with instability and in some cases can increase the deformity (7–13). Pedicle screw fixation has been utilized to stabilize the spine in these instances; however, the use of fixation without other attempts at postural reduction has had limited success in restoring the anatomical lumbosacral angle (6,14,15). This chapter is not an argument for justifying reduction of spondylolisthesis, but rather a description of a unique technique for spondylolisthesis reduction when indicated.

A new spinal fixation system (SpineLink, EBI, Parsippany, NJ, USA) with polydirectional screws and modular links was recently introduced. The independent linking of multiple vertebral fixation points has been termed "intrasegmental" fixation. The intrasegmental nature of the fixation eliminates the need for intraoperative contouring and cutting of the rods and plates. The addition of extended polydirectional screws and StepLinks, along with the development of an attachable spondylolisthesis reduction jack, affords the surgeon the ability to internally fix the spine and reduce the spondylolisthesis by manipulating two unconnected instrumented segments. The corrective forces that can be applied to the spine with this system are (a) extension, (b) distraction-compression, and (c) translation, to achieve the desired reduction.

SURGICAL TECHNIQUE

The reduction technique for spondylolisthesis can be performed regardless of the number of vertebral levels fused. Described here is the surgical technique for a two-level posterior fusion of L4 to the sacrum with reduction of an L5-S1 spondylolytic spondylolisthesis.

After a complete decompression of L5, soft tissue and intervertebral disc space release, and any bone resection needed, the segmental instrumentation is applied to the spine using the standard technique for the polydirectional pedicle screw insertion and link placement. To facilitate application of the links and the subsequent reduction, the

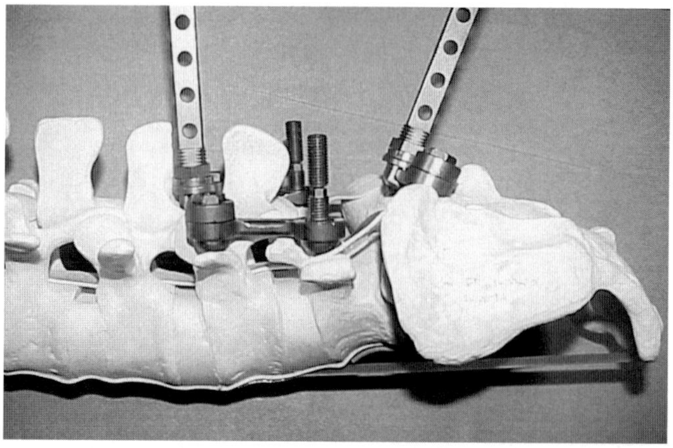

FIG. 20.1. Machine-threaded portion of polydirectional pedicle screws at L4–L5 are oriented perpendicular to floor, while at S1, the screw heads are angled caudally to match the slip angle. The spondy reduction instrument is attached to the transverse links on L4 and S1 by securing the reducer arm assemblies.

machine-threaded portion of the polydirectional screws at L4 and L5 is oriented perpendicular to the floor. The machine-threaded portion of S1 screw is angled caudally in the sagittal plane to match the slip angle determined by preoperative radiographic measurements (Fig. 20.1). This angle can be reproduced using a goniometer, which is included with the instrumentation. With the S1 pedicle screws in position, the caliper is used to measure the interscrew distance and an appropriately sized standard link is used to transversely connect the S1 screws. This link is provisionally maintained in position with end caps and lock nuts. The caliper is used to measure the distance between the L4 and L5 pedicle screws on both sides, and an appropriately chosen standard link is then used to affix the L4 and L5 screws ipsilaterally. This is done bilaterally. The interscrew distance between L4 is then measured with the caliper, and a standard link is used to link the L4 screws transversely. The transverse link is locked into position with lock nuts. Temporary end caps and lock nuts are applied to provisionally lock the construct to the L5 pedicle screws. To allow reduction to proceed, no link is applied at this point to connect L5 to the sacrum.

The spondylolisthesis reduction instrument (or "spondy reduction instrument") is now applied by firmly affixing the two "reducer arm" assemblies to the transverse links at L4 and S1. These outriggers are placed at the midportion of the transverse link and secured to the transverse link with a speed wrench (Fig. 20.1). The reduction maneuver, in conjunction with spinal cord monitoring, is then started by bringing the two reducer arms into parallel position (Fig. 20.2). This effectively extends the spine to correct the flexion deformity. Distraction (or compression) can also be applied independently at any time during the procedure as needed. Once the reducer arms are parallel, the slotted "reducer distraction bar" and the "reducer lever assembly" are applied and secured with the reducer thumb screws to the reducer arms, forming a parallelogram (Fig. 20.3). The assembly of the spondy reduction instrument is now complete and the final reduction maneuver to correct for translation of the L5 vertebrae is performed. This is achieved by applying a downward force to the caudal handle while lifting upward on the cephalad handle. This maneuver will reduce the vertebral translation between L5 and the sacrum.

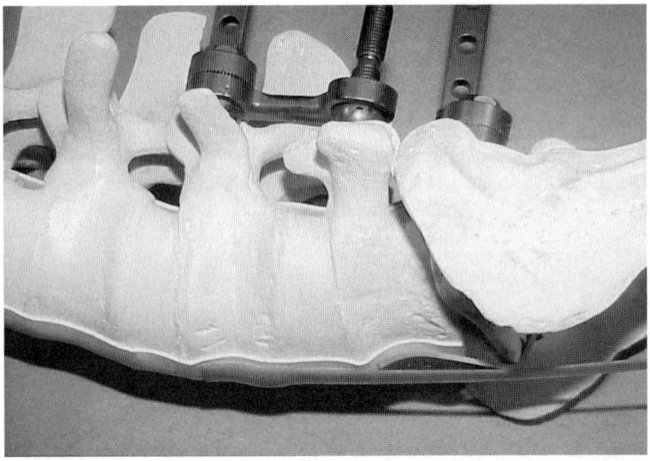

FIG. 20.2. L5-S1 is left uninstrumented to allow reduction to proceed. The reduction maneuver is begun by moving the two reducer arm assemblies into parallel position, which extends the spine and corrects for the flexion deformity.

When performing the reduction maneuver, great care and attention need to be directed to the L5 root and intraoperative spinal cord monitoring. Once the reduction is completed, the spondy reduction instrument is locked into position with the "reducer locking rod" to maintain the reduction (Fig. 20.4).

To complete the instrumentation and maintain the reduction, the two independent segments of the spine (the sacrum and L4–L5) are then intrasegmentally connected. This is achieved by using the caliper to determine the distance between L5 and S1 (Fig. 20.5). The caliper measures longitudinal distance as well as any residual vertebral translation

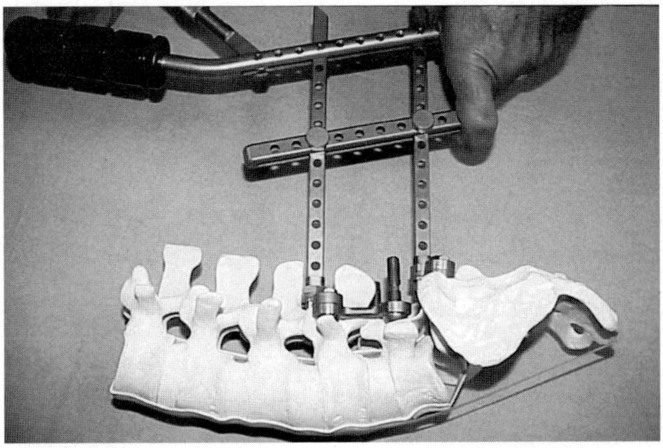

FIG. 20.3. The reduction maneuver continues with the attachment of the slotted reducer distraction bar and the spondy reducer lever handle to the reducer arms. Distraction can be applied and maintained by fixing the parallelogram. Translation of the vertebrae is then performed by placing downward force to the caudal handle and lifting upward on the cephalad handle.

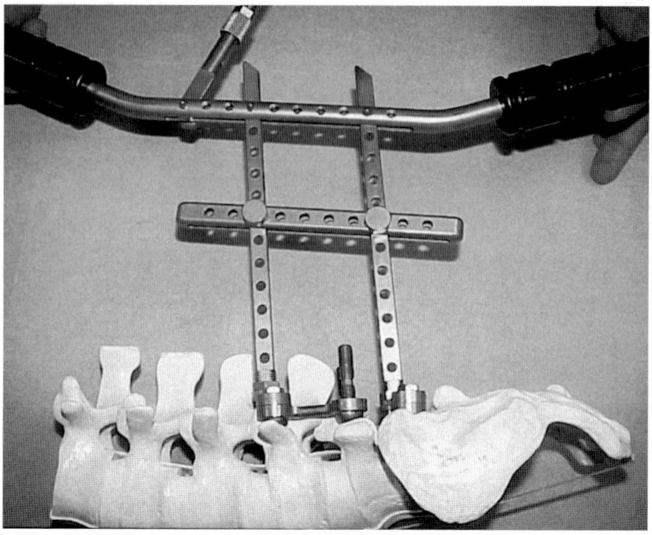

FIG. 20.4. With the reduction complete, the Spondy Reduction Instrument is locked into position by means of the reducer locking rod to maintain the reduction. Direct observation of the L5 nerve root and intraoperative monitoring is used to assess the nerve roots.

that may result in a step-off between S1 and L5. The end caps and lock nuts that were provisionally securing L5 and the sacrum are removed on one side and replaced with the appropriately sized standard or StepLink and lock nuts. This maneuver is then repeated on the contralateral side. Once assembly is complete, all lock nuts are provisionally tightened

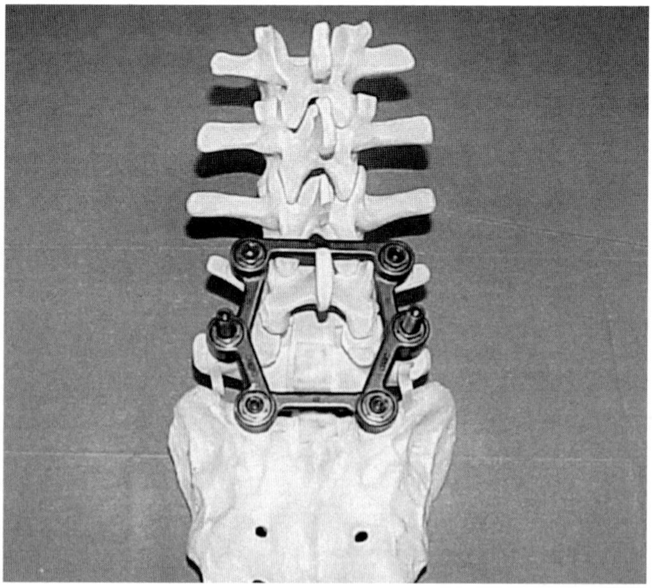

FIG. 20.5. The two instrumented segments of the spine (sacrum and L4–L5) are intrasegmentally connected. The components of the spondy reduction instrument are removed in reverse order.

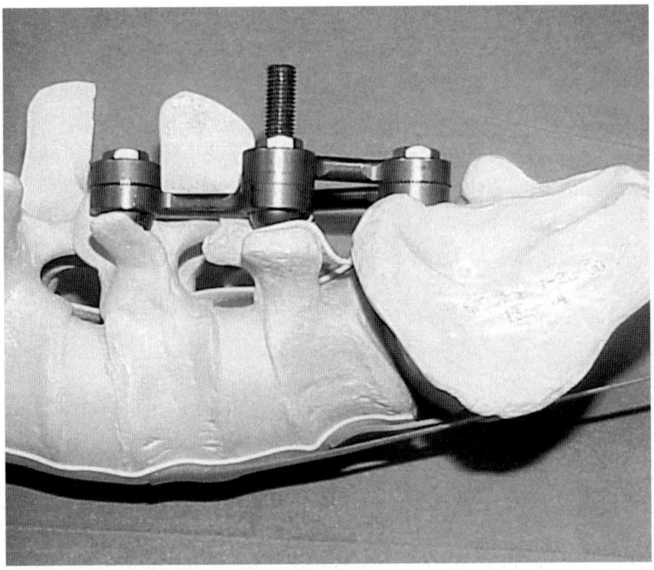

FIG. 20.6. Lateral view of completed instrumentation of L4 to S1 maintaining the reduction. After final tightening of the lock nuts with the torque wrench, the threaded extension of the L5 screw head is removed. Decortication and graft application can be performed at the surgeon's discretion either prior to or after instrumentation.

and then finally tightened with a torque wrench and doubly torqued. The spondy reduction instrument is then removed in reverse order (Fig. 20.5). The threaded extension of the L5 screw is then sheared off at the scored mark.

Although the technique described above is for the reduction itself, decortication and graft application can be performed at the surgeon's discretion either prior to or after instrumentation (Fig. 20.6). The technique may also be performed using a one-level construct involving only L5-S1. In a one-level fusion application, a link is applied transversely to interconnect the L5 pedicle screws. Closure and postoperative management are performed according to the surgeon's standard protocol.

RESULTS

The technique as described allows for open reduction when indicated in cases of severe spondylolisthesis using intrasegmental fixation (Fig. 20.7). Four patients have undergone this procedure with no intra-operative or postoperative complications. Anatomical decompression has been achieved in all cases with variable relief of symptoms. The patient with the longest follow-up (15 months) is free from ongoing back pain or leg pain, is neurologically intact, and has returned to normal activity. All patients are being followed prospectively at 3, 6, 12, and 24 months with anteroposterior (A-P) and lateral radiographs, the Oswestry Disability Index (ODI), and 36-item Short Form Health Survey (SF-36) outcome instruments. These outcome measurements will be reported subsequently when a sufficient number of the surgical patients have reached 24 months follow-up.

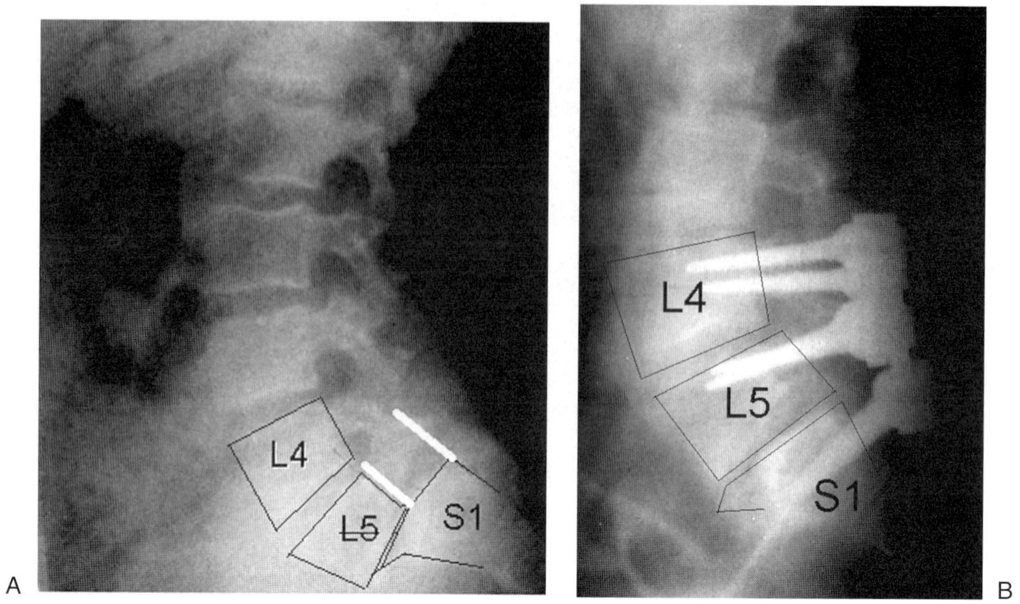

FIG. 20.7. A: Preoperative lateral radiograph of high-grade spondylolisthesis L5-S1. **B:** Post-operative lateral radiograph of L5-S1 spondylolisthesis reduction with intrasegmental fixation and posterolateral fusion stabilizing.

DISCUSSION

Surgical correction of spondylolisthesis may create instability and in some cases recurrence of deformity. Rigid pedicle screw fixation will stabilize the spine in these instances but has limited ability to restore anatomical alignment. Advantages of intrasegmental fixation in these patients can include improved biomechanical strength at each level of fixation, which allows restoration of anatomical alignment and maintenance of the patient's normal lordosis.

Intrasegmental fixation is predicated on the ability to link or manipulate multiple vertebral fixation points. Applying this concept to spondylolisthesis reduction enables the surgeon to reduce the spine regardless of the number of levels that are fused. Three distinct reduction forces—extension, distraction-compression, and translation—can be applied independently to the spine in a controlled fashion by using an attachable spondy reduction instrument to restore alignment. Once the two independently instrumented segments are reduced to the desired position, they are linked together to maintain the reduction. The reduction technique described provides the surgeon a controlled method to restore spinal anatomy, thereby offering improved clinical benefits to patients presenting with this complex condition.

REFERENCES

1. Bridwell KH, Sedgewick TA, O'Brien MF, et al. The role of fusion and instrumentation in the treatment of degenerative spondylolisthesis with spinal stenosis. *J Spinal Disord* 1993;6(6):461–472.
2. Fabris DA, Costantini S, Nena U. Surgical treatment of severe L5-S1 spondylolisthesis in children and adolescents: results of intraoperative reduction, posterior interbody fusion, and segmental pedicle fixation. *Spine* 1996;21:728–733.

3. Fischgrund JS, Mackay M, Herkowitz HN, et al. Degenerative lumbar spondylolisthesis with spinal stenosis: a prospective, randomized study comparing decompressive laminectomy and arthrodesis with and without spinal instrumentation. *Spine* 1997;22(24):2807–2812.
4. Henderson ED. Results of surgical treatment of spondylolisthesis. *J Bone Joint Surg Am* 1966;48:619–642.
5. Albert TJ, Jones AM, Balderston RA. Spinal instrumentation. In: Rothman RH, Simeone FA, ed. *The Spine*. Philadelphia: W.B. Saunders; 1992:1777–1800.
6. Hirabayashi S, Kumano K, Kuroki T. Cotrel–Dubousset pedicle screw system for various spinal disorders: merits and problems. *Spine* 1991;16(11):1298–1304.
7. Dandy DJ, Shannon MJ. Lumbo-sacral subluxation. *J Bone Joint Surg Br* 1971;53:578–595.
8. Davis IS, Bailey RW. Spondylolisthesis: long-term follow-up study of treatment with total laminectomy. *Clin Orthop* 1972;88:46–49.
9. Grobler LJ, Moe JH, Winter RB, et al. Loss of lumbar lordosis following surgical correction of thoracolumbar deformities. *Orthop Trans* 1978;2:239.
10. Matthiass HH, Heine J. The surgical reduction of spondylolisthesis. *Clin Orthop* 1986;203:34–44.
11. Newton PO, Johnston CE II. Analysis and treatment of poor outcomes following in situ arthrodesis. *J Pediatr Orthop* 1997;7:754–761.
12. Riley P, Gillespie MB. Severe spondylolisthesis: results of posterolateral fusion. *Ortho Trans* 1985;9:119–120.
13. Schoennecker PL, Cole HO, Herring JA, et al. Cauda equina syndrome after in situ arthrodesis for severe spondylolisthesis at the lumbosacral junction. *J Bone Joint Surg Am* 1990;72:369.
14. Kostuik JP, Errico TJ, Gleason TF. Techniques of internal fixation for degenerative conditions of the lumbar spine. *Clin Orthop* 1986;203:219–231.
15. Steffee AD, Sitkowski DJ. Reduction and stabilization of grade IV spondylolisthesis. *Clin Orthop* 1988; 227:82–89.

21

Spondylolisthesis Stabilization and Reduction through MIS Approach

Anthony P. Fabrizi, Mino Zucchelli, and Andrea Barbanera

We can define minimally invasive surgery (MIS) as a procedure that allows less extensive manipulation of surrounding tissues than a conventional open one while accomplishing the same goals and objectives at the target structure. In spine surgery, minimal access surgery for the treatment of lumbar disc disease is by no means a new concept; many procedures have been developed for the purpose of achieving a less destructive surgery: percutaneous laser disc decompression (1,2); percutaneous endoscopic laser discectomy (3); percutaneous nucleotomy (4,5). Endoscopic discectomy was proposed in 1997 by Foley and Smith (6) to allow a decompression of a nerve root even in the case of bony decompression with minimal tissue trauma through a direct visualization of the structures.

Minimally invasive surgery also found an application in reducing tissue damage in fusing procedures that, when performed in open surgery, are associated with lengthy hospital stays (intense postoperative pain), significant costs (7), and not marginal morbidity for patients caused by the muscle dissection and retraction and soft tissue injury occurring during standard lumbar fusion procedures (8–10). Kahanovitz et al. reported that in a long-term strength assessment postoperatively of patients who had undergone back surgery, "every strength parameter tested except male isokinetic flexion strength showed at least a 30% decrease when compared with normal values" (11).

In light of the evidence, we consider muscle damage a possible cause of long-term postoperative back pain, which may be due to vertebral instability of the adjacent segments as consequence of the decrease in muscle strength.

We present our experience with a minimally invasive spine procedure that allows a posterior stabilization of the vertebral segments through only two small, symmetric, paravertebral wounds. This technique is based on standard spinal techniques but moves beyond them to minimize iatrogenic injury (avoiding stripping and cutting muscles) while still achieving the traditional goals of spinal surgery.

Analyzing the surgical steps, the first one is represented by the individuation of some surgical landmarks (Fig. 21.1): Then, under radioscopic guidance (A-P and L-L control), the trocar is introduced in the pedicle (Fig. 21.2). After tissue dilatation (Fig. 21.3), the pedicle is prepared for the screw and the first screw is placed.

Next, to prepare the adjacent level, a Cobb is inserted along previously placed shaft and moved laterally under x-ray control until the adjacent pedicle is reached. This maneuver is repeated two or three times to assure that the space is free before inserting the trocar in the upper level through insert the second screw (Fig. 21.4).

Before the insertion of the connecting bar, the removal of all muscle and soft tissue (performed with a high-speed drill under fluoroscopic control) is needed, and inside the facet joints, we insert some bone to promote a posterolateral fusion (Fig. 21.5).

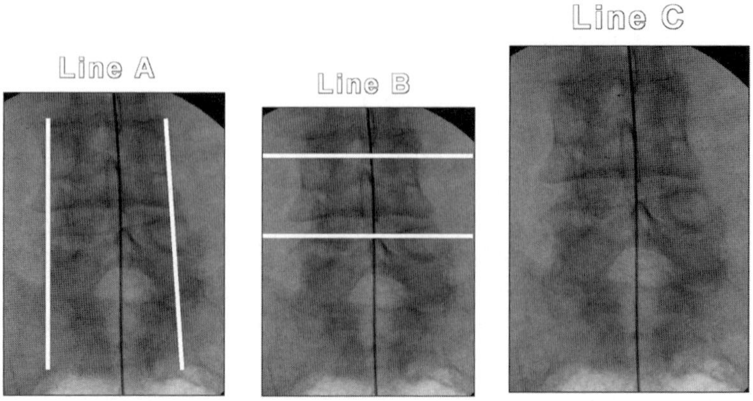

FIG. 21.1. Individuation of surgical landmarks before the skin incision. **A:** The lateral border of the pedicles. **B:** The upper limits of the pedicles. **C:** The oblique trajectory through the pedicle to the intersection of (B) at (A). There is the correct marking (*red line*) for incision.

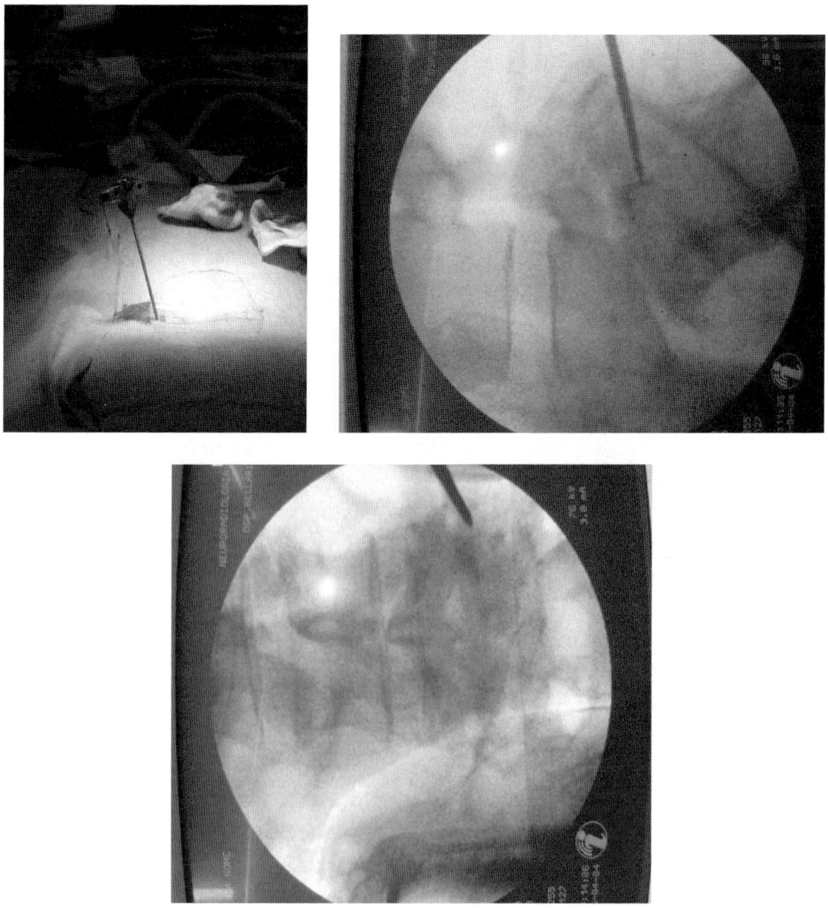

FIG. 21.2. Introduction of the trocar in the pedicle under radioscopic guidance.

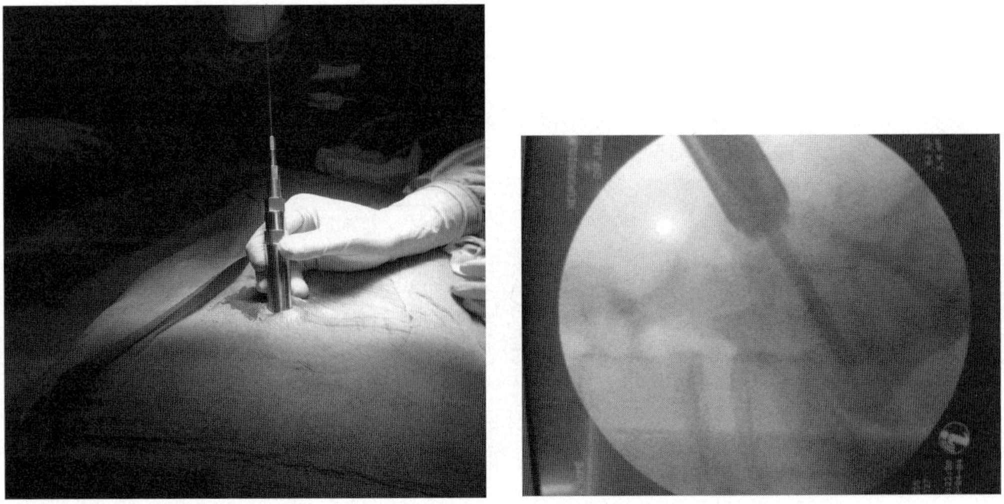

FIG. 21.3. Tissue dilatation to prepare the pedicle for the screw insertion.

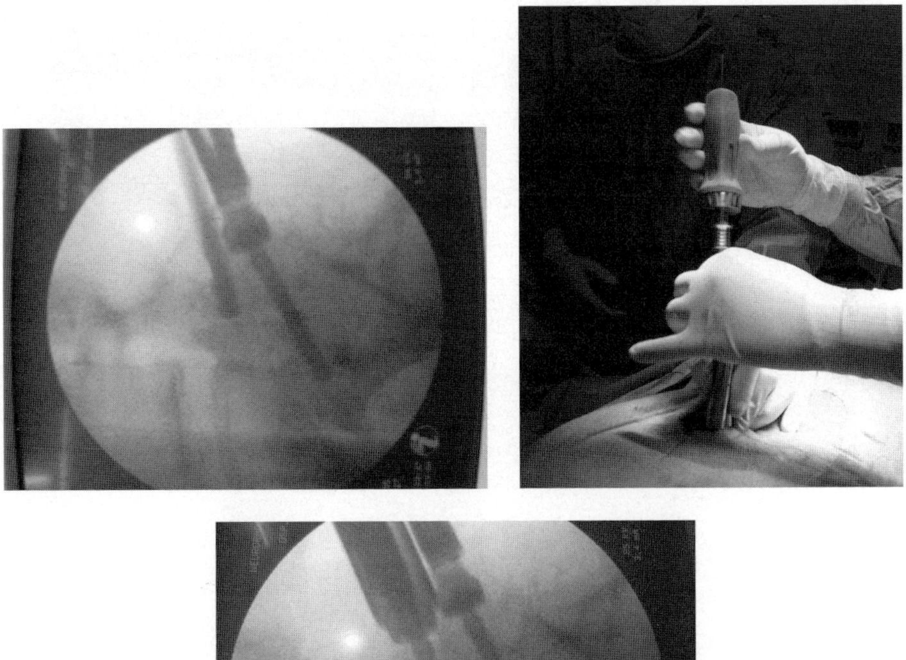

FIG. 21.4. Insertion of a second screw through a trocar inserted in the upper level.

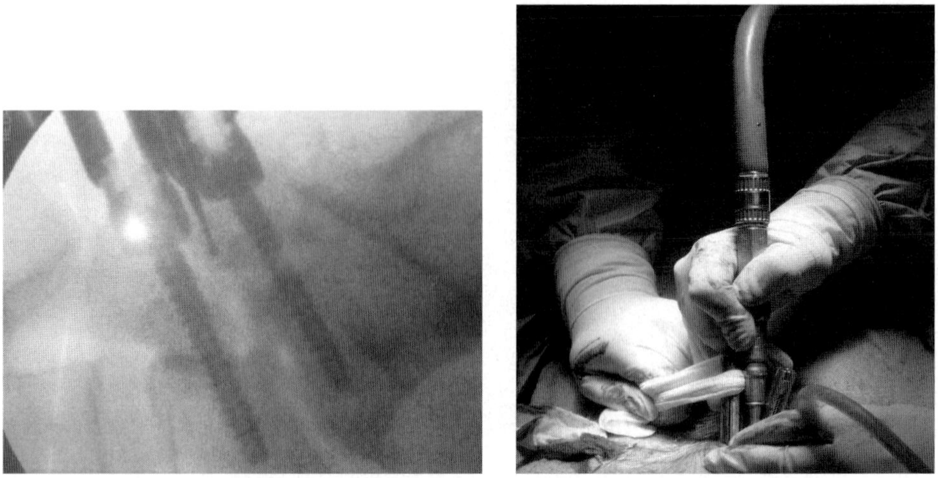

FIG. 21.5. Removal of all muscle and soft tissue (performed with a high-speed drill under fluoroscopic control) before the insertion of the connecting bar.

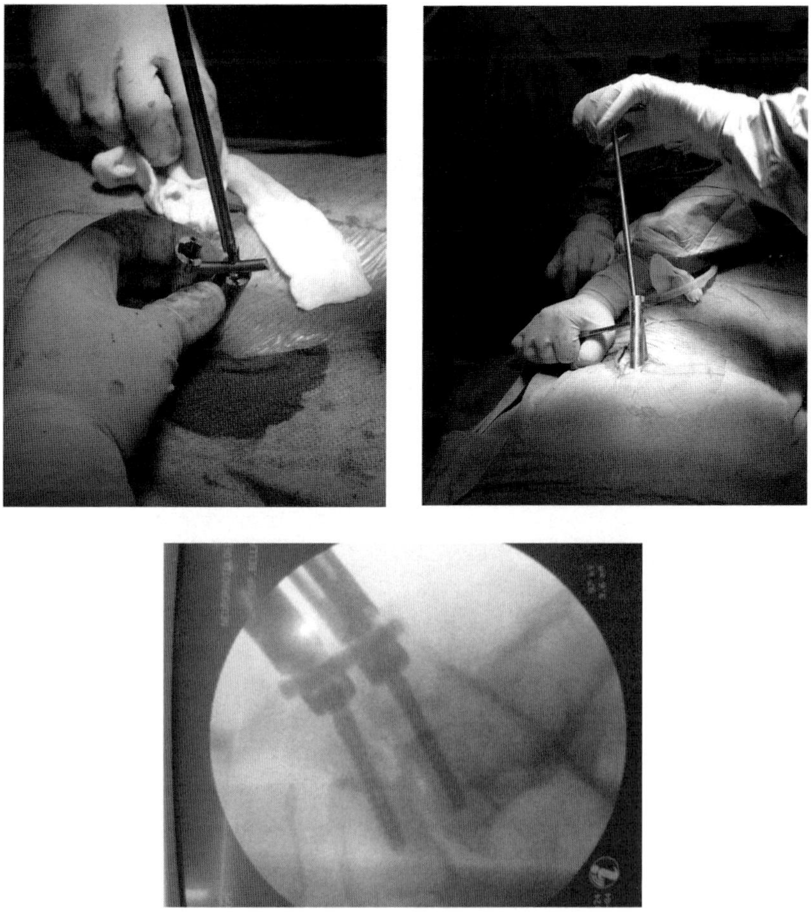

FIG. 21.6. Insertion and locking of the connection bar.

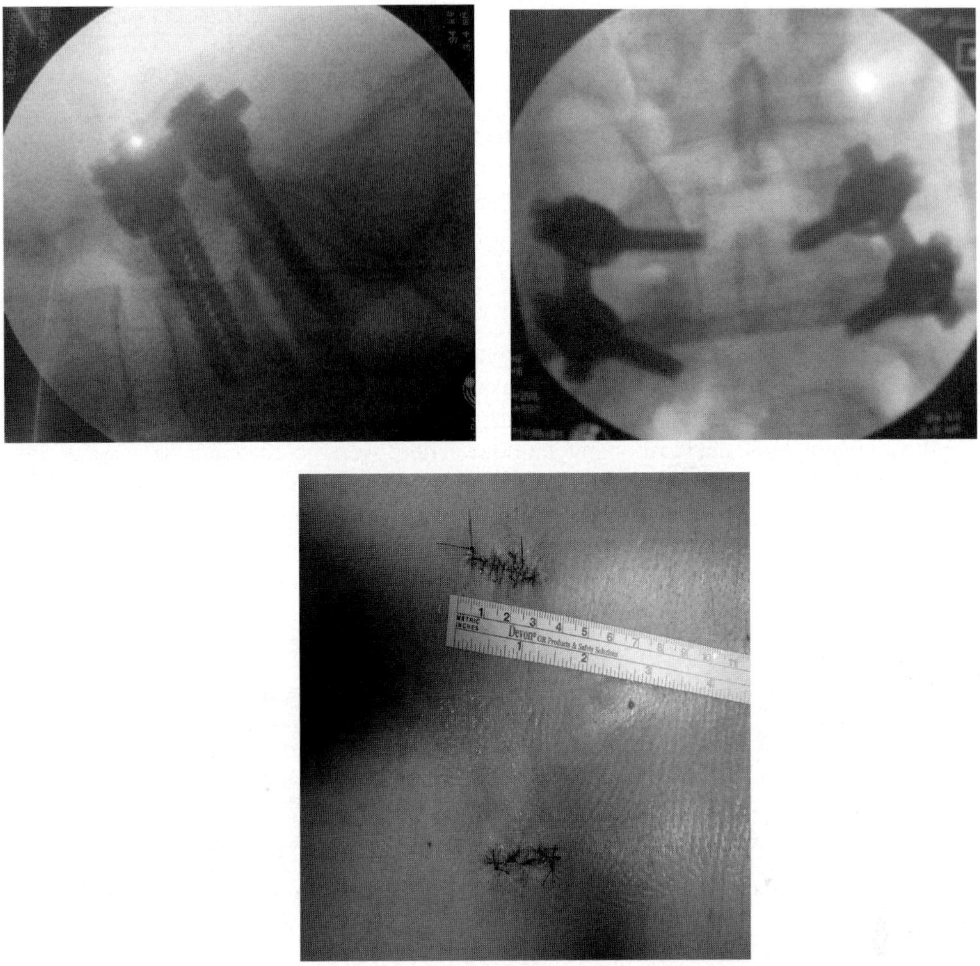

FIG. 21.7. Skin closing with a conventional aesthetic suture after contralateral screw and bar placement and intraoperative fluoroscopic control.

After its length is measured, the connection bar is inserted and locked with the insertion of the locking screw (Fig. 21.6). After contralateral screw and bar placement and intraoperative fluoroscopic control, the skin is closed with a conventional aesthetic suture (Fig. 21.7).

We treated 24 patients (mean age 37 years of age), 16 males and 8 females, 14 were operated in L5-S1, 8 in L4–L5, 1 in L3–L4, 1 from L4 to S1 (two levels).

In 15 patients, we performed a posterolateral fusion in addition; 9 cases underwent to intersomatic arthrodesis.

The results are summarized in Table 21.1. It is clear that the fusion rate is almost the same of the open procedures, but the hospitalization period and the blood loss are dramatically smaller than for the conventional procedure. Regarding the time spent in operating room for the procedure, we think that the improvement of the surgeons' skill with this technique will shorten the surgical time.

All the patients underwent pain assessment with the Visual Analog Score (VAS), and the results are summarized in Table 21.2. The pain was lower from the first days postoperatively compared to the pain measured in patients who have undergone open procedures,

TABLE 21.1.

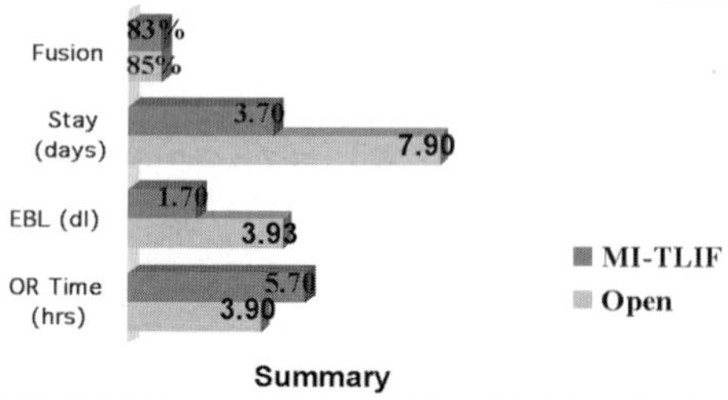

TABLE 21.2.

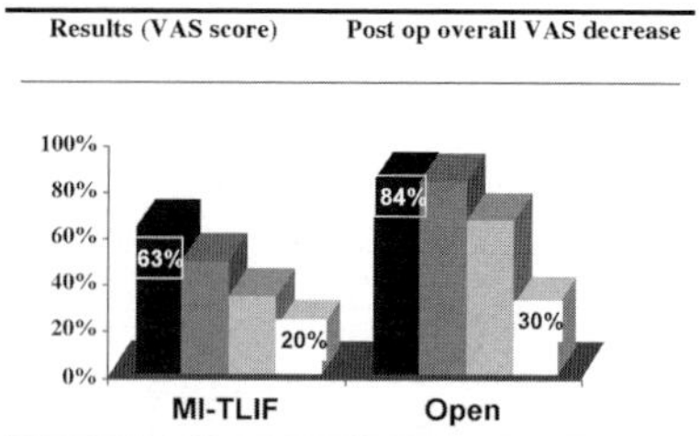

and also the use of narcotic drugs was lower than following conventional procedures. In conclusion, patients undergoing minimally invasive lumbar interbody fusion report less post- and perioperative pain, require less narcotics, ambulate earlier, and are discharged earlier than those treated by a standard open technique. There were no complications in our cases and minimal blood loss during operation. In nine cases, we performed a 360 degree fusion with the addition of an intersomatic arthrodesis during the same surgical time.

We think that, as more surgeons become experienced in this minimally invasive technique, it should become the new gold standard in vertebral stabilization.

REFERENCES

1. Casper GD, Hartman VL, Mullins LL. Percutaneous laser disc decompression with the holmium: YAG laser. *J Clin Laser Med Surg* 1995;13:195–203.
2. Choy DS. Percutaneous laser disc decompression (PLDD): twelve years' experience with 752 procedures in 518 patients. *J Clin Laser Med Surg* 1998;16:325–331.
3. Boult M, Fraser RD, Jones N, et al. Percutaneous endoscopic laser discectomy. *Aust N Z J Surg* 2000; 70:475–479.
4. Kotilainen E, Valtonen S. Long-term outcome of patients who underwent percutaneous nucleotomy for lumbar disc herniation: results after a mean follow-up of 5 years. *Acta Neurochir (Wien)* 1998;140:108–113.
5. Marks RA. Transcutaneous lumbar diskectomy for internal disk derangement: a new indication. *South Med J* 2000;93:885–890.
6. Foley KT, Smith MM, Rampersaud YR. Microendoscopic discectomy. In: Schmidek HH, ed. *Operative Neurosurgical Techniques: Indications, Methods, and Results*. 4th edition Philadelphia: W.B. Saunders Co.; 2000.
7. Thomsen K, Christensen FB, Eiskjaer SP, et al. 1997 Volvo Award winner in clinical studies: the effect of pedicle screw instrumentation on functional outcome and fusion rates in posterolateral lumbar spinal fusion: a prospective, randomized clinical study. *Spine* 1997;22:2813–2822.
8. Gejo R, Matsui H, Kawaguchi Y, et al. Serial changes in trunk muscle performance after posterior lumbar surgery. *Spine* 1999;24:1023–1-28.
9. Kawaguchi Y, Matsui H, Tsuji H. Back muscle injury after posterior lumbar spine surgery: a histologic and enzymatic analysis. *Spine* 1996;21:941–944.
10. Styf JR, Willen J. The effects of external compression by three different retractors on pressure in the erector spine muscles during and after posterior lumbar spine surgery in humans. *Spine* 1998;23:354–358.
11. Kahanovitz N, Viola K, Gallagher M. Long-term strength assessment of postoperative post discectomy patients. *Spine* 1989;14(4):402–403.

22

The Economics of Spondylolysis

Rikke Soegaard and Finn Bjarke Christensen

The methodology and adaptation of health economics has emerged rapidly over the past decades. From cost-of-illness studies, which describe the economic impact of a disease, through cost-benefit, cost-utility, and cost-effectiveness evaluations, which analyze costs against consequences and thus provide a decision-analytic approach in determining which intervention that provides the best value for money. The aim of the present chapter is to (a) introduce the basics of health economic methodology relevant to spondylolysis, (b) present a selection of recent studies applying this methodology, and (c) describe the opportunities in applied health economics as seen from Denmark.

A BRIEF INTRODUCTION TO THE METHODOLOGY

The Cost-of-Illness Approach

The burden of a disease to society can be estimated in economic terms by the cost-of-illness approach. Although this method has substantial limitations because it returns only an absolute point measure of costs, which is rarely comparable between societies or repeated measurements, this approach can be useful to visualize potentials for research efforts or simply to awaken politicians.

Basic considerations of a cost-of-illness study are (a) whether to adapt prevalence-based or incidence-based data, (b) whether to take a top-down or bottom-up approach, and (c) which cost categories to include. Costs are defined by "opportunity costs," not to be confused by expenditures, which are only relevant to financial analyses (e.g., budget impact analyses). An opportunity cost reflects the value of a resource in the best alternative use (e.g., should a surgeon choose to perform an operation free of charge, the cost would still be the value of the surgeon's time spent although the expenditure for salary would be zero).

In conducting or evaluating a cost-of-illness study, all consequences associated with the disease should be identified, measured, and valuated. Hence, the costs occurring in the health care sector, other sectors, and the patient and family sphere (e.g., transportation for treatment activities, medication, time spent, etc.) should be included. In practice, however, cost categories most often comprise the costs directly associated with the disease and occurring in the health care sector (so-called direct costs of prevention, diagnostics, treatment, and rehabilitation), production loss from absenteeism or disability, and finally, the value of informal care.

Cost-Effectiveness, Cost-Utility, and Cost-Benefit Approaches

Because of a lack of consensus regarding the definition of economic evaluation several studies are indexed as economic evaluations although in practice they are cost descriptions or cost analyses.

Drummond defines an economic evaluation from two criteria: (a) there should be a comparison of two or more alternatives and (b) both costs (inputs) and consequences (outputs) of the alternatives should be examined (1). If one of these criteria is not fulfilled, the evaluation is considered partial and should be termed "description" or "analysis" instead of "evaluation."

The main purpose of economic evaluation is to provide a decision-analytic foundation for the decision makers who prioritize efficiency in health care. Very often, the experimental intervention at hand is an intervention that is obviously both more effective and more costly than the usual regimen. Thus, we want to document the cost-effectiveness (alternatively cost-utility or cost-benefit) of the new intervention to establish an argument for implementing it in everyday clinical practice.

In practice, we have to identify, measure, and valuate all resources consumed in relation to the interventions at hand. This measure of total costs is put up against consequences and, thus, a ratio of cost-consequences is obtained. The higher the ratio between costs and consequences, the more efficient is the intervention. However, the meaningful ratio one should be concerned about is the *incremental* cost-consequence ratio, which describes the *additional* costs and the *additional* consequences one intervention imposes over another. The argument here is, of course, that we do not develop an intervention from scratch but rather, we enhance or extend the usual regimen to gain additional effect. The question is: Are we willing to accept the incremental cost-effectiveness ratio (ICER) for obtaining the additional effect? Most often, the average cost-effectiveness ratio (the first effect units) is far more attractive than the incremental (the last effect units). For example, the first 10 points gain in a scale of function ability or pain is obtainable by an average of x per point whereas the following point is obtainable by a cost of multiple times the x per point. The principle of the average and the incremental cost-effectiveness ratio (ICER) is illustrated in Figure 22.1.

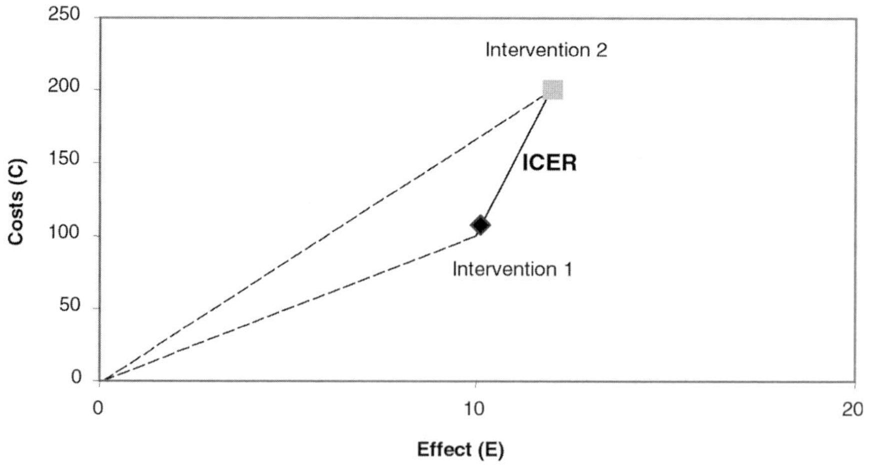

	Costs (C)	Effect (E)	C/E ratio	ΔC	ΔE	*ICER* ΔC/ΔE ratio
Intervention 1	100	10	10	-	-	-
Intervention 2	200	12	12	100	2	50

FIG. 22.1. The incremental cost-effectiveness ratio (ICER).

TABLE 22.1. *Four methods for economic evaluation*

Costs	(Monetary Unit)	Consequences
Cost-minimization	√	—
Cost-effectiveness	√	Effect (physical units measured by means of the Dallas Pain Questionnaire, Low Back Pain Rating Scale, Oswestry Disability Index, or SF-36)
Cost-utility	√	Quality of life (Health-Related Quality-of-Life by, e.g., EQ-50 (35)
Cost-benefit	√	Willingness-to-pay (monetary unit)

To set up an economic evaluation, the first step is to decide upon the perspective relevant to the purpose of the study (that of the recipients of the study, who are often the decision makers). From a theoretical viewpoint, it is difficult to vote against a societal perspective because the consequences are most often not isolated within a department, a hospital, or the health care sector. However, societal costs are often rather difficult to estimate with reasonable precision. The solution often seen is to report both the health care sector perspective (costs occurring in the health care sector) and the societal perspective (health care sector costs plus societal costs of production loss, patient costs, and family costs).

The method used for measuring consequences (output) distinguishes among the types of economic evaluation as illustrated in Table 22.1. The evaluation is defined as a cost-effectiveness when consequences are measured in physical units, which is most often the case in the field of spine research evaluation, by means of e.g., using the Dallas Pain Questionnaire (2), Low Back Pain Rating Scale (3), Oswestry Disability Index (4), SF-36 Health Survey (5) or global health assessments. Should consequences be expressed as generic health-related quality-of-life measures (e.g., quality-adjusted life years, QALYs), the evaluation is defined as a cost-utility. Finally, if consequences are measured in monetary units that reflect the patient's willingness to pay for the consequences of the intervention provided, the evaluation is defined as cost-benefit. Put another way, the choice is a question of comparability between studies; cost-effectiveness measures allow for disease-specific comparisons (if there is consensus about effect measures), whereas the other types of measures are generic. In economic evaluation, hybrid types are often seen. Especially, a fourth type is commonly used: the cost-minimization analysis. This method is relevant if the consequences of two or more interventions have already been compared and do not differ significantly although the resources needed to accomplish the output differ. Here, the purpose is to determine which intervention demands the least costs to accomplish the output.

In conclusion, the cost-effectiveness evaluation allows for allocation of resources within one specific field (e.g., conservative versus surgical treatment in chronic low back pain), and the cost-utility approach allows for allocation within different fields of health (e.g., hip replacements versus kidney transplants), whereas the cost-benefit approach allows for allocation among different sectors in society (e.g., traffic controls versus trauma facilities). Important to recognize, however, is the fact that these studies still leave it to the decision makers to prioritize ethics and, especially in relation to the cost-effectiveness approach, to put a value on the health effects attained. Given these limitations, economic evaluations arc useful tools in determining which interventions offer the best value for money, and as this discipline emerges, the methodology is continuously being improved. Because of increasing health care costs and scarcity of resources, governments and societies are increasingly demanding evidence not only for the clinical effect, but no less for the cost-effectiveness, of various health treatments and procedures—a fact that is underlined by the World Health Organization in the text of the Bone and Joint Decade 2000–2010 announcement (6,7). Hence, economic evaluation is a need rather than an option in modern health scientific research.

For further reading, Drummond et al. (1,8) or Gold et al. (9) among others, provide comprehensive introductions to health economic evaluation. Alternatively, Korthals-de Bos et al. very recently published an overview focused in spinal disorders (10).

APPLIED HEALTH ECONOMICS IN SPONDYLOLYSIS

Applied Cost-of-Illness Methodology

Several studies have investigated the economic burden of back pain to society (11–18). In a recent review by Maetzel and Li, the socioeconomic burden of low back pain is concluded equal to the burdens of depression, heart disease, or diabetes (19). Another significant conclusion by Maetzel and Li is that the costs of low back pain are characterized by a heavily right-skewed distribution. Hence, those 5% to 9% of patients who manifest chronic pain account for 65% to 85% of costs (19).

Maniadakis and Gray (16) have conducted a cost-of-illness study in the United Kingdom concluding that the direct medical costs of back pain amount to US$4.2 billion and the associated production loss and value of informal care amount to US$27.5 billion (1998 prices). In total, these figures are equal to 1.43% of the British gross national product. This state-of-the-art study is probably one of the most comprehensive to date and takes advantage of a national survey of 6,000 adults with regard to both prevalence of back pain and related service utilization. Service utilization was validated by relevant sources (e.g., registries and statistics of medical societies), and national cost estimates per item were multiplied (e.g., 7.5 million consultations with a surgeon at US$36 per consultation) (16). The estimation of production loss however, is somehow controversial. Maniadakis and Gray faced the methodologic discrepancies by presenting two different, but commonly used approaches (a) the human capital method, in which production loss is estimated from days of absenteeism and disability multiplied by the earning potential of the person not contributing to production, and (b) the more conservative friction method, in which sick leave of a person is only considered significant if no other person can replace him or her, and thus only a limited period of friction is multiplied by the earning potential. Maniadakis and Gray found that the human capital approach yielded the estimate of US$27.5 billion and the friction approach yielded the estimate of US$12.9 billion. Health economists do not agree on which is the correct approach, and the approach chosen may depend on the purpose of the study.

A critical point of the Maniadakis and Gray study is reflected in the study by Lou et al. (15), who investigated direct medical costs of back pain in the United States. Lou et al. conclude, upon a regression analysis, that direct medical costs due to back pain comprise US$90.7 billion, but of this total only US$26.3 billion are incremental costs related to back pain. Evidently, caution should be taken in concluding that the full resource consumption in back pain patients is allocatable solely to the disease of back pain.

Table 22.2 shows national costs of back pain in five countries estimated by either a selected cost study or in combination with a Health Technology Assessment. Direct costs are defined as costs directly related to prevention, diagnostics, treatment, and rehabilitation, which are occurring in the health care sector. Indirect costs are defined as and limited to production loss. Again, one should be very cautious in comparing studies among

TABLE 22.2. *The medical costs of low back pain in Sweden, Denmark, the Netherlands, United Kingdom, and the United States of America*

		Costs (US$, 1998 price-year)				
	Population[a]	Direct costs per inhabitant	Direct costs (millions)	Indirect costs ($ millions)	Total ($ millions)	Year of measurement
Sweden[b,c] (36)	8.87	46.91	416	4,601	5,017	1995
Denmark[b,c] (37)	5.35	45.38	243	1,508	1,751	1996
The Netherlands[c,d] (18)	16.07	32.19	517	6,191	6,708	1991
UK[b] (16)	59.07	71.21	4,206	27,495	31,701	1998
USA(11,15)	291.04	90.37	26,300	39,900–52,500	66,200	1997–1998

Note: Direct costs are medical costs occurring in the health care sector that are directly related to prevention, diagnostics, treatment, and rehabilitation. Indirect costs are defined as production loss.
[a]Million inhabitants 2002 (38).
[b]Monetary conversion to US$ by OECD's Purchasing Power Parity (29).
[c]Costs are converted to price-year 1998 by annual rate of 5%.
[d]Indirect costs comprise US$4.1 million of informal care.

nations due to methodologic differences. However, the high costs seen in the figures of direct costs per U.S. inhabitant (US$ in the price-year 1998) have support from studies comparing international rates of surgery, which conclude that the United States has the highest costs (20,21). The relatively low figures of the Netherlands might be biased due to the measurement- and cost-year (1991). It could be that the incidence of the disease, the associated absenteeism, or the definition of disability has increased over the years, and further it could be questionable to project costs over such a relatively long period (from 1991 through 1998).

Applied Cost-Benefit, Cost-Utility, and Cost-Effectiveness Methodology

A literature search within the framework of the databases of Centre for Reviews and Dissemination (CRD)—a sister organization to the Cochrane Collaboration, which is focused in health economic evaluation—returned 31 hits when searching by the Medical Subject Headings (MeSH) term "back pain" in the NHS Economic Evaluation Database. Of these 31 studies, only four were considered economic evaluations upon review by the CRD commissioned health economists. A similar search on U.S. National Library of Medicine's PubMed returned 104 hits from a search with the MeSH terms "back pain" and "cost-benefit," and looking through the abstracts it was obvious that a considerable number of these studies were also not economic evaluations but rather partial analyses.

In a recently published study, Fritzell et al. (22) evaluated nonsurgical treatment versus three surgical approaches of lumbar spinal fusion in a cost-effectiveness model using a randomized, controlled design. This truly important study is probably the first to conduct an economic evaluation in a randomized design that investigates the cost-effectiveness of spinal fusion. The authors concluded the probability of surgery being cost-effective over nonsurgical treatment to increase with the value decision makers put on effect units (e.g., the value of one gained unit of functional ability). The authors' conclusion was based upon four outcome measures and thus, four incremental cost-effectiveness ratios: cost per unit of (a) global improvement, (b) function, (c) net return to work, and (d) back pain. This study further demonstrated state of the art concerning the handling of uncertainty in estimates which is another controversial issue in economic evaluation. Given that the cost-effectiveness ratio consists of both stochastic clinical effects and stochastic cost estimates, which are both covering true unknown values, the calculation of confidence intervals becomes a challenge. Fritzell et al. adopted a bootstrap method. The basic assumption is that the collected data are representative and hence, the method prescribes repeated sampling to mimic a process of sampling from the entire population (23). Further to the handling of variation related to the sampling, the remaining uncertainty can be explored by applying sensitivity analysis (8). With regard to this issue, Fritzell et al. explored the impact of an underestimation of costs for rehabilitation, minute cost in surgery, and ignorance of the cost of family support.

Unfortunately, in the study by Fritzell et al., the resource utilization was measured retrospectively, which could have introduced recall bias. Another, yet more controversial issue arises from the fact that such economic retrospective evaluation necessarily relies on the sampled population and sample size from the original clinical trial. Most often, economic evaluation, in fact, requires a larger sample size than was calculated for the clinical trial (24). Cost variation in back pain has been found to be relatively wide even compared to variation in clinical outcomes (19,20).

Other economic evaluations have been conducted using a randomized design. Skouen et al. (25) compared extensive and light multidisciplinary treatment programs to usual (nonprotocolized) treatment in conservative treatment of chronic low back pain. The light multidisciplinary program was found cost-effective compared to the extensive, but only in male patients. The costs were measured in a top-down manner that did not differentiate between interventions and single-supplier-based treatment. Although this method might not have caused significant bias in this particular study, the validity of such a method is indeed debateable. In addition, this study measured the effect based solely upon productivity gain estimated by mean income, and no secondary measures of clinical effect. This may be problematic due to different incentives of return-to-work among patients.

A study similar to that of Skouen et al. (25) was reported by Moffett et al. (26), who evaluated progressive exercise compared to usual care in a mixed population of subacute and chronic low back pain. Moffett et al. concluded that the exercise program was superior to usual care upon a variety of effect measures. Although this seems to be a relevant conclusion due to clinical effect, the cost analysis does not provide findings that allow for conclusions about cost-effectiveness of the exercise intervention. The costs were calculated upon retrospective questionnaires in combination with a cost diary (returned by patients at the 6- and 12-month follow-up). No significant difference was found between groups, although a tendency toward reduced service utilization in the exercise group of £24 (95% confidence interval −30;78) was suggested. Also, the societal costs of days off work were acknowledged, but unfortunately the authors did not report the method for valuation.

Goossens et al. (27) investigated cognitive extensions of an operant regimen by either individual therapy or group discussion in a sample of patients suffering chronic low back pain. Goossens et al. concluded that the addition of a cognitive rehabilitation element was cost-effective in general and further they concluded that group therapy was superior to individual therapy. This study introduced, very impressively, a cost diary to measure service utilization in a prospective manner. The patients were asked to register their service utilization during a 12-month period of follow-up. One might question the compliance of such protocol, especially, should the compliance have been differentiated among randomization groups, this would have caused severe bias to findings. Also, it should be mentioned that this study suffered a 43% dropout.

In conclusion, we need to face three crucial issues when planning to supplement clinical trials by economic evaluations: (a) how to establish a valid and precise method for measuring costs of an intervention without unbalanced requirements of effort; (b) how to measure extrainstitutional service utilization during fairly long periods of follow-up and without serious bias; and finally (c) how to handle insufficient power when adapting a sample size calculated for the purpose of a clinical study. The following section of this chapter discusses this challenge as seen from a clinical spine research unit in Denmark.

THE ECONOMICS OF SPONDYLOLYSIS IN DENMARK

Investigating the cost-effectiveness of an intervention should be a balancing act between theory and common sense. In theory, all related resources should be identified, measured, and valuated. In practice, one has to discuss the significance of the components of the interventions at hand. Also, one might take an incremental perspective where only activities *additional* to the usual regimen are measured. This approach is obviously applicable only when a certain range of activities is similar between interventions. The advantage is a substantial time saving, but also improved precision of the estimates.

How to Provide a Valid Cost Estimate?

All costing represents an estimate with a certain level of precision and further, all costing *is* biased. The interesting question is to what extent estimates are biased. The level of precision is derived from the method of costing, which can range from microcosting (measuring each single component of resource use) through a non-disease-specific average cost (average cost of bed days regardless of procedures). Microcosting obviously provides the most precise estimate but is very time consuming however (and almost impossible in this arena), whereas the average-cost-approach provides very little information. In between those endpoints is the case-mix grouping system adapted in many countries (e.g., Norway, Sweden, the United Kingdom, the United States, France, Germany, and Denmark among others).

In Denmark, patients gain access to basic treatment at any hospital of their own choice by referral from their general practitioner (or acute via the casualty department). Cross-country payments are calculated by means of the case-mix system. Continuous validation of diagnostic grouping and the service utilization associated is ongoing in collaboration between the Danish National Board of Health and the medical societies. Table 22.3 shows the costs of common procedures in relation to the treatment of chronic low back pain.

An admission for the purpose of an instrumented spinal fusion in a patient diagnosed with isthmic spondylolisthesis has a cost equivalent to US$19,837. Additionally, the diagnostic regimen might include initial ambulatory visit upon referral, x-ray, magnetic

TABLE 22.3. *Costs of operative regimens at Danish public hospitals (2004)*

	Bed days included (maximum)	Costs (US$, 2004 price-year))
Instrumented	23	19,837
Noninstrumented	26	13,295
Removal of instrumentation	9	3,503

Source: The Danish National Board of Health's case-mix system DRG (Diagnosis Related Grouping). Available at http://www.sst.dk (28). Costs are total hospital costs.

resonance imaging (MRI) scan, and a comprehensive preoperative examination. These activities add a cost of US$988 (28). Finally, the follow-up regimen might include one visit for the purpose of x-ray and four outpatient visits to the ambulatory, which in total equals US$1,112 (28). The grand total of direct hospital costs of a standard regimen of lumbar spinal fusion amounts to US$21,937. Compared to other health care services, such regimen equals 880 daytime visits to a general practitioner, 570 treatments of exercise therapy at a physiotherapist, 656 chiropractic clinical treatments, 176 consultations with a psychologist, or 94 days of sick leave. It is evident that such service utilization has significant impact on the overall cost-consequence ratio of the treatment regimen of chronic low back pain.

Although the case-mix system provides a major advantage in providing a very easy-to-adapt cost estimate, we advise caution in using such an approach. In general, the case-mix system estimates have been found to be in line with estimates of more valid approaches such as microcosting, only when mean duration of admission is equal to national mean (within the case-mix group) (39). Another (often adapted) cost estimate is that provided by the hospital's financial department. This estimate is most often calculated from average non-disease-specific costs, and hence it could be even more imprecise and invalid than that of the case-mix system.

In Denmark, the case-mix system has divided the whole health care sector into less than 500 groups of case-mix estimates. Given the known variation in chronic low back patients concerning age, gender, diagnosis, treatment modalities, and the varying outcomes, costing is indeed a lot more complex and the parameters mentioned might constitute serious bias. In this light, we are at the moment investigating patient-individual cost-effectiveness to gain knowledge about predictors of treatment costs and cost-effectiveness. The goal is to establish an algorithm for costing, which is based upon patient-individual activity-flow. Such an application of the method of *activity-based-costing* reflects a bottom-up approach close to microcosting, and thus the challenge is to avoid unrealistic demands for registering each single component related to the treatment regimen. We approach this challenge by encircling valid indicators of activity-flow, which along with the quality assurance registrations (monitoring of clinical effect) can be registered in a database and applied as a syntax of unit costs that calculates the total estimate of in-hospital service utilization.

Should Extrahospital Service Utilization Be Measured?

Eriksen et al. investigated health service utilization in a sample of 10,066 adults with regard to chronic, nonmalignant pain (31). Nineteen percent (1,871 individuals) in this sample reported chronic pain, and this subgroup was found to have an increased health service utilization of 25% compared to those reporting no chronic pain (31). Further, the group reporting chronic pain scored significantly lower on all subscales of the SF-36 instrument (5) and were found to have twice as high odds of having at least one day of absence from work due to illness. These results, which are similar to those found in international studies of musculoskeletal diseases and also specifically in back pain (20,32), demonstrate the importance of a relevant perspective that is often a multisectored, including both hospital and primary health-care services. Chronic pain (and its relief) has wide consequences affecting both multisectored service utilization and productivity as well as the health-related life-quality of the individual. The question is to what extent those categories are relevant to an economic evaluation in chronic low back pain.

Investigating the cost-effectiveness of a cost-heavy surgical technique, it can be justifiable to stick to hospital costs alone. However, in most cases, ignorance of service utilization in the primary health care sector would downgrade the decision-analytic impact and relevance. Multisectored investigations are, of course, resource demanding and introduce a problem of how to measure this extrainstitutional service utilization in a valid and relatively precise manner. Cost diaries and retrospective questionnaires are commonly used as described above. However, they should be applied with great caution in chronic low back pain, especially when investigations are characterized by long follow-up periods, because recall bias and compliance would be very difficult to control.

The Danish health scientific arena has a variety of registries in both the primary and secondary health care sector. These registers provide high-quality data that, although antecedent, are collected in a prospective manner and are of relatively high validity. Further, a central person register provides the opportunity to collect multiple-register data alongside clinical trials. Although these data can be fairly costly, doing so is of great importance to future scientific investigations.

Recently, we investigated the effect of extending our in-hospital rehabilitation regimen with a behavioral element of "back cafés" (group meetings) or extended exercise therapy (33). Evidently, both extensions were more costly per patient than the usual regimen although their purpose were ultimately to improve cost-effectiveness. To control for extra hospital service utilization, we applied register data of patients' service utilization in the primary health care sector. The extension of back cafés to the usual regimen generated cost savings of service utilization in the primary health care sector amounting to nearly 4 times the incremental costs of extending the regimen (34).

CONCLUSION

Medical resources are finite, and economic evaluations for the purpose of decision making in health care must become an integral part of outcome research. Maximizing health care quality and minimizing costs are inseparable goals. Costly new interventions and treatment modalities are constantly introduced, but they need to be proven equal or superior to clinical practice via well-controlled clinical cost-effectiveness studies.

REFERENCES

1. Drummond MF. *Methods for the Economic Evaluation of Health Care Programmes*. Oxford: Oxford University Press; 1997.
2. Lawlis GF, Cuencas R, Selby D, et al. The development of the Dallas Pain Questionnaire: an assessment of the impact of spinal pain on behavior. *Spine* 1989;14:511–516.
3. Manniche C, Asmussen K, Lauritsen B, et al. Low Back Pain Rating scale: validation of a tool for assessment of low back pain. *Pain* 1994;57:317–326.
4. Fairbank J. Use of Oswestry Disability Index (ODI). *Spine* 1995;20:1535–1537.
5. Ware J. *SF-36 Health Survey: Manual and Interpretation Guide*. Boston: Nimrod Press;1993.
6. Bjorklund L. The Bone and Joint Decade 2000–2010: inaugural meeting 17 and 18 April 1998, Lund, Sweden. *Acta Orthop Scand* 1998(suppl) 281:67–80.
7. The bone and joint decade 2000–2010 for prevention and treatment of musculo-skeletal disorders. Lund, Sweden, April 17–18, 1998. Proceedings. *Acta Orthop Scand* 1998(suppl) 281:1–86.
8. Drummond MF, McGuire A, ed. *Economic Evaluation in Health: Merging Theory with Practice*. Oxford: Oxford University Press; 2001.
9. Gold MR, Siegel JE, Russell LB, et al., ed. *Cost-Effectiveness in Health and Medicine*. New York: Oxford University Press; 1996.
10. Korthals-de Bos I, van Tulder M, van Dieten H, et al. Economic evaluations and randomized trials in spinal disorders: principles and methods. *Spine* 2004;29:442–448.
11. Frymoyer J, Duret C. The economics of spinal disorders. In: Frymoyer JW, ed. *The Adult Spine: Principles and Practice*. Philadelphia: Lippincott–Raven; 1997:143–150.

12. Gobel H. [Epidemiology and costs of chronic pain syndromes exemplified by specific and unspecific low back pain]. *Schmerz* 2001;15:92–98.
13. Hemmila HM. Quality of life and cost of care of back pain patients in Finnish general practice. *Spine* 2002;27:647–653.
14. Hutubessy RC, van Tulder MW, Vondeling H, et al. Indirect costs of back pain in the Netherlands: a comparison of the human capital method with the friction cost method. *Pain* 1999;80:201–207.
15. Luo X, Pietrobon R, Sun SX, et al. Estimates and patterns of direct health care expenditures among individuals with back pain in the United States. *Spine* 2004;29:79–86.
16. Maniadakis N, Gray A. The economic burden of back pain in the UK. *Pain* 2000;84:95–103.
17. Pai S, Sundaram LJ. Low back pain: an economic assessment in the United States. *Orthop Clin North Am* 2004;35:1–5.
18. van Tulder MW, Koes BW, Bouter LM. A cost-of-illness study of back pain in the Netherlands. *Pain* 1995;62:233–240.
19. Maetzel A, Li L. The economic burden of low back pain: a review of studies published between 1996 and 2001. *Best Pract Res Clin Rheumatol* 2002;16:23–30.
20. Andersen CK, Søgaard J, Gyrd-Hansen D. [Hvad koster ryg- og bevægeapparatslidelser samfundet og "kasserne"]. Odense Universitet, Odense, 1996.
21. Cherkin DC, Deyo RA, Loeser JD, et al. An international comparison of back surgery rates. *Spine* 1994; 19:1201–1206.
22. Fritzell P, Hagg O, Jonsson D, et al. Cost-effectiveness of lumbar fusion and nonsurgical treatment for chronic low back pain in the Swedish Lumbar Spine Study: a multicenter, randomized, controlled trial from the Swedish Lumbar Spine Study Group. *Spine* 2004;29:421–434.
23. Efron B, Tibshirani RJ. *An Introduction to Bootstrap*. New York: Chapman and Hall; 1993.
24. Willan AR, O'Brien BJ. Sample size and power issues in estimating incremental cost-effectiveness ratios from clinical trials data. *Health Econ* 1999;8:203–211.
25. Skouen JS, Grasdal AL, Haldorsen EM, et al. Relative cost-effectiveness of extensive and light multidisciplinary treatment programs versus treatment as usual for patients with chronic low back pain on long-term sick leave: randomized controlled study. *Spine* 2002;27:901–909.
26. Moffett JK, Torgerson D, Bell-Syer S, et al. Randomised controlled trial of exercise for low back pain: clinical outcomes, costs, and preferences. *BMJ* 1999;319:279–283.
27. Goossens ME, Rutten-Van Molken MP, et al. Health economic assessment of behavioural rehabilitation in chronic low back pain: a randomised clinical trial. *Health Econ* 1998;7:39–51.
28. The Danish National Board of Health [database and e-publication on the Internet]. The Danish National Board of Health: Casemix.int. c2004. [Cited Aug. 19, 2004]. Available from: http://www.sst.dk/Planlaegning_og_behandling/DRG/Takster aspx?lang=da.
29. Organisation for Economic Co-operation and Development. Purchasing Power Parities and Real Expenditures—1999 Benchmark Year. OECD Report 7, 2002.
30. The Danish National Health Insurance Board [Takstkortoversigt]. The Danish National Health Insurance Board, The Danish National Board of Health, 2002.
31. Eriksen J, Jensen MK, Sjogren P, et al. Epidemiology of chronic non-malignant pain in Denmark. *Pain* 2003;106:221–228.
32. Woolf AD, Pfleger B. Burden of major musculoskeletal conditions. *Bull World Health Organ* 2003;81:646–656.
33. Christensen FB, Laurberg I, Bunger CE. Importance of the back-cafe concept to rehabilitation after lumbar spinal fusion: a randomized clinical study with a 2-year follow-up. *Spine* 2003;28:2561–2569.
34. Soegaard R, Christensen FB, Lauerberg, I, et al. Lumbar spinal fusion patients' demands to the primary health sector: evaluation of three rehabilitation protocol: a prospective randomized study. *Eur Spine J* 2005, June 4.
35. Brooks R. EuroQol: the current state of play. *Health Policy* 1996;37:53–72.
36. The Swedish Council on Technology Assessment in Health Care) Back pain. *Int J Technol Assess Health Care* 2000;16:929–943.
37. Andersson GB. Epidemiological features of chronic low-back pain. *Lancet* 1999;354:581–585.
38. WHOSIS [database on the Internet]. World Health Organization (WHO): WHO Statistical Information System (WHOSIS). [cited Aug. 9, 2004]. Available from: http://www3 who int/whosis.
39. Larsen J, Skjoldborg US. Comparing systems for costing hospital treatments: The case of stable angina pectons. *Health Policy* 2004;67:293–307.

23

Video-Assisted ALIF with Cage and Anterior Plate Fixation for L5-S1 Spondylolisthesis

S. Aunoble, D. Hoste, B. Bley, Y. Basso, L. Villet, F. Liquois, P. Donkersloot, and J. C. Le Huec

Anterior lumbar interbody fusion (ALIF) has become a widespread technique since the 1990s, when metallic cages were first used for interbody fusion (1). In comparison with the use of autologous bone grafts (2–6), the use of interbody fusion cages has improved fusion rates and clinical results (7). The anterior approach prevents epidural fibrosis and posterior muscle damage, and it can help prevent adjacent level disease after spinal fusion (8).

However, an increased rate of pseudarthrosis is associated with the use of a stand-alone anterior lumbar interbody fusion technique because the cage provides insufficient initial stability. In those cases, posterior stabilization can be added (9–12). Most certainly in patients with isthmic spondylolisthesis, complementary posterior fixation can be helpful in achieving fusion. The combination of anterior plate fixation and an interbody fusion cage provides better vertebral stabilization (13). The latter approach permits a single-stage surgery with improved fusion rates.

We report on the clinical and radiographic results in a series of 20 patients with an isthmic spondylolisthesis at the level L5-S1 of Grade 0 or 1 according to the classification of Meyerding. All patients were operated by means of an anterior retroperitoneal video-assisted approach (14). In every case, we used an interbody fusion cage and the Pyramid anterior plate fixation (Medtronic USA).

MATERIALS AND METHODS

We performed a prospective study on 20 patients, who underwent anterior lumbar interbody fusion at spinal level L5-S1. Patients were operated between February 2001 and March 2003. The Medtronic Sofamor Danek (Memphis, TN, USA) materials: Pyramid anterior plate, combined in 15 cases with a Union cage and in five cases with a Lordotec cage. Autologous bone graft from the iliac crest was used in all cases.

The patients were 11 women and nine men with a mean age of 44 years and 2 months (range 31 to 65 years). All suffered from single-level L5-S1 degenerative disc disease. They complained of chronic, severe low back pain resistant to conservative treatment for more than 6 months. All patients had an isthmic spondylolisthesis at the level L5-S1.

Two patients had a medical history of previous posterior decompressive spine surgery, and one patient had a L4-S1 posterior arthrodesis with persistent discogenic pain assessed by a positive provocative discography at the L5-S1 level only. Preoperative magnetic resonance imaging (MRI) revealed Modic type 0 changes in two cases, type 1 in 13 cases, and type 2 in five cases.

Clinical and Radiographic Evaluation Criteria

Clinical data were collected preoperatively, at 6 weeks and at the 6-, 12-, and 24-month postoperative follow-up. Complication analysis includes the intraoperative and immediate postoperative period.

Clinical results were measured by means of the Oswestry Disability Index (ODI) and the visual analogue scale (VAS) for back and leg pain. The appearance of sacroiliac joint pain or posterior facet pain was registered.

At each visit, we obtained plain frontal and lateral radiographs at the L5-S1 level and lateral radiographs of the entire lumbar spine. Fusion was defined as the absence of a peri-implant lucency surpassing more than 50% of the total implant surface, a translation equal to or less than 3 mm, and the absence of implant breakage. Measurements of the L5-S1 intervertebral disc height led to the detection of cage subsidence into the vertebral endplates. Lumbar lordosis at the L1-S1 and L5-S1 level and sacral slope were found, leading to a global lumbar sagittal balance analysis.

Patients were operated by two surgeons (LH and PD). All measurements were performed by an independent surgeon. Radiographs were analyzed and measured by means of a graduated goniometer.

Clinical and radiographic information was stored using the File Marker Pro 5/0 program. The aortocaval bifurcation positioning and feasibility of an anterior approach were indicated by means of angio magnetic resonance imaging (MRI) performed in every patient.

In the procedure, patients are placed in supine position with slight hyperlordosis and the legs spread. Autologous bone harvesting is performed through a mini-incision on the left iliac crest.

A horizontal, left paramedial incision of about 8 cm is chosen. The anterior rectus sheath is split vertically, and the muscle is retracted laterally. The rectus muscle is freed from his posterior sheet. The retroperitoneal space is then reached between the fascia transversalis and the peritoneum. The superior anterior iliac spine is palpated. The psoas muscle is identified and retracted. The peritoneal sac is bluntly pushed aside allowing the surgeon to progressively clear out the retroperitoneal working space. A 10-mm cold-light endoscope coupled to a Tri-CCD screen is put in place. Through direct visual and endoscopic control, the left iliac artery and vein are located and dissected. Identification of the left ureter, which is left to the posterior peritoneal sheath, is performed. The peritoneum is further bluntly dissected from the anterior surface of the lumbar spine, being careful not to disturb the superior hypogastric plexus. We continue lateral dissection between the left and right iliac artery and vein, superior dissection ends at the aortic bifurcation. We thus obtain a triangular working space corresponding to the anterior surface of the intervertebral disc. Coagulation of the median sacral vessels is performed. An EndoRing orthostatic valve device is put in place by means of two pins in the L5 vertebral body and one pin in the S1 vertebral body (Fig. 23.1). The anterior longitudinal ligament is opened and discectomy is performed, permitting a release of the disc space and restoration of the intervertebral disc height. Subchondral bone is freshened up and, after trial implant, a definitive interbody fusion cage filled with spongeous autologous bone grafts is put in place. In a final step, the anterior Pyramid plate is applied through double screw fixation in S1 and single screw fixation in L5. Backing out of the screws is prevented

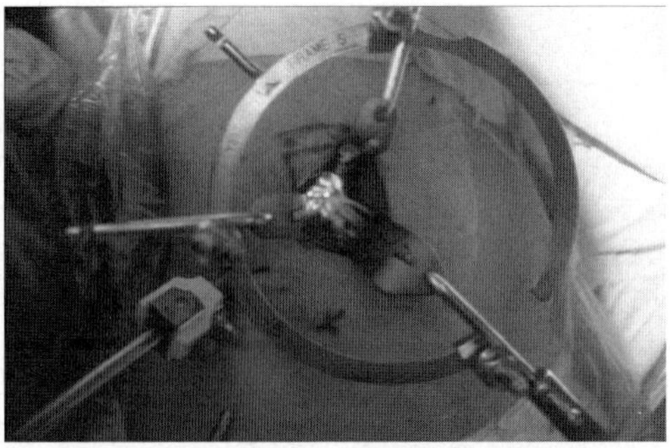

FIG. 23.1. Video-assisted L5-S1 retroperitoneal approach: Per operative view of the operating field.

by a locking plate (Fig. 23.2). The plate is made of titanium; it is triangular with smooth angles and a posterior lip on the back of the plate. This shape fits well in the vessels' bifurcation in the majority of cases as demonstrated with our angio MRI analysis in this series (Fig. 23.3).

The average hospital stay is 5 days. In the postoperative period, no drainage is used. A soft lumbar brace is applied, and the patient can start ambulation the day after surgery. The soft brace is recommended for 6 weeks.

Statistics

Pre- and Postoperative Oswestry Disability Index scores were analyzed using the Student T-test.

RESULTS

Anterior lumbar interbody fusion with cage and anterior plate fixation was feasible in every patient.

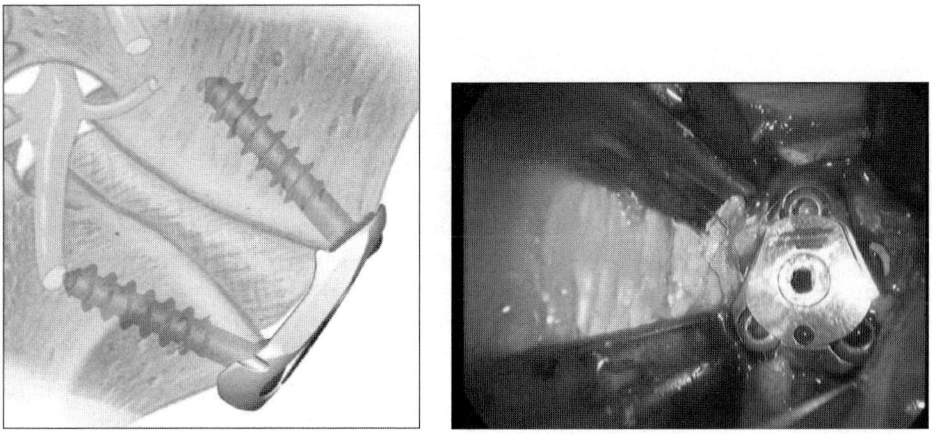

FIG. 23.2. Scheme of the plate on lateral view and per operative view of the plate with screw locking mechanism.

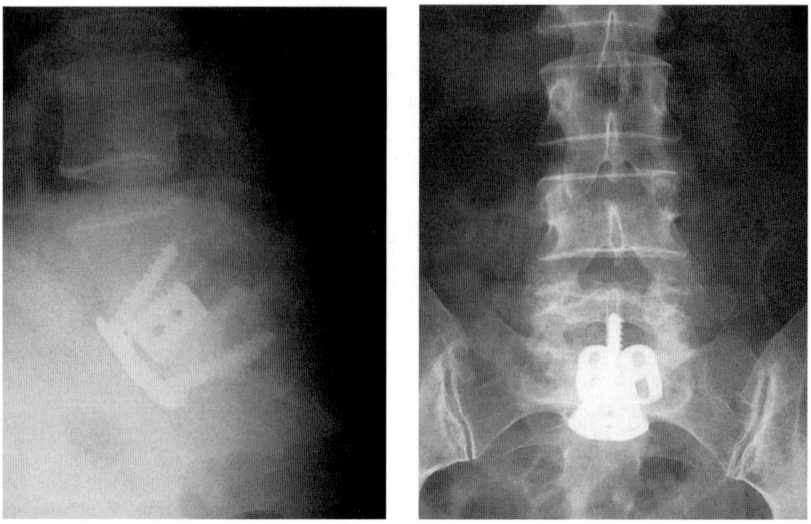

FIG. 23.3. Postoperative AP and lateral radiography of Grade 1 spondylolisthesis operated with anterior lordotic cages and pyramid plate.

Complications

Vascular Complications. One vascular complication was noted. It involves a minor lateral injury to the left common iliac vein. The hole was clipped, and the procedure was continued without further problems. Deep venous thrombosis was not encountered.

No Retrograde Ejaculation. None of the nine male patients suffered from retroejaculation.

Donor Site Problems. One superficial wound infection that necessitated prolonged local aseptic dressings occurred. There were no lesions of the lateral femoral cutaneous nerve. However, a hypoesthesia in the region of the lateral cutaneous nerve was noted in six patients. After 1 year, there was a clear recuperation of sensibility in all patients but one.

Wound Problems. One case of superficial wound dehiscence occurred and was treated with local dressings. Abdominal wall herniation was not seen.

Clinical Results

Mean follow-up was 26.2 months (range 12 to 48 months). All patients but two, who sent us their questionnaires and radiographs by mail, were followed at the outpatient-clinic.

Oswestry Disability Index Score. Mean preoperative score was 57% (range 16% to 82%). With a mean ODI score of 30% at the 6-week follow-up consultation, there was a statistically significant improvement ($p < 0.0001$). At the last follow-up visit, the mean ODI score was 21% (range 0 to 50%). This amelioration is also statistically significant in comparison with the 6-week follow-up scores ($p < 0.05$).

Low Back Pain. Two patients suffered from invalidating chronic low back pain with ODI scores at the last visit comparable to their preoperative score (24% and 46%). The first case is a clear problem of adjacent level disease. The L4–L5 disc was degenerated before the surgery with a black disc without Modic change. This overweight patient has a clear sagittal imbalance with a high incidence angle, and this could be the reason for a higher constraint on the superior level. The second patient had undergone a posterior arthrodesis earlier in his medical history, and he presented with a pseudarthrosis. (See discussion later in the chapter.)

Posterior Facet Pain. Two patients presented with severe posterior facet pain. In both cases, an increase of more than 13 degrees in local lumbar lordosis could be measured on postoperative radiographs. Both patients were helped by fluoroscopic controlled, local corticosteroid infiltrations at the levels L4–L5 and L5-S1, and they had a complete relief of pain at last follow up.

Radicular Pain. Two patients suffered from L5 and/or S1 radicular pain. Both had previous posterior decompressive spine surgery in their medical history and complained preoperatively of similar pain. In one case, the patient described a bilateral sciatica without specific pattern. Nevertheless, that patient's ODI score improved from 82% to 28% after the procedure described here.

Sacroiliac Joint Pain. Two patients complained of sacroiliac joint pain. Treatment consisting of physiotherapy and local anti-inflammatory infiltrations resulted in consistent improvement.

Radiographic Results

The average slippage of 19% was reduced to 5% postoperatively and became stable with time. At the last visit, no hard wear failure or interbody fusion cage subsidence or migration was seen. Only in the case of pseudarthrosis could a clear peri-implant lucency be noted. The two patients suffering from posterior facet pain showed an increase in local L5-S1 lordosis of more than 10 degrees.

The two patients with sacroiliac joint pain demonstrated an undercorrection of a vertical sacrum on pre- and postoperative radiographs. Those two as well as the two patients with low back pain and the two with residual radicular pain each underwent computed tomography (CT), which confirmed solid fusion in every case.

One patient had no pain relief and was reoperated for posterior pedicular screw fixation and grafting. Pseudarthrosis was obvious even after posterior instrumentation and anterior transperitoneal revision was performed with removal of the interbody fusion cage and iliac crest bone graft packing altogether. Propioni bacterium acnes was found and held responsible for the anterior nonunion. The revision surgery together with a prolonged antibiotics treatment was successful and the ODI score at 2 years (1 year after revision) is 18%.

DISCUSSION

Since the work of Crock (15) in 1970, the anterior retroperitoneal approach to the lumbar spine has been well described. The anterior approach has many advantages in comparison with the posterior approach. It offers direct access to the intervertebral disc and permits, by means of a thorough discectomy, the total removal of the chemical and mechanical nociceptive stimulation (16–18).

The anterior approach avoids muscle damage and neurologic risks inherent to the posterior approach. The posterior approach to the spine induces muscle denervation and atrophic changes (19) that can lead to persistent low back pain and prolonged postoperative rehabilitation (20–22).

The development of new technologies has led to the introduction of the concept of minimally invasive spine surgery. At the lumbar level, the anterior approach can be performed in a laparoscopic transperitoneal way (23,24) or in a minimally invasive, video-assisted retroperitoneal way (25). The laparoscopic technique includes an elevated risk of lesions to the upper hypogastric plexus with consequent retroejaculation in the male patient. According to some research papers, this risk accounts for 10% of the cases (26), ranging from 5.1% (27) to 16.2% (28). This laparoscopic technique is also associated with a non-negligible number of open conversions due to inadequate exposure or due to vascular and/or visceral injuries. The latter accounts for 10% to 20% of the cases in the literature (27,29).

The miniopen, video-assisted retroperitoneal anterior approach was first described by Onimus in 1996 (30). The video support permits a mini-incision, and it facilitates the dissection of the front of the lumbar spine. This technique is very well adapted to L5-S1 anterior arthrodesis. In fact, we were always able to gain access to the L5-S1 level, and the cage and anterior plate fixation could always be put in place.

The feasibility of this technique was confirmed by Capellades et al. (31). In a MRI-based study concerning the position of the aortocaval bifurcation, they observed a well-disposed position of the great vessels in relation to the L5-S1 level in 90% of the cases. The use of the endoscope permits a smaller incision and a better illumination of the operating field; the improvement in visualization is important even in obese patients. The endoscope offers better visual control to the surgeon, because at any given moment the endoscope can be reoriented or approached in the operating field.

Few papers report on this video-assisted anterior approach. Brau (32) reports 3.8% severe complications in a total of 686 procedures, of which 242 concern the L5-S1 level. Surgery to the L5-S1 level was in Brau's series always feasible, except in one revision case for posterior cage position. He reports one case of retroejaculation.

Concerning our series, we mentioned one partial lesion to the left common iliac vein (accounting for 3.3% of complications). This partial lesion was clipped by the surgeon, and the procedure was consequently brought to a good end.

Stand-alone ALIF with interbody fusion cage remains a controversial procedure issue in spine surgery. In cases of isthmic spondylolisthesis, an additional fixation is indispensable. Before leading to fusion, an arthrodesis has to be stable over time (34) and in all planes (33). Many authors believe that the stand-alone ALIF procedure doesn't give a satisfying stabilization due to a loss of stability over time (9–11). Kettler et al. (35) and Lund et al. (36) describe a postoperative stability loss as a result of tension loss in the annulus fibers and bone density loss in the adjacent vertebrae, responsible for the subsidence of cages into the vertebral endplates. The stabilization function depends also on the way the cage was brought into place. Oxland and Lund (9) and Rathonyi et al. (10) showed that ALIF is associated with instability in extension. Le Huec et al. (37), in a biomechanical study, demonstrated that lumbar interbody fusion through a lateral approach induces an axial rotation instability. The addition of an anterolateral plate augmented the stability in all plans. In another biomechanical study, Dickman and Le Huec (38) found that the use of an anterior plate in ALIF procedures at the level L5-S1 rendered a significant higher stability in comparison with the stand-alone procedure. This augmented stability was comparable with the use of cage and pedicular screw fixation. Bozkus et al. concluded the same in their study (39). We can conclude that for an optimal stabilization, a complementary act is necessary.

Pedicular screw fixation through a classic posterior approach seems to annihilate all the advantages of the anterior approach. Recently, a percutaneous technique for pedicular screw fixation, called Sextant, was described (40,41). It is an elegant alternative to additional anterior interbody fusion in cases of failure. Nevertheless, this technique involves a second-stage surgery that may be difficult in cases of spondylolisthesis, where access to the pedicles sometimes can be very difficult.

The use of the anterior Pyramid plate is convenient because conflicts with the great vessels can be avoided through its low-profile and triangular contours. Biomechanically, the

Pyramid plate benefits from a very solid cortical anchorage perpendicular to the distraction forces. Finally, there is no need to enlarge the approach for achieving plate fixation.

In a prospective randomized study on 286 patients, Burkus et al. (42) recently showed that the use of stand-alone cage filled with a sponge drenched in rhBMP-2 leads to very high fusion rates. Burkus et al. don't use complementary fixation, and they conclude that the use of corticocancellous autografts is no longer necessary in using a cage with rhBMP-2. Nevertheless, there are no patients with isthmic spondylolisthesis in their series. In our experience we haven't seen any complications in autologous bone harvesting at midterm. We should also mention that, for the moment, the use of bone morphogenetic proteins in daily practice is very difficult due to their elevated cost.

With a minimum follow-up of 1 year, ODI scores improved in 18 of 20 patients. The poorer clinical results seem to be more influenced by the position of the arthrodesis than the technique itself. In fact, during the surgery it is very hard to manipulate the sacrum in relation to the lumbar spine (43), and every nonoptimal lumbosacral position can lead to prolonged postoperative lumbosacral pain. In our study, two patients suffered from posterior facet pain due to increased lumbosacral lordosis. Two patients described sacroiliac joint pain due to increased vertical sacral slope and attempted correction in the sacroiliac joint, which resulted in overcorrection. Finally, there was one patient with clear adjacent level disease. Lumbar sagittal balance was abnormal in this patient.

VAS for back pain significantly improved from 6.5 to 2.7, and VAS for leg pain improved from 6.2 to 3.4. Satisfaction rate was 90%. All active patients, except for two, were back to work at an average of 5.5 months (range 6 weeks to 1 year).

The clinical results are very satisfying but typically seem to be more nuanced in cases of previous posterior spine surgery, psychologic problems, and workers' compensation.

CONCLUSION

In the treatment of low-grade isthmic spondylolisthesis, anterior plate fixation in combination with an interbody fusion cage filled with autologous bone grafts permits an efficient and durable stabilization over time. Results from our series of 20 patients with spondylolisthesis Grade 0 or 1 operated through an anterior, video-assisted, retroperitoneal approach indicate that the approach is a good alternative with a very low complication rate.

At a minimum follow-up of 1 year, following the radiographic criteria chosen, solid fusion at the L5-S1 level was reached in all patients but one. Clinical results are very satisfying. We recommend the use of an interbody fusion cage in combination with anterior plate fixation to achieve lumbosacral arthrodesis through an anterior approach.

REFERENCES

1. Sacks S. Anterior interbody fusion of lumbar spine. *J Bone Joint Surg Br* 1965;47:211–223.
2. Ray CD. Threaded titanium cages for lumbar interbody fusions. *Spine* 1997;22:667–680.
3. Kuslich SD, Ulstrom CL, Griffith SL, et al. The Bagby and Kuslich method of lumbar interbody fusion, history, techniques, and 2-years follow-up: results of a United States prospective, multicenter trial. Spine 1998;23:1267–1279.
4. Hacker RJ. Comparison of interbody fusion approaches for disabling low back pain. *Spine* 1997;22:660–666.
5. Weiner BK, Fraser RD. Spine update: lumbar interbody cages. *Spine* 1998; 23:634–640.
6. Zdeblick TA, Phillips FM. Interbody cage device. *Spine* 2003;28(15S):S2–S7.
7. Vamvaniij V, Fredrickson BE, Thorpe JM, et al. Surgical treatment of internal disc disruption: an outcome study of four fusion techniques. *J Spinal Disord* 1998;11:375-382.
8. Penta M, Sandhu A, Fraser RD. Magnetic resonance imaging assessment of disc degeneration 10 years after anterior lumbar interbody fusion. *Spine* 1995;20:743–747.
9. Oxland TR, Lund T. Biomechanics of stand-alone cage and cage in combination with posterior fixation. *Eur Spine J* 2000;9(suppl 1):S95–S101.

10. Rathonyi GC, Oxland TR, Gerich U, et al. The role of supplemental translaminar screws in anterior lumbar interbody fixation: a biomechanical study. *Eur Spine J* 1998;7(5):400–407.
11. Tencer AF, Hampton D, Eddy S. Biomechanical properties of threaded inserts for lumbar interbody spinal fusion. *Spine* 1995;20(22):2408–2414.
12. Pavlov PW, Spruit M, Havinga M, et al. Anterior lumbar interbody fusion with threaded fusion cages and autologous bone grafts. *Eur Spine J* 2000;9:224–229.
13. Bozkus H, Chamberlain RH, Perez Garza LE, et al. Biomechanical comparison of anterolateral plate, lateral plate, pedicle screws-rods for enhancing anterolateral lumbar interbody cage stabilisation. *Spine* 2004; 29:635–641.
14. Le Huec JC, Aunoble S, Magendie J, et al. Video-assisted anterior approach to the spine. Ed. Elsevier, Surg. Techniques Orthop Trauma, 2003, 55-060-D-10.
15. Crock HV. A reappraisal of intervertebral disc lesions. *Med J Aust* 1970;1:983-989.
16. Kuslich SD, Ulstrom CL, Michael CJ. The tissue origin of low back pain and sciatica. *Orthop Clin North Am* 1991;22:181–187.
17. Mooney V. Where is the pain coming from? *Spine* 1987;12:54–59.
18. Weinstein J, Claverie W, Gibson S. The pain of discographie. *Spine* 1988;13:1344–1348.
19. Olivier CW, Greenough CG. The role of lumbar paraspinal surface electromyography in low back pain. *J Bone Joint Surg Br* 1994;76(suppl):44.
20. Kahanovitz N, Viola K, Gallagher M. Long term strength assessment of postoperative diskectomy patients. *Spine* 1989;14:402–403.
21. Beimborn DS, Morrissey MC. A review of the literature related to trunk muscle performance. *Spine* 1998;13: 655–660.
22. Rantanen J, Hurme M, Falck B, et al. The lumbar multifidus muscle five years after surgery for a lumbar intervertebral disc herniation. *Spine* 1993;18:568–574.
23. Mathews HH, Evans MT, Molligan HJ, et al. Laparoscopic discectomy with anterior lumbar interbody fusion: a preliminary review. 1995;20:1797–1802.
24. Zucherman JF, Zdeblick TA, Bailey SA, et al. Instrumented laparoscopic spinal fusion. *Spine* 1995;20:2029–2035.
25. Mayer HM. A new microsurgical technique for minimally invasive anterior lumbar interbody fusion. *Spine* 1997;22:691–700.
26. Sasso RC, Burkus JK, Le Huec JC. Retrograde ejaculation after anterior lumbar interbody fusion. *Spine* 2003; 28:1023–1026.
27. Regan JJ, Yuan H, McAfee PC. Laparoscopic fusion of the lumbar spine: minimally invasive spine surgery: a prospective multicenter study evaluation open and laparoscopic lumbar fusion. *Spine* 1999;24:402–411.
28. LT-CAGE lumbar tapered fusion device. Memphis, TN: Medtronic Sofamor Danek. PMA Number P970015. FDA application approved September 28, 2000.
29. Liu JC, Ondra SL, Angelos P. Is laparoscopic ALIF a useful minimally invasive procedure? *Neurosurgery* 2002;51(suppl 2):155–158.
30. Onimus M, Papin P, Gongloff S. Extraperitoneal approach to the lumbar spine with video assistance. *Spine* 1996;21(21):2491–4249.
31. Capellades J, Pellise F, Rovira A, et al. Magnetic resonance anatomic study of iliocava junction and left iliac vein positions related to L5-S1 disc. *Spine* 2000;25:1695–1700.
32. Brau SA. Mini-open approach to the spine for anterior lumbar interbody fusion: description of the procedure, results and complications. *Spine J* 2002;2:216–223.
33. Nibu K, Panjabi MM, Oxland T, et al. Multidirectional stabilizing potential of BAK interbody spinal fusion system for anterior surgery. *J Spinal Disord* 1997;10(4):357–362.
34. Moeini SM, Nasca RJ, Lemons JE, et al. Intervertebral spacer as an adjunct to anterior lumbar fusion. *J Spinal Disord* 1998;11(2):129–135.
35. Kettler A, Wilke HJ, Dietl R, et al. Stabilizing effect of posterior lumbar interbody fusion cages before and after cyclic loading. *J Neurosurg* 2000;92(1 suppl):87–92.
36. Lund T, Oxland TR, Jost B, et al. Interbody cage stabilisation in the lumbar spine: biomechanical evaluation of cage design, posterior instrumentation and bone density. *J Bone Joint Surg* 1998;80(2):351–359.
37. Le Huec JC, Liu M, Skalli W, et al. Lumbar lateral interbody cage with plate augmentation: in vitro biomechanical analysis. *Eur Spine J* 2002;11:130–136.
38. Dickman C, Le Huec JC. Biomechanical comparison of anterior plate with interbody cage and four pedicle screws-rods for enhancing lumbar interbody fusion. Orthopaedic Meeting of Salt Lake City, 2001.
39. Bozkus H, Chamberlain RH, Perez Garza LE, et al. Biomechanical comparison of anterolateral plate, lateral plate, and pedicle screws-rods for enhancing anterolateral lumbar interbody cage stabilization. *Spine* 2004;29(6):635–641.
40. Foley KT, Gupta SK. Percutaneous pedicle screw fixation of the lumbar spine. Preliminary clinical results. *J Neurosurg* 2002;97(suppl 1):7–12.
41. Foley KT, Gupta SK, Justis JR, et al. Percutaneous pedicle screw fixation of the lumbar spine. *Neurosurg Focus* 2001;10(article 10):1–8.
42. Burkus JK, Gornet MF, Dickman CA, et al. Anterior lumbar interbody fusion using rhBMP-2 with tapered interbody cages. *J Spinal Disord* 2002;15(5):337.
43. Lazennec JY, Ramare S, Arafati N, et al. Sagittal alignment in lumbosacral fusion: relations between radiological parameter and pain. *Eur Spine J* 2000;9:47–55.

24

Posterior Lumbar Interbody Fusion (PLIF) in Spondylolisthesis

P. Suchomel, P. Barsa, and P. Buchvald

Despite a large number of patients with lumbar spondylolisthesis treated surgically worldwide, it remains controversial whether reduction of the slip is advantageous and what type of fusion offers the best outcome to surgical candidates (1–3).

Good or acceptable results are described for simple posterolateral fusion (4,5), posterior instrumented fusion (6), and anterior and circumferential procedures (7) without slip reduction. The aim of contemporary surgical treatment is, however, not only fusion, but also fusion in physiologic position.

Interbody location has some theoretical advantage over posterolateral fusion. The Wolf law says that osteointegration potential is superior in grafts placed under compression. Interbody position of the bone graft is therefore ideal because the anterior and middle spinal columns bear 80% of the spinal load, compared to 20% borne by the posterior elements. Interbody location further provides 90% of the vertebral osseous contact area; also, the vascular bed, mandatory for osteoinduction, is more abundant in the interbody region. Higher potential to form solid bone mass is not the only advantage of interbody grafts and spacers. They also help to further restore disc space height, optimize sagittal balance, and in some cases also adjust coronal alignment (8–11). Posterolateral fusion has only very limited potential to do this.

The commonest methods of achieving lumbar interbody fusion are anterior lumbar interbody fusion (ALIF) with or without posterior instrumentation and posterior lumbar interbody fusion (PLIF) or transforaminal lumbar interbody fusion (TLIF) supplemented by transpedicular stabilization. Advocates of anterior approach argue that it provides a better anterior column support and a superior contact for osteointegration (11,12). Opponents are defending one-stage posterior surgery with good nerve root decompression and posterior lumbar interbody fusion (13). The type of olisthesis appears to be important in determining both the type of fusion that should be implemented and the desirability of slip reduction. The status of sagittal profile of the lumbopelvic junction seems to be of a major importance in determining the risk of further slip progression (14), especially in cases with insufficiency of the hook and catch posterior retaining mechanism (15). Surgical indication is usually based on intractable pain that has failed to respond to conservative management and/or neurologic deficit in adults. However, in adolescents with dysplastic types of spondylolisthesis, the risk of slip progression can be sufficient to warrant surgical intervention (3–16). Inability to walk or work under load and cosmetic consequences should not be underestimated when considering surgery (17).

We reviewed our series to assess the outcome of different methods with further subgroup analysis of isthmic spondylolisthesis treated with instrumented PLIF and reduction of slip.

MATERIAL AND METHODS

Over a period of 8 years (1994–2002), 113 patients were operated for spondylolisthesis in our department. Isthmic type was present in 63 patients (55.7%), degenerative in 43 patients (38%), and other types in 7 (6.2%). All the patients had indications for surgery following failure of at least 1 year of conservative treatment (with the exception of those with progressive neurologic deficit, who were operated earlier).

Most cases (83) were fused with PLIF: 2 allograft, 13 autograft, 68 Prospace (titanium Plasmapore coated prismatic cage). Autograft ALIF was performed in 29 cases, exclusively in patients with degenerative spondylolisthesis. Posterolateral fusion was performed only once. All cases were instrumented.

A subgroup of 48 patients with Meyerding Grade 1–3 isthmic spondylolisthesis, treated with posterior transpedicular fixation and Prospace cage (Aesculap, Germany) without any bone addition, was analyzed further. Low back pain (93.75%), radiculopathy (95.8%), and neurologic deficit (45.8%) were the most frequent indications for surgery.

SURGERY

Patients were positioned prone on pillow supports on a radiolucent table with slight flexion of the hips and knees. The standard midline posterior approach was used to reach the lower lumbar spine. Prior to introduction of the screw, a one-piece Gills laminectomy was usually performed. The exiting nerve roots were fully decompressed and the medial surface of pedicles clarified. Pedicular screws (6 mm) of a Socon internal fixator (a fixation device manufactured by Aesculap in Germany) were introduced under lateral fluoroscopy and direct visualization of the medial pedicular cortex. Entry points were at the lateral facet surface-transverse process junction in order to avoid upper joint capsule damage. Screws were inserted with appropriate medial angulation and parallel to the upper end plate. Sacral screws were directed slightly obliquely and convergent to the condensed bone in the promontory. In few cases of "hollow sacrum," drilling through promontory bone was necessary.

Connecting clamps and rods were assembled on the screw heads. The spondylolisthesis reduction instrument SRI (Aesculap) was connected to the internal fixator (Fig. 24.1). At the beginning of procedure, a discectomy was performed to facilitate distraction of the collapsed disc space (Fig. 24.2). This was achieved through the application of distractive forces via the adjacent pedicle screws and/or with a Steffee interbody persuader. Further distraction was achieved during slip reduction (Fig. 24.3). A wide decompression enabled the completion of disc material removal as well as control of the stretch of neural elements. In the overdistracted position thus achieved, there is enough space to introduce posterior dowel or cage.

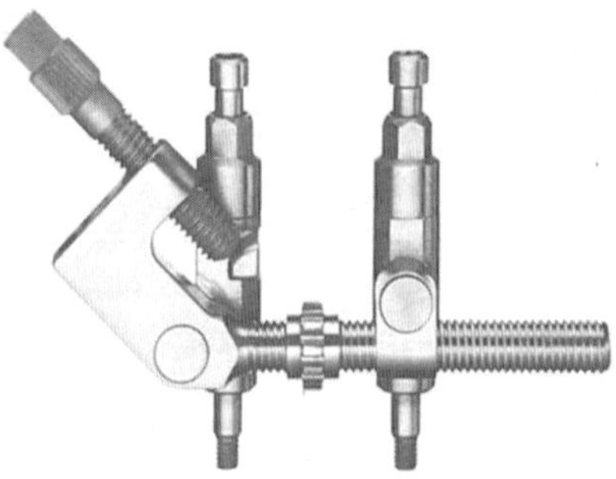

FIG. 24.1. Spondylolisthesis reduction instrument (SRI) (Aesculap).

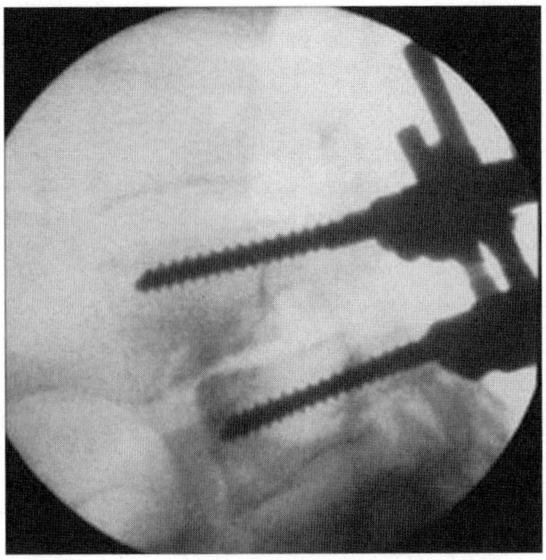

FIG. 24.2. Beginning of distraction by means of pedicular screws and SRI.

Prospace spacers are available as either quadrangular (Fig. 24.4) or lordotic (5 degrees). Asymmetrical lordotic cages are introduced with parallel surfaces and turned to distract the anterior column in target position. Finally, distraction is released without changing the reduction force. The correction of slip angle is then achieved by simple release or by forced compression over the fulcrum of cage. Slight angle corrections with respect to preoperative planning are possible before final tightening of the internal fixator.

On average, patients were mobilized on the second postoperative and discharged from hospital on the ninth postoperative day. External bracing was not used.

FOLLOW-UP AND RESULTS EVALUATION

Data of patients in the study were collected retrospectively. Clinical and radiologic follow-up were conducted immediately after operation, at discharge from hospital and 6 weeks, 6 months, 1 year, and 2 years after the operation. Presence of isodense bony bridges over

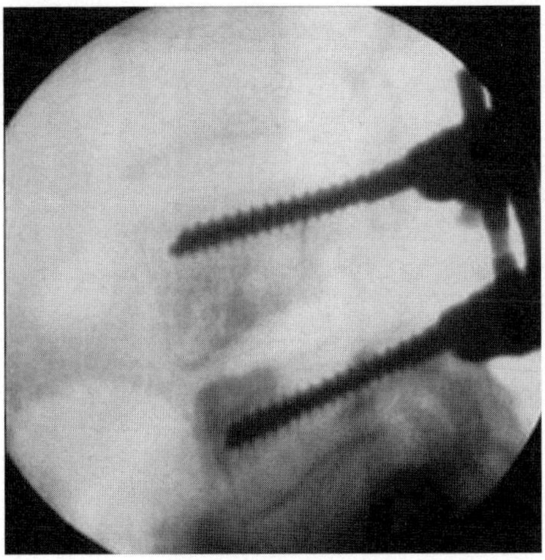

FIG. 24.3. Distracted and reduced L4–L5 spondylolisthesis.

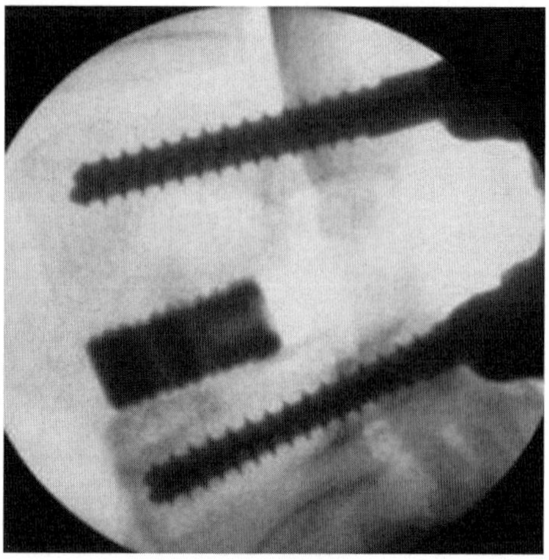

FIG. 24.4. Prospace (Aesculap) spacer in final position.

the implanted motion segment was interpreted as an indicator of fusion. Long-term stability was defined by the absence of segmental movement, no "halo" surrounding the cage and stable implants.

RESULTS

In the analyzed cohort of patients with isthmic spondylolisthesis, a complete reduction was achieved in 43 cases (89.6%). Perioperative complications (dural tear, excessive bleeding, etc.) were present in 8.3%. The infection rate was 2%. Two-year follow-up data was available for 35 (73%) patients. According to Odom criteria, 28 patients (80%) had excellent or good outcome, 5 (14.3%) had no change in clinical status, and 2 were worse. In one case removal of the hardware was required. A complete bony bridging was present in 15 cases, and 18 were stable. The fusion and long-term stability rate was evaluated at 94%.

DISCUSSION AND CONCLUSION

Spondylolisthesis, recognized as an obstacle to labor already in the 18th century, was precisely anatomically described by Rokitanski, a Czech pathologist working at University of Vienna, for the first time in 1839 (18). Kiwisch and Seifert, German physicians working in Prague, used the term spondylolisthesis in 1851, and Kilian in 1854 made this term well known (18).

Naturally, classification attempts arose with increasing knowledge of this pathology. The first classification was offered by Neugebauer in 1888 (18,19). A more comprehensive system was suggested by Newman in 1963 (20) and modified, together with Wiltse, in 1975 (21). Although this classification has been the most commonly used, it was criticized by Marchetti and Bartolozzi (16) for mixing etiologic and anatomical factors and not considering an acquired process on dysplastic background. The latter classification based on etiologic factors is becoming more and more popular, but the Wiltse and Newman system is still widely accepted.

Indications for surgery are usually based on intractable back pain failing conservative treatment, neurologic deficit, and inability to walk for long distances or work under load (1,3,17).

Most of our patients are referred by neurologists and therefore in this cohort, the neurologic deficit appears more prevalent than in other series. Another indication for surgery can include a risk of further slippage, even though the clinical picture may not be so imperative (22,23). This scenario is defined by shear force across the disc space and the capability to resist it. Especially in dysplastic adolescent types, the risk of further slip is approximately 30% (3). The shear is created by impairment of spinopelvic balance and the resistance produced by the "hook and catch" posterior mechanism (14–24).

In our series of patients with isthmic spondylolisthesis (Wiltse), we have included also patients with low dysplastic (Bartolozzi) changes. The balance and pelvic parameters were not routinely measured until 2002. All patients underwent a single-stage procedure via a posterior approach involving a wide decompression, reduction, PLIF, and pedicle screw fixation.

First attempts to reduce spondylolistheses were closed reductions followed by noninstrumented fusions (17). Unsatisfactory results and the discomfort caused by preoperative traction and postsurgical long-term cast immobilization led to the development of internal corrective devices (1,25). The Harrington rods and Lugue instrumentation were not stable enough to retain the corrected positions achieved by ligamentotaxis. Unpredictable reduction range defined by previous mobility of the slip and a high frequency of neurologic complications caused further development of surgical techniques. The discovery of pedicular screws is considered as a breakthrough in the philosophy of spondylolisthesis treatment. René Louis used anterior reduction and transvertebral fusion secured with pedicular system in 1973 (1), but the real posterior reduction bolt screw was developed by Matthias and Heine in 1986 (17) and popularized by Steffee in the late 1980s. Temporary external fixation devices for gradual slip reduction (22) replaced afterward with internal fixation devices were used especially in high-grade slips (12,26,27).

High morbidity rates after multistage operations used so far inspired restrictive indications for reduction (7). Currently available single-level systems simplifying these procedures also popularized the efforts to achieve physiologic alignment of the spine, especially in adolescents, a cohort in which adaptive changes in the entire spine can be expected (11–13).

Slip reduction maneuver has to counteract the forces that have created the deformity. Not only should the translation be reduced but also the height of disc should be restored and the slip angle corrected (14–28). This is possible by gradually applying forces in opposite directions. Three-dimensional adjustability of reduction instrument is necessary to counteract anterior translation, decreased disc height, and kyphotization of slipped vertebra. This goal can be achieved with posterior single-level reduction devices like the SRI, which gives surgeons ability to distract, reduce the slip, and change the slip angle all at once.

According to the literature, posterolateral fusion as a support of instrumentation for spondylolisthesis often fails (11,12,21), and despite the lack of evidence-based data, it seems that interbody fusion (ALIF or PLIF) creates a more reliable form of support through the anterior column. Anterior procedure provides very good fusion results, but it requires a two-stage or second surgery that increases the surgical risks considerably. Posterior procedure with wide decompression has the benefit of being simple, however, and the neural elements can be directly visualized. Results are comparable, especially when cages with higher load-bearing capacity are used.

Morphologic evaluation of fusion can be difficult, and the only definitive fusion criterion available is direct bony bridging of the fused interspace (Fig. 24.5). With metal spacers, this is hard to establish and may take years to become evident. Therefore, other supporting

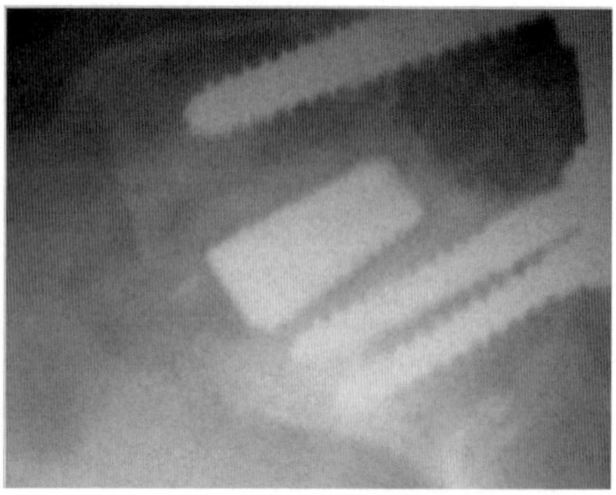

FIG. 24.5. Fusion after 1.5 years.

criteria of good outcome have been developed. These include no segmental movement, no halo around the cage, and stability of implants. This means that radiologic evidence of fusion is not the only outcome criterion, and results should be described in terms of fusion and/or long-term stability.

CONCLUSIONS

In isthmic spondylolisthesis, the nerve roots are predominantly compromised in narrow foramina. Simple distraction or reduction can cause further compression with undesirable neurologic deficit. Removal of fibrous tissue generated in isthmic defect as well as enlargement of foramina is necessary prior to reduction of olisthesis. Extensive posterior nerve root decompression following the removal of lamina is the simplest method of achieving this goal. The created space is usually large enough for introduction of an interbody cage from behind (PLIF) under direct visualization of neural elements. Final compression of interbody implants can be achieved by means of pedicle screw fixation. The slip angle can be adjusted to respect the spinopelvic alignment. In our experience, the above technique with use of titanium cages and no bone addition produces sufficiently effective results in 2-year follow-up.

REFERENCES

1. DeWald RL. Spondylolisthesis. In: Bridwell KH, DeWald RL, ed. *The Textbook of Spinal Surgery*. 2nd edition. Philadelphia: Lippincott–Raven; 1997:1201–1210.
2. Fredrickson BE, Baker D, McHolick WJ, et al. The natural history of spondylolysis and spondylolisthesis. *J Bone Joint Surg Am* 1984;66:699–707.
3. Lonstein JE. Spondylolisthesis in children. *Spine* 1999;24:2640–2648.
4. Ishikawa S, Kumar J, Torres BC. Treatment of dysplastic spondylolisthesis. *Spine* 1994;19:1691–1696.
5. McGuire RA, Amundson GM. The use of primary internal fixation in spondylolisthesis. *Spine* 1993;18:1662–1672.
6. Ricciardi JE, Pflueger PC, Isaza JE, et al. Transpedicular fixation for the treatment of isthmic spondylolisthesis in adults. *Spine* 1995;20:1917–1922.
7. Poussa M, Schlenzka D, Seitsalo S, et al. Surgical treatment of severe isthmic spondylolisthesis in adolescents. *Spine* 1993;18:894–901.
8. Cagli S, Crawford NR, Sonntag VKH, et al. Biomechanics of grade I degenerative lumbar spondylolisthesis. Part 2: treatment with threaded interbody cages/dowels and pedicle screws. *J Neurosurg (Spine 1)* 2001;94:51–60.
9. Crawfors NR, Cagli S, Sonntag VKH, et al. Biomechanics of grade I degenerative lumbar spondylolisthesis. Part 1: in vitro model. *J Neurosurg (Spine 1)* 2001;94:45–50.
10. Cunningham BW, Lewis SJ, Long J. Biomechanical evaluation of lumbosacral reconstruction techniques for spondylolisthesis. *Spine* 2002;27:2321–2327.
11. Harms J, Jeszenszky D, Stolze D, et al. In: Bridwell KH, DeWald LD, ed. *The Textbook of Spinal Surgery*. 2nd edition. Philadelphia: Lippincott–Raven; 1997:1337–1347.

12. Spruit M, Pavlov PW, Leitao J, et al. Posterior reduction and anterior lumbar interbody fusion in symptomatic low-grade adult isthmic spondylolisthesis: short-term radiological and functional outcome. *Eur Spine J* 2002;11:428–433.
13. Klöckner C. Surgery for severe spondylolisthesis and spondyloptosis. *Orthop and Trauma* 2002;1:47–59.
14. Hanson DS, Bridwell KH, Rhee JM, et al. Correlation of pelvic incidence with low- and high-grade isthmic spondylolisthesis. *Spine* 2002;27:2026–2029.
15. Curylo LJ, Edwards C, DeWald RW. Radiographic markers in spondyloptosis. *Spine* 2002;18:2021–2025.
16. Marchetti PG, Bartolozzi P. Classification of spondylolisthesis as a guideline for treatment. In: Bridwell KH, DeWald LD, ed. *The Textbook of Spinal Surgery.* 2nd edition. Philadelphia: Lippincott–Raven; 1997.
17. Edwards CC. Reduction of spondylolisthesis. In: Bridwell KH, DeWald RL, ed. *The Textbook of Spinal Surgery.* 2nd edition. Philadelphia: Lippincott–Raven; 1997;1317–1335.
18. Newell RLM. Spondylolysis: an historical review. *Spine* 1995;20:1950–1956.
19. MacNab I. Spondylolisthesis with an intact neural arch: the so-called pseudo-spondylolisthesis. *J Bone Joint Surg Br* 1950;32:325–333.
20. Newman PH. The etiology of spondylolisthesis. *J Bone Joint Surg Br* 1963;45:39–59.
21. Wiltse LL, Newman PH, MacNab I. Classification of spondylolisis and spondylolisthesis. *Clin Orthop* 1976;117:23–29.
22. Boos N, Marchesi D, Zuber K, et al. Treatment of severe spondylolisthesis by reduction and pedicular fixation. *Spine* 1993;18:1655–1661.
23. Dick WT, Schebel B. Severe spondylolisthesis: reduction and internal fixation. *Clin Orthop* 1988;(232):70–79.
24. Hu SS, Bradford DS, Transfeldt EE, et al. Reduction of high-grade spondylolisthesis using Edwards instrumentation. *Spine* 1996;21:367–371.
25. Abdu WA, Wilber RG, Emery SE. Pedicular transvertebral screw fixation of the lumbosacral spine in spondylolisthesis. *Spine* 1994;19:710–715.
26. Gaines RW. The l5 vertebrectomy approach for the treatment of spondyloptosis. In: Bridwell KH, DeWald RL, ed. *The Textbook of Spinal Surgery.* 2nd edition. Philadelphia: Lippincott–Raven; 1997;1357–1370.
27. Luk KDK, Chow DHK, Holmes A. Vertical instability in spondylolisthesis. *Spine* 2003;28:819–827.

25

Treatment of Adult, Low-Grade, Isthmic Spondylolisthesis: What Is the Evidence?

A. W. J. Vreeling, W. C. H. Jacobs, and M. de Kleuver

Low-grade isthmic spondylolisthesis in adults occurs in approximately 5% of the population and is frequently a relatively benign disease entity. The degree of anterior slippage in isthmic spondylolisthesis can be rated using four grades, according to Meyerding (1), but the relation between the degree of listhesis and the level of complaints such as low back pain and sciatica remains somewhat unclear. For example, in a considerable number of asymptomatic patients, the spondylolytic defect and associated slip are discovered during routine x-rays taken for other reasons. This is one of the reasons why specific treatment for isthmic spondylolisthesis is still not completely clarified.

WHAT ARE THE THERAPEUTIC OPTIONS?

Some patients can benefit from conservative treatment including physical therapy, braces, or pain medication. With regard to surgical treatment there are several different options, of which posterolateral fusion with instrumentation is generally considered to be the gold standard of treatment. Table 25.1 lists some of the most common procedures with some of the positive and negative aspects of each treatment, respectively.

Because of the many controversies regarding the optimal treatment strategy, a systematic review of the literature was performed, which is reported in this chapter. The aim of the study was to determine which surgical technique provides the best clinical and radiologic outcome in adult patients with low-grade lumbar isthmic spondylolisthesis. A secondary aim was to find out for each of the fusion techniques described what the clinical and radiologic results were, what degree of reduction of the spondylolisthesis was achieved with the procedure and what loss of this correction occurred postoperatively. Of further interest were the lordotic angles before and after the surgical procedure, adjacent segment degeneration, as well as associated complications.

METHODS

To obtain all the relevant literature, we used a sensitive search in the most common databases of published literature: the Cochrane Database of randomized controlled trials (2004 issue 1), Current Contents (1996 to March 2004), Medline (through PubMed; 1966 to March 2004), and Embase (through March 2004).

The search strategy was adopted for the different databases. We made no restrictions on language or date. From the articles that were selected, the references were screened for further articles.

TABLE 25.1. *Some of the most common procedures with some of the positive and negative aspects of each treatment*

Treatment	Theoretical and practical considerations
Uninstrumented posterolateral fusion	Simple and safe No support of anterior column No reduction of slip possible Possibility of higher risk of pseudoarthrosis
Instrumented posterolateral fusion	No anterior column support Reduction possible Expensive implants
Posterolateral instrumented fusion with posterior lumbar interbody fusion (PLIF)	Good anterior column support Stable construction Technically difficult Possibility of more neurologic complications Expensive
Posterolateral instrumented fusion with anterior lumbar interbody fusion (ALIF) (Fig. 25.2)	Good anterior column support Stable construction Few neurologic complications Two operative procedures needed Expensive
Direct decompression (Gill procedure)	Addresses root pain only Destabilizes the spine

All articles were selected by two independent reviewers. The selection was not blind but during selection of the titles and abstracts, the rest of the information was masked. The articles were selected on basis of title and abstract with the following criteria:

The intervention(s) used had to include at least one surgical intervention. Type of instrumentation used, the performance of a decompression, and the possible intention to reduce the listhesis had to be stated in the article. Some studies did not mention all of these minimal criteria. These studies were included but were used as a separate group in the best evidence synthesis.

The indication for surgery had to be adult low-grade (Grade 1 and 2, or <50%) isthmic spondylolisthesis at one lumbar level that did not respond to conservative treatment. The study population had to include a minimum number of 10 patients. When the isthmic spondylolisthesis group was a subgroup (<95%) of a study population, results for this subgroup had to be given.

Outcome parameters had to be a radiologic, clinical, or functional measure. For example, the 36-item Short-Form Health Survey (SF-36), Western Ontario MacMaster (WOMAC), or Oswestry Disability Index (ODI) questionnaires; pain scores; accomplished fusion rates; and complications. The selected articles had to be published in peer-reviewed journals.

METHODOLOGIC QUALITY ASSESSMENT

The methodologic quality of the selected articles was assessed by the same two independent reviewers and was scored according to the criteria described by van Tulder (3,4) and by Cowley (5).

ANALYSIS

For evidence on the best treatment available, only the randomized controlled trials (RCTs) found in the search were used. Best evidence synthesis was performed stratified for studies meeting at more than 50% as opposed to those meeting 50% or less of the

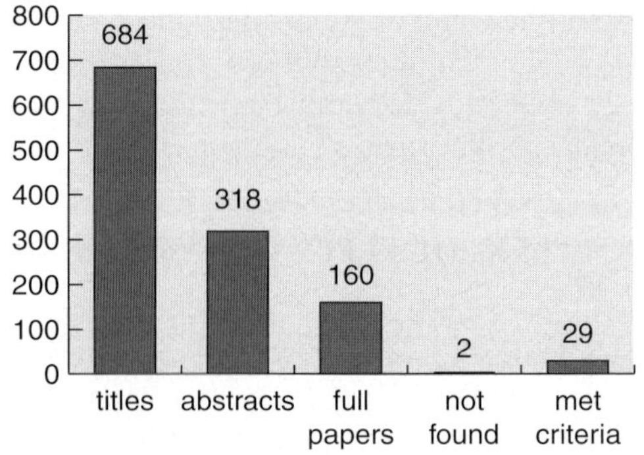

FIG. 25.1. Search results.

quality criteria on the van Tulder list. Evidence regarding the effect of the treatments found was based on the nonrandomized studies.

RESULTS

Search Results

The database searches yielded 684 articles, of which eventually only 29 articles could be included in the present review (Fig. 25.1). Most articles were excluded because it was clear from the title or abstract that the topic of the article was not relevant to the objective of the review. Others were excluded because the type of spondylolisthesis was not appropriate or was unknown, no subgroup results were given, the report did not contain original data, or the study included fewer than 10 patients. Eight studies were prospective RCTs that were used for the best surgical treatment analysis.

The results for outcome after surgical treatment were based on the remaining 21 noncontrolled studies, which included 24 patient groups. Among these were 4 prospective consecutive studies and 17 retrospective studies divided in 11 consecutive and 6 nonconsecutive

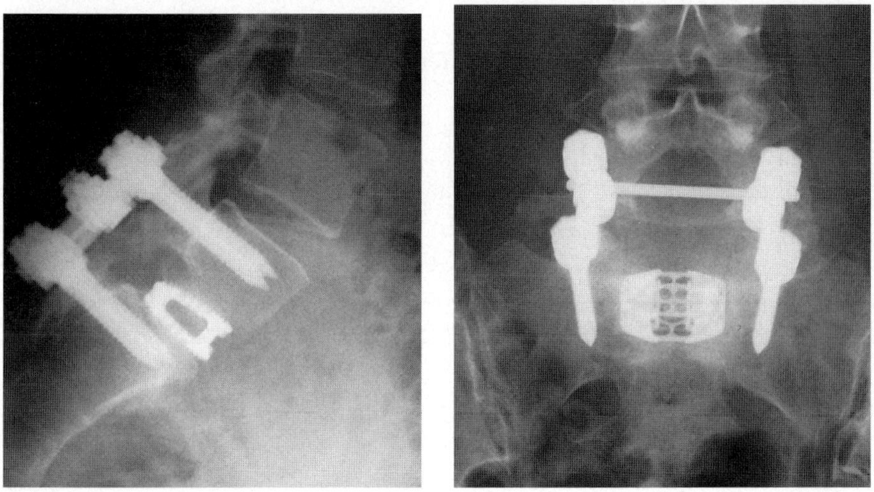

FIG. 25.2. Posterolateral instrumented fusion with ALIF.

studies. Three of the noncontrolled studies included a control group, but no effort was made to match the study groups on any variable, so these study groups are analyzed as separate patient groups. Of these 21 noncontrolled studies, 5 studies with 7 patient groups fulfilled the criteria of adequate treatment information and consecutive patient selection.

METHODOLOGIC QUALITY OF INCLUDED STUDIES

According to the van Tulder criteria, only 4 of the 8 randomized trials were rated as a "high quality" study. High quality according to the Cowley criteria was awarded to only two of the five noncontrolled studies.

THE BEST SURGICAL TREATMENT

The eight RCTs were used to determine which treatment could be considered the best surgical treatment. They all evaluated the effect of different techniques of posterolateral fusion. The role of instrumentation was investigated in four studies. Reduction of the listhesis was not used by McGuire (6) and France (7). It is unclear whether reduction of the listhesis was used in the studies by Moller (8) and Thomsen (9). The two studies from Moller (8) and Thomsen (9) were available for the best evidence synthesis.

In performing this best evidence synthesis, only the fusion rates can be compared. This is because items such as clinical outcome and complications are not reported for the isthmic spondylolisthesis subgroup by Thomsen (9).

The fusion rate in posterolateral fusion for the *non*instrumented group compared to the instrumented group was higher in both the Moller study (8) (78% vs. 65%) and Thomsen (9) 84% vs. 73%). The results were, however, not significant (Table 25.2).

Posterolateral fusion (PLF) combined with other modifications were compared in four studies (Table 25.3). These studies showed no beneficial effect of the addition of ALIF (10), decompression (11), or osteogenic protein (12). Evidence that PLF was superior to exercise alone was found in the article by Moller (13), but according to the methodologic criteria that paper is rated as a low-quality study.

OUTCOME AFTER SURGICAL TECHNIQUES

The 21 noncontrolled case series included 24 patient groups. Clinical outcome results and fusion rates were different for the different treatment protocols (Table 25.3). Posterolateral fusion was used in 15 groups.

Not all procedures intended to reduce the listhesis. Three studies reported adequately the preoperative, postoperative, and follow-up percentage of slip and lordotic angles (14–16). All three studies used posterolateral fusion. The average reduction achieved was

TABLE 25.2. *Posterolateral fusion with or without instrumentation*

Study	N	Decompression	Reduction	Clinical outcome – instr.	Fusion – instr.
Moller and Hedlund (8)	41/39	Mixed	?	66 vs. 83%	78% vs. 65%
Thomsen et al. (9)	19/16	Mixed	?	NR (subgroup)	84% vs. 73%
McGuire and Amundson (6)	14/13	Yes	N	NR	72% vs. 78%
France et al. (7)	11/16	?	N	63 vs. 62%	NR (subgroup)

NR, not reported.

TABLE 25.3. *Other comparisons*

Study	N	Postinstrumentation	Decompression	Reduction	Clinical outcome	Fusion
Carragee (11) PLF – decompression	8/12 10/12	Yes No	Random Random	No No	75% vs. 100% 60% vs. 91%	88% vs. 100% 70% vs. 100%
Johnsson et al. (12) PLF – OP1	10/10	No	No	No	80% vs. 70%	60% vs. 80%
Moller and Hedlund (8) PLF mix vs. exercise	77/34	Mixed	Mixed	Mixed	74% vs. 43%	NR
Christensen et al. (10) PLF instrumentation – ALIF	24/19	Yes	Mixed	Yes	n.s. (subgroup)	n.s. (subgroup)

NR, not reported.
n.s., not significant.

12.3%; average loss of reduction at follow-up was 5.9%. One study reported that the reduction was maintained at follow-up (17).

Preoperative lordotic angles were too heterogeneous to pool the results. None of the 29 publications reported degeneration of adjacent segments. Not all articles reported adequately the number of complications. Those that did contained a wide variety of complications such as neurologic symptoms, instrument failure, and infections (Table 25.4).

DISCUSSION

Isthmic spondylolisthesis is not uncommon and can cause complaints such as low back pain and sciatica. Many different options are available including conservative and surgical treatment. The goal of surgical intervention is to achieve pain reduction by a solid fusion between the vertebra affected. This fusion can be achieved through a posterior, anterior, or combined approach. Supplementary instrumentation, decompression, or reposition of the listhesis can be considered.

Theoretical advantages of supplementary pedicle screw fixation are the ability to correct the deformity and to reduce the listhesis. The rigid fixation is expected to give better fusion rates.

TABLE 25.4. *Complications*

Treatment (N)	Clinical outcome good or excellent	Fusion rate	Complications	
			Neurologic	Other
PLF (378) 12 cohorts, 0 good Q	60%–98%	81%–100%	5	20 screw complications 13 infections
ALIF (186) 8 cohorts, 0 good Q	85%–94%	47%–90%	7	1 infection 24 other
PLIF (174) 3 cohorts, 1 good Q	45%	80%–95%	23	1 infection 18 other
Endoscopic foraminal decompression alone 1 good Q cohort	79%	NA	—	2 revisions

NA, not available.

Disadvantages include the extra costs, a more extensive surgical trauma, and the risk of neurologic complications because of misplaced pedicle screws. Besides, it has been speculated that rigid fixation may increase the pseudoarthrosis rate because of stress-shielding.

These phenomena all have been studied extensively, and results have been published in many articles. The results are very inconsistent, however, and no systematic review of the literature has been available. Therefore, this systematic review of the literature was performed.

To determine the best treatment available, only RCTs were reviewed. We were unable to identify the best surgical treatment for adult low-grade isthmic spondylolisthesis. Posterolateral fusion was the most studied, but it could not be proven to be superior or inferior to a circumferential fusion. Supplemental decompression, osteogenic protein-1 (OP1), or instrumentation could not be shown to be superior, and some results suggest that all three are in fact inferior to PLF alone.

Some studies with control groups were identified, but these could not be used as controlled trials because there was no report on any attempt being made to match the patient groups. Consecutive patient selection or sufficient information about the treatments applied was no selection criteria for the RCTs because the randomization process maintains an equal distribution among the groups whatever the criteria has been.

For the outcome after surgical treatment, we used nonrandomized studies with consecutive patient selection. We did not include the results from the RCTs in this analysis because the rigorous selection criteria usually applied in RCTs can produce selection bias in the results, and therefore, RCTs do not allow for a valid assessment of treatment outcomes and complication rates in general.

A weak point about the noncontrolled studies is that, although they may mention consecutive patient selection, they usually include patients indicated for a certain treatment ("consecutive treatment selection"). When there are multiple treatment options available, a preceding selection process has allocated patients to treatments according to their diagnosis. Although the studies may mention consecutive patient selection, they might be applying some form of bias. Ideally, all patients with a certain diagnosis should be included.

A critical note can be placed by this present study, therefore, allowing for the possibility of selection bias in these consecutive treatment series when assessing the outcome after surgical treatment.

The intention of the review was to perform a meta-analysis. This was not possible because of the heterogeneity of the treatments used.

Despite a relatively large number of studies available (eight RCTs and five adequate cohorts), we could not determine the best treatment or outcomes of different surgical techniques. This is partly due to the poor quality of the studies. However, another reason is the large number of confounding variables with respect to individual patients, such as degree of neurologic compromise and individual lumbopelvic parameters (18). These factors all influence outcome, and given the available numbers of patients in spine surgery, they will always disturb the results. Surgical treatment continues to be based on empirical data, the surgeon's preference, and the individual patient's characteristics. Hard scientific evidence is still not available.

CONCLUSIONS

Implications for Practice

Posterolateral fusion appears to be the generalized gold standard for the treatment of adult isthmic low-grade lumbar spondylolisthesis. This is the case although there is not much scientific evidence to support this choice. One randomized trial has shown superior results for PLF as compared to conservative treatment (exercises). Supplemental to PLF, there is still no evidence to support the use of posterior instrumentation. Decompression has not proven to be necessary (and may be detrimental) but may be used in the clinical setting in case of root pain.

The role of sagittal alignment and the related possible benefits of reduction (and therefore also instrumentation) of the listhesis have not been adequately studied. This is immensely important, as these factors may be confounding variables that have made it impossible for us to determine the optimum surgical treatment strategy, and they may well influence long-term outcome.

Implications for Research

Based on this study, we recommend that an RCT be conducted comparing the following three surgical interventions:

1. Uninstrumented PLF without reduction (control group)
2. Reduction with modern instrumented PLF
3. Reduction with modern instrumented PLF with anterior column support.

ACKNOWLEDGMENTS

We would like to thank Dr. R. Schrijnemakers and the Dutch Cochrane Centre for assisting in the literature search.

REFERENCES

1. Meyerding HW. Spondylolisthesis. *Surg Gynec Obstet* 1932;54:371–378.
2. Scaduto AA, Gamradt SC, Yu WD, et al. Perioperative complications of threaded cylindrical lumbar interbody fusion devices: anterior versus posterior approach. *J Spinal Disord Tech* 2003;16(6):502–507.
3. van Tulder MW, Assendelft WJ, Koes BW, et al. Method guidelines for systematic reviews in the Cochrane Collaboration Back Review Group for Spinal Disorders. *Spine* 1997;22(20):2323–2330.
4. van Tulder M, Furlan A, Bombardier C, et al. Updated method guidelines for systematic reviews in the Cochrane Collaboration back review group. *Spine* 2003;28(12):1290–1299.
5. Cowley DE. Prostheses for primary total hip replacement: a critical appraisal of the literature. *Int J Tech Assess Health Care* 1995;11(4):770–778.
6. McGuire RA, Amundson GM. The use of primary internal fixation in spondylolisthesis. *Spine* 1993;18(12):1662–1672.
7. France JC, Yaszemski MJ, Lauerman WC, et al. A randomized prospective study of posterolateral lumbar fusion. Outcomes with and without pedicle screw instrumentation. *Spine* 1999;24(6):553–560.
8. Moller H, Hedlund R. Instrumented and noninstrumented posterolateral fusion in adult spondylolisthesis: a prospective randomized study: part 2. *Spine* 2000;25(13):1716–1721.
9. Thomsen K, Christensen FB, Eiskjaer SP, et al. 1997 Volvo Award winner in clinical studies. The effect of pedicle screw instrumentation on functional outcome and fusion rates in posterolateral lumbar spinal fusion: a prospective, randomized clinical study. *Spine* 1997;22(24):2813–2822.
10. Christensen FB, Hansen ES, Eiskjaer SP, et al. Circumferential lumbar spinal fusion with Brantigan cage versus posterolateral fusion with titanium Cotrel—Dubousset instrumentation: a prospective, randomized clinical study of 146 patients. *Spine* 2002;27(23):2674–2683.
11. Carragee EJ. Single-level posterolateral arthrodesis, with or without posterior decompression, for the treatment of isthmic spondylolisthesis in adults: a prospective, randomized study. *J Bone Joint Surg Am* 1997;79(8):1175–1180.
12. Johnsson R, Stromqvist B, Aspenberg P. Randomized radiostereometric study comparing osteogenic protein-1 (BMP-7) and autograft bone in human noninstrumented posterolateral lumbar fusion: 2002 Volvo Award in clinical studies. *Spine* 2002;27(23):2654–2661.
13. Moller H, Hedlund R. Surgery versus conservative management in adult isthmic spondylolisthesis: a prospective randomized study: part 1. *Spine* 2000;25(13):1711–1715.

14. Markwalder TM, Saager C, Reulen HJ. "Isthmic" spondylolisthesis: an analysis of the clinical and radiological presentation in relation to intraoperative findings and surgical results in 72 consecutive cases. *Acta Neuro Wien* 1991; 110(3–4):154–159.
15. Kaneda K, Satoh S, Nohara Y, et al. Distraction rod instrumentation with posterolateral fusion in isthmic spondylolisthesis. 53 cases followed for 18–89 months. *Spine* 1985;10(4):383–389.
16. Suk SI, Lee CK, Kim WJ, et al. Adding posterior lumbar interbody fusion to pedicle screw fixation and posterolateral fusion after decompression in spondylolytic spondylolisthesis. *Spine* 1997;22(2):210–219.
17. Spruit M, Pavlov PW, Leitao J, et al. Posterior reduction and anterior lumbar interbody fusion in symptomatic low-grade adult isthmic spondylolisthesis: short-term radiological and functional outcome. *Eur Spine J* 2002; 11(5):428–433.
18. Labelle H, Roussouly P, Berthonnaud E, et al. Spondylolisthesis, pelvic incidence, and spinopelvic balance: a correlation study. *Spine* 2004;29:2049–2054.

26

Progression and Surgical Management of Isthmic Spondylolisthesis in Adults

Yizhar Floman

Although isthmic spondylolisthesis is often referred to as a congenital anomaly, it is well documented that spondylolysis usually evolves long after birth; between the ages of 5 and 8 years, and that the development of spondylolisthesis may begin up to the age of 20 years (1). Spondylolisthesis is present in about 6% of the population aged 20 years (2). A stress or a fatigue fracture through the pars interarticularis is probably the basic lesion leading to the development of isthmic spondylolisthesis (3). Despite the fact that the condition usually originates before adulthood, only 23% of children and adolescents are symptomatic; among the 23% are especially those with high-grade slips (4). Many adults are unaware of their spondylolisthesis until the fourth or fifth decade of life (5). If spondylolisthesis is a lesion that characteristically develops in late childhood or adolescence and seldom after the age of 20 years, why is this lesion clinically silent in early adulthood, and why does it become symptomatic after the third or fourth decade? What is the mechanism that leads this dormant lesion in the lumbar spine to manifest itself, and what is the best surgical solution for symptomatic adult isthmic spondylolisthesis? These questions will be addressed throughout the following chapter.

The intervertebral disc and the posterior elements, including the facet joints and the spinal ligaments, all play an important role in stabilizing the spinal motion segment. The facet joints determine the direction of movement of the spinal motion segment, whereas the intervertebral disc determines the extent of motion. Anterior translatory motion is mainly resisted by the paired facet joints, the pars interarticularis, and the intervertebral disc (6). The vertical sum of the forces affecting the spine results in 80% anterior column compression and 20% anteriorly directed shear forces (7).

In the presence of a bilateral pars interarticularis defect, spondylolisthesis occurs as a result of anterior shear forces acting parallel to the disc space at the slip level. There are higher anterior shear forces at the lumbosacral junction due to the obliquity of the L5-S1 disc. Because of the pars defect, the facet joints are no longer able to resist the anterior shear forces, and the intervertebral disc becomes the main structure resisting these forces and maintaining the stability of the spinal motion segment. As long as the disc retains its normal biochemical and biomechanical properties, the spinal motion segment will remain stable, despite the presence of mild slip and the loss of the resistance to anterior shear forces that is normally provided by the facet joints.

Although Friberg (8) contended that adult isthmic spondylolisthesis is hypermobile and unstable, several in-vivo radiologic studies have demonstrated Grade 1 to 2 isthmic lumbosacral spondylolisthesis in adults as being stable (9–11). Penning and Blickmann (9) studied sagittal plain motion in 24 individuals with lumbosacral spondylolisthesis who underwent radiography in various positions. No abnormal sagittal translatory motion at the lumbosacral level was detected in any of the x-rays taken. Pearcy and Shepherd (10) used biplanar radiography to study symptomatic patients with Grade 1 to 2 lumbosacral olisthesis and found decreased motion at the lumbosacral level in flexion, extension, lateral bending, and axial rotation as well as in coupled motions. They detected no forward or backward translation greater than 2 mm; they also noted that translation in persons with symptomatic lumbosacral olisthesis was not larger than translation occurring in a healthy control group. The only significant difference between olisthetic individuals and controls was a decrease in flexion and extension at the lumbosacral level. Pearcy and Shepherd (10) therefore questioned the contention that mild adult lumbosacral spondylolisthesis is mechanically unstable. However, they could not rule out the role of muscle splinting in providing mechanical stability to the lumbosacral slip. More recently, Axelsson et al. (11) studied adult patients with mild spondylolisthesis and matched controls by means of roentgen stereophotogrammetry, which is the most accurate radiographic method currently available for measuring intervertebral motion. They failed to find any difference in the sagittal or vertical axis motion between the spondylolisthetic individuals and the controls. The transverse translatory motion was negligible in both groups (11). Thus, three independent radiographic investigations attested to the stability of adult low-grade isthmic spondylolisthesis (9–11).

The fate of mild isthmic spondylolisthesis in individuals who sustain major trauma to the lumbar spine may also attest to the stability of this lesion. Since isthmic lumbosacral slip occurs in about 6% of the population, it is not uncommon for some of these individuals to sustain a traumatic lumbar vertebral fracture. The incidental occurrence of lumbar spine fractures in individuals with preexisting mild lumbosacral slip may be considered as being a simulated in-vivo biomechanical experiment that tests the stability of lumbosacral spondylolisthesis. Seven such cases were retrieved among 300 patients with thoracolumbar spine fractures who were managed during a 10-year period at one institution (12). All seven patients had a Grade 1 spondylolisthesis; five had sustained a lumbar burst fracture, and two had a lumbar compression fracture. The lumbosacral slip in all of them was judged to be old, preexisting the lumbar fracture, as evidenced either by a positive previous history of a slip, by dating the lesion with a 99 m-Tc-MDP bone scan, or by operative findings at the slip level. No evidence was found in any of these seven cases to indicate that the lumbosacral slip was affected by the major lumbar trauma. These cases serve to illustrate that a lumbosacral spondylolisthesis can absorb vertical compression forces as well as considerable anterior shear forces without demonstrable evidence of damage. This in-vivo "experiment" sheds some light on the biomechanics of mild lumbosacral olisthesis and lends support to the notion that mild olisthesis is mechanically stable.

What then are the sources of back and leg pain in adults with mild or moderate lumbosacral spondylolisthesis? Symptoms are usually the results of disc degeneration or herniation above the slip level, or a result of disc degeneration at the slip level (i.e., the lumbosacral level). It is reasonable to assume that the integrity of the disc at the slip level plays a key role in the stability of the lumbosacral articulation in the presence of a bilateral pars defect. As long as this disc maintains its structural and functional integrity, the lumbosacral articulation will be stable and will not generate painful stimuli, while its degeneration will eventually lead to adult slip progression. As the slip increases, anterior shear forces will increase as well, leading to further disc degeneration and further slip progression. Slip progression generates painful stimuli of instability and associated spinal stenosis (5).

Until recently, there has been little mention in the literature of progression of lumbosacral spondylolisthesis in adults (5). On the contrary, while slip progression before

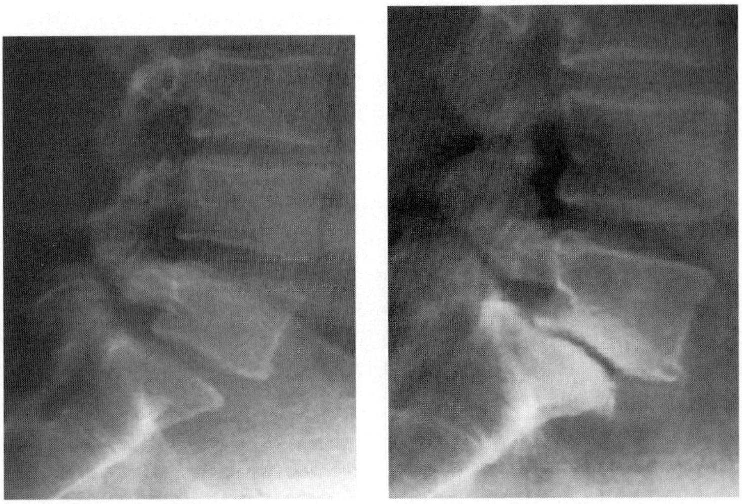

A B

FIG. 26.1. A: Lateral x-ray of the lumbar spine in a 34-year-old man. Note the isthmic spondylolisthesis at the L5-S1 level. **B:** Same patient at age 47. Note the disc degeneration at the L5-S1 level and the increase in the amount of vertebral slip.

skeletal maturity has been adequately recorded, its occurrence in adults has been questioned (13–15). Slip progression in adults does occur, however (Figs. 26.1 and 26.2). Floman (5) reported on the progression of isthmic spondylolisthesis after skeletal maturity in 21 patients between the ages of 32 and 60 years. Documented slip progression ranged between 8% and 30% and occurred over a period of 3 to 20 years. In most cases, slip progression started after the age of 30 years. The increased olisthesis was always associated with degenerative disc disease at the slip level. Disc degeneration increased anterior shear forces, giving rise to increased olisthesis. Unlike lumbosacral adult slip

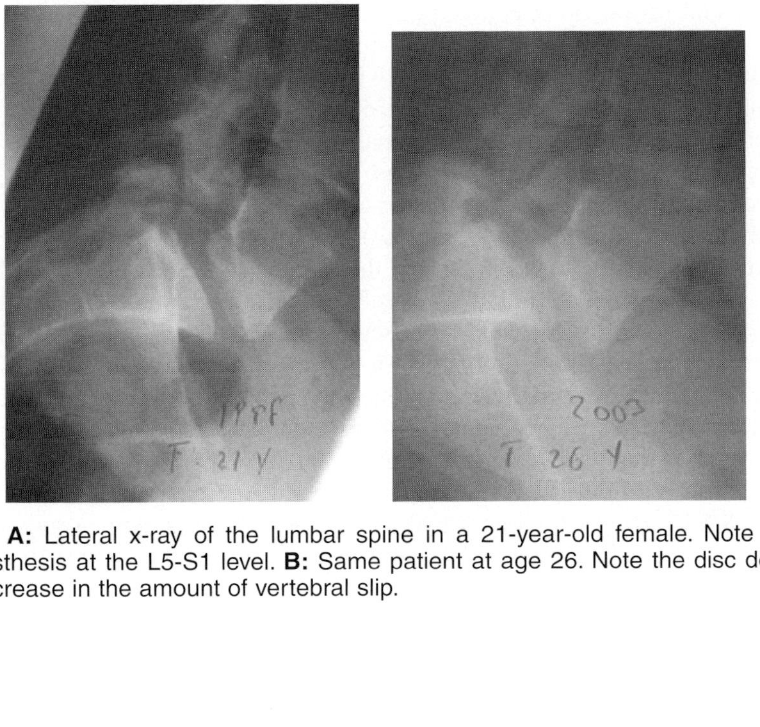

A B

FIG. 26.2. A: Lateral x-ray of the lumbar spine in a 21-year-old female. Note the isthmic spondylolisthesis at the L5-S1 level. **B:** Same patient at age 26. Note the disc degeneration and the increase in the amount of vertebral slip.

progression, progression of L4–L5 isthmic olisthesis in adult life is better documented in the literature (15).

Ample evidence in the literature suggests that disc degeneration is the key to converting a stable spondylolisthesis into an unstable, progressing slip. The classical teaching was that disc degeneration and herniation occur at the level above the slip (16). It was Farafan et al. (17) who correctly stressed that disc degeneration below the pars defect occurred as a result of rotatory and anteriorly directed shear forces. Disc degeneration at the slip level may start as early as adolescence (18). Sarasta (19) found that spondylolisthesis was associated with disc degeneration, especially after the age of 40 years and that slip increase was associated with disc degeneration. Fredrickson et al. (20) as well as Danielson et al. (21) conducted research on long-term follow-up of spondylolisthesis and concluded that the disc had an important role in buffering the instability imposed by the anterior shear forces and the pars defect.

In conclusion, the concurrent occurrence of adult slip progression and disc degeneration at the slip level explains how an asymptomatic developmental lesion may become symptomatic (5). Although nonoperative treatment should always be tried first, operative treatment for symptomatic isthmic spondylolisthesis in adults was shown to be superior to physiotherapy (22,23). It remains unclear, however, which surgical strategy should be adopted, because there is limited scientific evidence to guide decision-making.

PATIENTS, METHODS, AND RESULTS

Between January 1999 and November 2003, the author operated on 25 adult patients with symptomatic lumbar or lumbosacral isthmic slip; the patients' ages ranged between 28 and 62 years (average 47 years). Spondylolisthesis was present at the L5-S1 level in 21 patients and at the L4–L5 level in 4 patients. One patient had spondylolisthesis at both the L4–L5 and L5-S1 levels. Two patients had a Grade 1–2 slip, 15 had Grade 2, seven had Grade 3, and one had Grade 3–4 slip.

Nine patients underwent posterior decompression with pedicle screw instrumentation and posterolateral fusion, an operative plan reserved for patients who had mild to moderate slips with marked disc space narrowing. Thirteen patients underwent posterior decompression and pedicle screw fixation with the addition of posterior lumbar interbody fusion (PLIF) or transforaminal lumbar interbody fusion (TLIF), an operative strategy reserved for slips with relatively preserved disc space height and for cases where slip reduction was performed (10 patients) (Figs. 26.3 and 26.4). Three patients underwent decompression and fixation with sacral transdiscal screw fixation ending in the L5 body, an approach reserved for patients who had moderate slips accompanied by advanced degenerative changes with complete loss of the disc space height.

At a mean follow-up of 32 months (range 16 to 64 months), x-rays revealed no evidence of instrumentation failure or frank pseudarthrosis. Patient outcome was excellent in 13 patients (marked pain relief, no need for treatment, and return to work status), good in 10 patients (significant pain relief, occasional medication intake), and unchanged or poor in 2 patients. The mean preoperative Oswestry Disability Index (measured in 11 patients) was 49 and dropped to 12 after surgery (range 0–30). The mean preoperative visual analog scale (VAS) for back pain was 7.3 and dropped to 1.6 after surgery (range 0–3). The mean preoperative VAS for leg pain was 8 and dropped to 1 after surgery (range 0–4). One patient had a transient foot drop and another had a wound infection that resolved with antibiotic treatment.

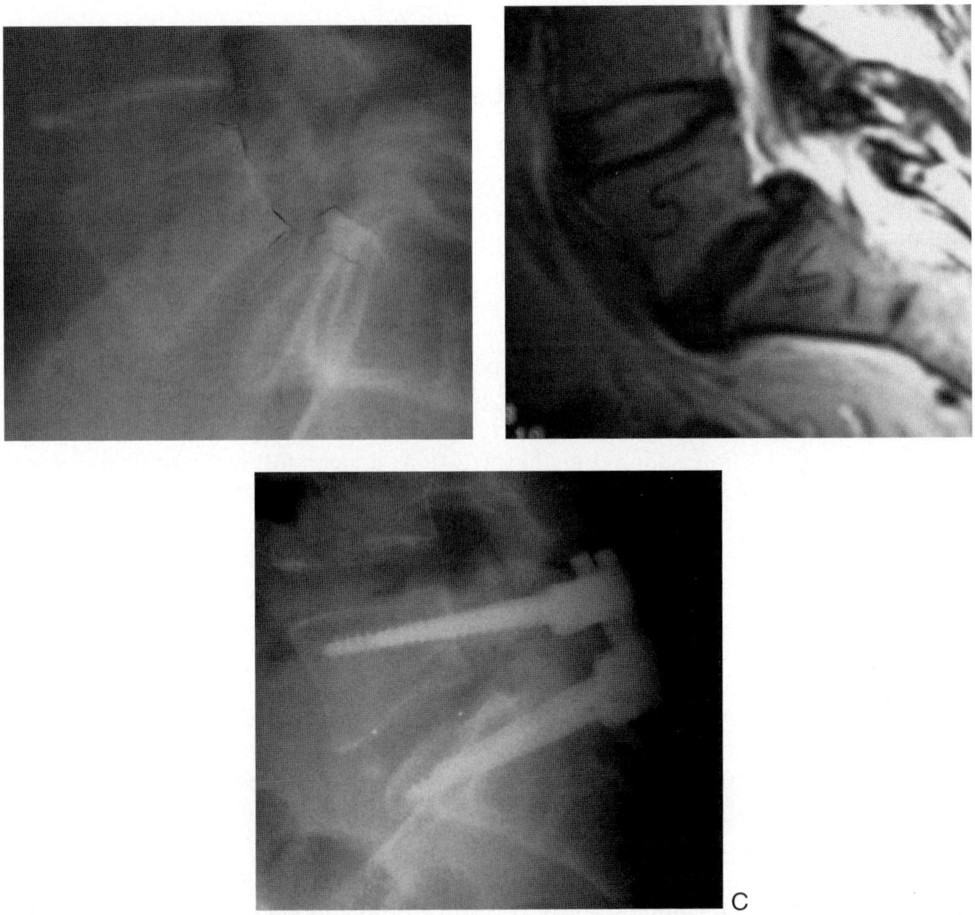

A B C

FIG. 26.3. A: Lateral x-ray of the lumbar spine in a 31-year-old male with symptomatic isthmic spondylolisthesis at the L5-S1 level. **B:** Sagittal T2 MRI. Note the disc degeneration at the slip level. **C:** Same patient after fixation with VSP and Brantigan cage.

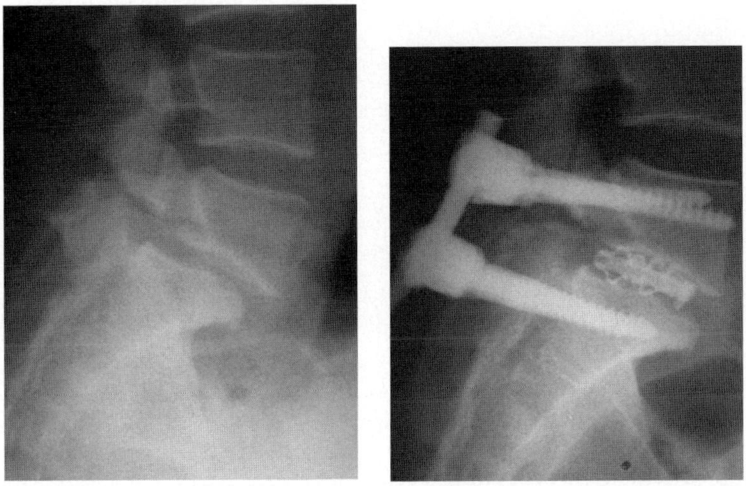

A B

FIG. 26.4. A: Lateral x-ray of the lumbar spine in a 40-year-old female with symptomatic isthmic spondylolisthesis at the L5-S1 level. **B:** Same patient after slip reduction and fixation with SOCON instrumentation and B-Twin TLIF cage.

DISCUSSION

Moller and Hedlund (22) conducted a randomized prospective clinical trial and reported a high success rate of in-situ posterolateral fusion in adults with low-grade slips. One hundred eleven patients were randomly allocated to either an exercise program or posterolateral fusion. At a minimum 2-year follow-up, the patients who underwent surgical fusion had statistically superior results on both the Disability Rating Index and the visual analog scale (22). Moller and Hedlund (22) concluded that posterolateral fusion is a method supported by evidence-based medicine standards to reduce back pain and functional disability in adult isthmic spondylolisthesis. They also reported that the results of noninstrumented fusion were as good as those attained with instrumentation (23). Ekman et al. recently published the long-term results of posterolateral fusion in adult patients with isthmic spondylolisthesis (24). At a mean follow-up of 9 years (range 5 to 13 years), the global assessment was significantly better for the surgical group than for the nonoperated group. Specifically, 76% of the surgical group were "much better" compared to only 50% of the control group ($p = 0.015$). Gill's decompression was carried out in two thirds of the patients reported by Moller and Hedlund (all with sciatic pain) both in the noninstrumented and the instrumented groups (personal communication). This author's own experience using decompression and fusion to treat adult isthmic spondylolisthesis is similar. In contrast, Carragee (25) considers it to be futile to perform decompressive laminectomy in adults who have mild isthmic slip without neurologic signs since it does not improve the clinical outcome and may increase the rate of pseudarthrosis following noninstrumented spondylodesis. He adds, however, that combining decompressive laminectomy with pedicular screw fixation will provide better clinical results (25). Carragee's experience echoes earlier reports that decompression is not always mandatory in patients with radicular pain; posterolateral fusion alone will often eliminate radicular symptoms (26,27). The absolute indications for decompression in spondylolisthesis are symptomatic radiculopathy with motor deficit or sphincteric involvement.

There are numerous operative procedures for the surgical management of adult isthmic spondylolisthesis. Posterior fusion with or without decompression and with or without instrumentation, lumbar interbody fusion (anterior or posterior), and circumferential fusion have all been reported (25,27–30). For example, Verlooy et al. (31) prospectively studied 20 adult patients with low-grade isthmic spondylolisthesis who underwent PLIF without posterior instrumentation. Only 45% of the patients obtained an excellent or good clinical result at a mean follow-up period of 41 months. Ishihara et al. (29) studied 23 patients with isthmic spondylolisthesis who underwent anterior lumbar interbody fusion. The union rate was 83% at a mean follow-up period of 10 years. Even patients with solid fusion showed evidence of some loss of slip reduction and disc space height. The results of the latter two studies (29,31) clearly show that posterior instrumentation is probably important in obtaining a 90% rate of good to excellent clinical results, and that stand-alone PLIF and anterior lumber interbody fusion (ALIF) are not adequate surgical solutions.

There is a lack of objective evidence to indicate which is the best surgical technique. Kwon et al. (32) recently conducted a critical analysis of the literature dealing with the surgical treatment of adult isthmic spondylolisthesis and concluded that circumferential fusion probably provided the best clinical results. Indeed, combined anterior lumbar interbody fusion and posterolateral instrumentation and fusion have been reported to provide a good clinical outcome (28). The main drawback of the combined approach, however, is that it necessitates two separate surgical procedures. In addition, a major concern in young adult males is that the anterior approach can result in retrograde ejaculation.

By performing PLIF or TLIF with posterior instrumentation, the surgeon can achieve nerve root decompression and slip reduction if desired with a single posterior surgical approach. Brantigan and Neidre (33) studied 36 patients with isthmic spondylolisthesis who underwent PLIF with wedged carbon cages and posterior instrumentation. The authors reported a 97% fusion rate and 94% "clinical success." Madan and Boeree (34) retrospectively compared the outcome of patients with low-grade isthmic spondylolisthesis who underwent either posterolateral fusion or posterior lumbar interbody fusion in combination with posterior instrumentation. They found that posterolateral fusion was associated with a better outcome, although the PLIF group had higher fusion rates and better maintenance of slip reduction. Similarly, La Rosa et al. (35) studied 35 patients with low-grade slips who underwent either posterior fusion alone (18 patients) or in combination with PLIF (17 patients). Although maintenance of disc space height and slip reduction was poorer in the group without PLIF, clinical outcome was similar in both groups.

Is PLIF mandatory, or could unilateral TLIF with posterior instrumentation suffice for obtaining interbody fusion in adult low-grade isthmic spondylolisthesis? TLIF is associated with a lower incidence of postoperative radiculitis and is less time consuming and less expensive (36). Kwon et al. (37) found that TLIF with a Brantigan cage and posterior instrumentation was adequate for restoring disc height and slip reduction. Placing the fusion cage anteriorly could also induce adequate lordosis.

Should slip reduction be considered in low-grade adult isthmic slip? The advantages of slip reduction in conjunction with arthrodesis are numerous and include improved spine biomechanics, better nerve root decompression (usually by an indirect effect of the reduction), and better opportunity to obtain fusion since the fusion is no longer under the influence of tension and anterior shear forces. There are several distinct characteristics of adult low-grade isthmic spondylolisthesis. The slip angle is usually small, and these cases lack typical dysplastic changes, such as a rounded sacrum or trapezoidal L5 body. As a consequence, lumbosacral kyphosis, which is a major problem in high-grade slips, is usually absent in these cases. Slip reduction is therefore feasible and safe, and there is no need to exert powerful corrective forces during its execution. Although it is a controversial issue, even in the pediatric to adolescent age group, slip reduction is feasible and safe in adult patients with isthmic slips.

A transsacral, transdiscal vertebral fixation should be considered in cases of adult isthmic spondylolisthesis with complete loss of the disc space. Transsacral, transvertebral interbody fixation is a modification of the technique described by Smith and Bohlman (38), who performed posterior decompression and posterolateral arthrodesis in addition to the insertion of a fibular graft that was passed from the back of S1 through the L5-S1 disc and into the L5 body. They carried out this procedure successfully on 11 patients, most of them adults with high-grade slips accompanied by neurologic deficit including cauda equina syndrome. Esses et al. (39) and Rocca et al. (40) utilized the same technique with equally successful fusion rates and clinical improvement. In a similar fashion, the spondylolisthetic deformity is fixed in situ by advancing the S1 pedicle screw through the superior sacral end plate through the L5-S1 disc and into the L5 body (41). This approach provides immediate three-column fixation of the lumbosacral junction. It is a good method for salvage of a failed spondylolisthesis fusion and in cases of advanced disc degeneration at the slip level, where reduction is not feasible or is contraindicated. This technique may also allow partial reduction to be combined with transsacral interbody fixation (42,43).

TABLE 26.1. *Surgical options for low-grade adult isthmic spondylolisthesis*

Type of procedure	Advantages	Contraindications
In situ fusion without instrumentation	Technically simple, no "hardware"	If neural decompression is needed, L4–L5 slip
In-situ fusion with posterior instrumentation without interbody fusion	Decompression possible	Well-preserved disc space height at slip level
PLIF or TLIF with pedicular fixation with or without slip reduction	Higher fusion rates Restoration of normal anatomy and spinal alignment with reduction	Osteoporosis
Stand-alone PLIF or ALIF		Probably contraindicated
Transsacral, transdiscal fixation	In cases with complete disc space collapse or in salvage procedures	

SUMMARY

Several distinct characteristics are typical of adult low-grade isthmic spondylolisthesis. Because the slip is usually mild and is not accompanied by dysplastic changes and lumbosacral kyphosis, slip reduction is feasible, safe, and easy to accomplish. It is, however, mandatory to add interbody fusion in the form of PLIF or TLIF. While our clinical results suggest that interbody spondylodesis is a helpful adjunct in the surgical management of adult low-grade isthmic slip, more studies are required to establish an evidence-based consensus approach regarding the role of interbody arthrodesis. It is also important to study the role of in-situ arthrodesis in adults as well as the advantages of slip reduction.

Unlike the unpredictable outcome of arthrodesis in patients with degenerative disc disease, which is influenced by socioeconomic confounders among other factors, the outcome of surgery in adult isthmic spondylolisthesis is much more favorable and predictable. This kind of surgery is highly rewarding because it repairs mechanical instability and local spinal stenosis.

A summary of the surgical options currently available for managing low-grade isthmic spondylolisthesis in adults is provided in Table 26.1.

REFERENCES

1. Baker RD, McHollick W. Spondylolysis and spondylolisthesis in children. *J Bone Joint Surg Am* 1956; 38:933–934.
2. Hensinger RN. Spondylolysis and spondylolisthesis in children. In: Floman Y. *Disorders of the Lumbar Spine*. Rockville, MD: Aspen, 1990:553.
3. Wiltse LL, Widell EH, Jackson DW. Fatigue fracture: the basic lesion in isthmic spondylolisthesis. *J Bone Joint Surg Am* 1975;57:17–22.
4. Lafond G. Surgical treatment of spondylolisthesis. *Clin Orthop* 1962;22:175–179.
5. Floman Y. Progression of lumbosacral isthmic spondylolisthesis in adults. *Spine* 2000;25:342–347.
6. Troup JDC. Mechanical factors in spondylolisthesis and spondylolysis. *Clin Orthop* 1977;117:59–67.
7. Bergmark A. Stability of the lumbar spine: a study of mechanical engineering. *Acta Orthop Scand* 1989; 230(suppl):1–54.
8. Friberg O. Lumbar instability: a dynamic approach by traction-compression radiography. *Spine* 1987; 12:119–129.
9. Penning L, Blickmann JR. Instability in lumbar spondylolisthesis: a radiologic study of several concepts. *Am J Roentgenol* 1980;134:293–301.
10. Pearcy M, Shepherd J. Is there instability in spondylolisthesis? *Spine* 1985;10:175–177.
11. Axelsson P, Johnsson R, Stromqvist B. Is there increased intervertebral mobility in isthmic adult spondylolisthesis? A matched comparative study using roentgen stereophotogrammetry. *Spine* 2000;25:1701–1703.
12. Floman Y, Margulies JY, Nyska M, et al. Effect of major axial skeleton trauma on preexisting lumbosacral spondylolisthesis. *J Spinal Disord* 1991;4:353–358.
13. Laurent LE, Einola S. Spondylolisthesis in children and adolescents. *Acta Orthop Scand* 1964;31:45–64.

14. Fredrickson BE, Baker D, McHollick WJ, et al. The natural history of spondylolysis and spondylolisthesis. *J Bone Joint Surg Am* 1984:66:699–707.
15. Grobler LJ, Wiltse LL. Classification, non-operative and operative treatment of spondylolisthesis. In: Frymoyer JW, ed. *The Adult Spine: Principles and Practice*, 2nd edition. New York: Raven Press; 1997:1865–1921.
16. MacNab I. *Backache*. Baltimore Md: Williams & Wilkins; 1977:51.
17. Farafan HF, Osteria V, Lamy C. The mechanical etiology of spondylolysis and spondylolisthesis. *Clin Orthop* 1976;117:40–55.
18. Haraldsson S, Wilner S. A comparative study of spondylolisthesis in operations on adolescents and adults. *Arch Orthop Traum Surg* 1983;101:101–105.
19. Sarasta H. Long-term clinical and radiological follow-up of spondylolysis and spondylolisthesis. *J Pediatr Orthop* 1987;7:631–638.
20. Fredrickson BE, Baker D, Murtland A, et al. Spondylolisthesis: the natural history age 5–40. Presented at the North American Spine Society meeting. Monterey, CA, 1990.
21. Danielson BI, Frennered AK, Irstam LK. Radiologic progression of isthmic lumbar spondylolisthesis in young patients. *Spine* 1991;16:422–425.
22. Moller H, Hedlund R. Surgery versus conservative treatment in adult isthmic spondylolisthesis: a prospective randomized trial. Part 1. *Spine* 2000;25:1711–1715.
23. Moller H, Hedlund R. Instrumented and non-instrumented posterolateral fusion in adult spondylolisthesis: a prospective randomized study. Part 2. *Spine* 2000;25:1716–1721.
24. Ekman P, Moller H, Hedlund R. The long-term effect of posterolateral fusion in adult isthmic spondylolisthesis: a randomized controlled study. *Spine J* 2005;5:36–44.
25. Carragee EJ. Single-level posterolateral fusion, with or without posterior decompression, for the treatment of isthmic spondylolisthesis in adults: a prospective, randomized study. *J Bone Joint Surg Am* 1997;79:1175–1180.
26. Peek RD, Wiltse LL, Reynolds JB, et al. In situ arthrodesis without decompression for grade III and IV isthmic spondylolisthesis in adults have severe sciatica. *J Bone Joint Surg Am* 1989;71: 62–68.
27. de Loubresse CG, Bon T, Deburge A, et al. Posterolateral fusion for radicular pain in isthmic spondylolisthesis. *Clin Orthop* 1996;323:194–201.
28. Spruit M, Pavlov PW, Leitao J, et al. Posterior reduction and anterior lumbar interbody fusion in symptomatic low grade adult isthmic spondylolisthesis: a short term radiological and functional outcome. *Eur Spine J* 2002; 11:428–433.
29. Ishihara H, Osada R, Kanamori M, et al. Minimum 10-year follow-up study of anterior lumbar interbody fusion for isthmic spondylolisthesis. *J Spinal Disord* 2001;14:91–99.
30. Kim NH, Lee JW. Anterior interbody fusion versus posterolateral fusion with transpedicular fixation for isthmic spondylolisthesis in adults: a comparison of clinical results. *Spine* 1999;24:812–816.
31. Verlooy J, De Smedt K, Selosse P. Failure of a modified posterior lumbar interbody fusion technique to produce adequate pain relief in isthmic spondylolytic grade 1 spondylolisthesis patients: a prospective study of 20 patients. *Spine* 1993;18:1491–1495.
32. Kwon BK, Hilibrand AS, Malloy K, et al. A critical analysis of the literature regarding surgical approach and outcome for adult low-grade isthmic spondylolisthesis. *J Spinal Disord Techn* 2005;18 (suppl 1):S30–S40.
33. Brantigan JW, Neidre A, Toohey JS. The lumbar I/F cage for posterior lumbar interbody fusion with the variable screw placement system: 10-year results of a Food and Drug Administration clinical trial. *Spine J* 2003;3: 186–196.
34. Madan S, Boeree NR. Outcome of posterior lumbar interbody fusion versus posterolateral fusion for spondylolitic spondylolisthesis. *Spine* 2002;27:1536–1542.
35. La Rosa G, Conti A, Cacciola F, et al. Pedicle screw fixation for isthmic spondylolisthesis: does posterior lumbar interbody fusion improve outcome over posterolateral fusion? *J Neurosurg Spine* 2003;99:143–150.
36. Humphreys CS, Hodges S, Pathwadhan AG, et al. Comparison of posterior and transforaminal approaches to lumbar interbody fusion. *Spine* 2001;26:567–571.
37. Kwon BK, Berta S, Daffner SD, et al. Radiographic analysis of transforaminal lumbar interbody fusion for the treatment of adult isthmic spondylolisthesis. *J Spinal Disord Tech* 2003:469–476.
38. Smith MD, Bohlman HH. Spondylolisthesis treated by a single-stage operation combining decompression with in situ posterolateral fusion and anterior fusion. *J Bone Joint Surg Am* 1990;72:415–420.
39. Esses SI, Natout N, Kip P. Posterior interbody arthrodesis with fibular strut graft in spondylolisthesis. *J Bone Joint Surg Am* 1995;77:172–176.
40. Roca J, Ubierna MT, Caceres E, et al. One-stage decompression and posterolateral and interbody fusion for severe spondylolisthesis. *Spine* 1999;24:709–714.
41. Grob D, Humke T, Dvorak J. Direct pediculo-body fixation in cases of spondylolisthesis with advanced intervertebral disc degeneration. *Eur Spine J* 1996;5:281–285.
42. Smith JA, Deviren V, Berven S, et al. Clinical outcome of trans-sacral interbody fusion after partial reduction for high-grade L5-S1 spondylolisthesis. *Spine* 2001;20:2227–2234.
43. Bartolozzi P, Sandri A, Ricci M. One-stage posterior decompression-stabilization and trans-sacral interbody fusion after partial reduction for severe L5-S1 spondylolisthesis. *Spine* 2003;28:1135–1141.

27

Surgical Treatment of Degenerative Spondylolisthesis: Simple Decompression without Fusion

Gianluca Cinotti

Degenerative spondylolisthesis (DS) is a complex condition characterized by the forward slipping of a lumbar vertebra with an intact posterior arch. It can be asymptomatic and thus not require any treatment, or it can cause a wide spectrum of symptoms including low back pain, radicular pain, or both.

Surgical treatment of degenerative spondylolisthesis includes simple decompression, simple fusion, or decompression plus fusion. The latter, in recent years, has been considered the treatment of choice of DS since several studies have shown that higher percentages of satisfactory results are reported when fusion is added to decompression (1–6). Although it is certainly true that, overall, fusion increases the percentages of satisfactory results in patients with this condition, it is the author's opinion that the surgical treatment of DS should vary according to the clinical and radiologic findings and that simple decompression should be considered a possible option in selected patients with DS. The rationale for this assumption is based on several findings: (a) early studies showed that high percentages of patients submitted to simple decompression reported satisfactory results (7,8); (b) after decompression and fusion, high percentages of satisfactory results were also reported by patients with pseudarthrosis (4–9) probably meaning that decompression, rather than fusion, was the necessary treatment in these patients; (c) it is widely reported that fusion increases the perioperative and postoperative morbidity, operative time, need for blood transfusion, and risks for degenerative changes at adjacent levels (10,11). Therefore, if there are patients with DS for whom simple decompression may be successful, to add fusion should be considered an overtreatment. Last, and possibly most important, a manifest spinal instability, which requires fusion, is not always present in DS.

SPINAL INSTABILITY IN DS

Spinal instability is defined as the loss of the ability of the spine to maintain its pattern of displacement under loads with subsequent nerve compression, deformity, or pain. According to this, DS should be considered a condition of spinal instability. However, the degree of instability present in DS and whether such an instability is about the same in any patient with this condition are still open questions. The uncertainty on these issues is increased by the fact that the criteria to be used to detect an instability in the degenerated spine are still controversial.

Historically, radiologic and clinical criteria have been used to diagnose spinal instability. Radiologic criteria include flexion-extension radiographs and, more recently, computed tomography (CT) and magnetic resonance imaging (MRI) under axial loading. The latter may provide information on the degree of vertebral slipping occurring during standing, but the clinical relevance of the results needs further clarification.

The results of flexion-extension radiographs in DS patients have been reported using defined parameters to diagnose abnormal vertebral motion (12). The olisthetic vertebra was found to show abnormal angular motion in 48% of cases, abnormal sagittal translation in 48%, and both in 37%. However, it was also found that about one third of patients with DS (31%) showed vertebral motion within normal values.

Clinical symptoms related to spinal instability in DS include postural and standing low back pain. Radicular pain may also be present on standing or walking although, in DS patients, this symptom is more likely to be related to spinal stenosis than to spinal instability. The severity of low back pain may vary remarkably in each patient. It may be the predominant symptom, it can be equal to radicular pain, or it can be mild or even absent. It is extremely important to investigate carefully the presence and severity of low back pain, particularly in patients in whom flexion-extension radiographs do not show any evident hypermobility of the olisthetic vertebra. In these cases, in fact, the presence of low back pain may be the only finding suggesting that an occult spinal instability is present.

In general, the majority of patients with DS complain of low back pain with or without radicular pain. However, a minority of patients (about 20% to 30%) complain of radicular pain with no, or mild, low back pain.

In conclusion, even considering the known limitations in detecting spinal instability, there are clinical and radiologic findings suggesting that about one third of DS patients do not show evidences of manifest spinal instability.

SPINAL INSTABILITY IN DS AFTER DECOMPRESSION

Many surgeons advocate fusion for patients with DS, even if low back pain is not present preoperatively, because surgical decompression will increase spinal instability to such an extent that low back pain will be present postoperatively. There are no studies, however, supporting this statement.

Johnsson et al. reported the results of patients with DS submitted to wide laminoarthrectomy without fusion (13). They found that olisthesis was increased after surgery in 65% of cases but that this did not affect the surgical outcome. In other studies in which decompression was accomplished through less invasive surgical procedures, a progression of vertebral slipping was found in 0% to 32% of cases (14–16). However, in none of these studies did the progression of olisthesis influence the clinical result.

In general, the degree of instability after surgery is related to the extension of decompression and, to a lesser extent, to the orientation of the facet joints.

The extension of decompression depends on the amount of excision of the facet joints, lamina, and posterior ligaments. However, biomechanical studies have shown that only the degree of facet joint resection and the preservation (or not) of the posterior ligaments influence spinal stability after surgery (17). Therefore, the surgeon should try to preserve these anatomical structures as much as possible, keeping in mind that this should not compromise the effectiveness of decompression, which is the main goal of surgery. On the other hand, if the surgeon feels that a wide decompression is needed to free the nerve roots, it would be better to perform such a wide decompression along with spinal fusion rather than to risk a persistence, or recurrence, of symptoms due to a too narrow opening of the spinal canal.

On these grounds, the extension of decompression should be related to the type and severity of stenosis. The latter, in patients with DS, may involve the lateral portion of the spinal canal (on one side or bilaterally) or the central portion of the spinal canal. In both cases, stenosis can be mild, moderate, or marked. In patients with lateral stenosis and in those with mild central stenosis, decompression of the nervous structures can be performed adequately by undercutting the anterior portion of the facet joints through a bilateral or unilateral laminotomy preserving the posterior ligaments. Instead, in patients with central stenosis, particularly of moderate-marked degree, a total laminectomy is usually necessary to free the nerve roots. A marked olisthesis, which is not frequent in DS, often requires a central laminectomy since the nervous structures may also be compressed by the anterior slipping of the posterior vertebral arch, which should be removed together with the anteromedial portion of the facet joints.

In conclusion, decompression in DS may be performed through a total laminectomy, in case of moderate-severe central stenosis, or through a unilateral or bilateral laminotomy, in case of lateral stenosis or mild central stenosis. Since biomechanical and clinical studies (17,18) have shown that laminotomy, by avoiding the division of the interspinous and supraspinous ligaments, preserves spinal stability to a greater extent than central laminectomy, simple decompression is indicated when the nervous structures may be adequately free through a unilateral or bilateral laminotomy. When a central laminectomy is necessary, spinal fusion should be associated to decompressiom to avoid a symptomatic instability after surgery.

DS WITH ASSOCIATED CONDITIONS

It is not rare to find DS patients showing associated conditions at the olisthesic level, including disc herniation and, even more frequently, synovial cyst of the posterior joints. These conditions may be asymptomatic or be responsible for radicular pain rather than low back pain. In particular, they may increase a previously mild-moderate radicular pain or render symptomatic a previously asymptomatic DS. In the latter event, particularly if a herniated disc is present, the patient often complains of clinical symptoms that suggest the presence of a disc herniation rather than a DS.

In any case in which the associated condition is clearly responsible for the onset of symptoms, i.e., the DS was, per se, asymptomatic, it is indicated to remove the associate condition through a unilateral laminotomy without performing a concomitant fusion.

However, if a relevant low back pain was present before surgery or a wide discectomy has to be performed, it is better to inform the patient that a unilateral or a bilateral fusion will probably be needed.

OPERATIVE TREATMENT

Whatever support is used, the patient should be positioned on the operative table so that the abdomen is maintained free during the operation in order to avoid compression of large abdominal vessels and reduce intraoperative bleeding.

As previously reported, laminotomy should be the procedure of choice when simple decompression has been planned. If the surgeon feels that a wide laminectomy is needed, simple decompression is not indicated.

Laminotomy can be performed unilaterally or bilaterally, depending on the clinical symptoms. Usually, if radicular pain is unilateral, decompression can be performed on the symptomatic side and there is no need for a preventive decompression on the asymptomatic contralateral side. Once the interlaminar space has been exposed, a fenestration of the spinal canal is performed preserving the spinous process with the supraspinous and intraspinous ligaments. The ligamentum flavum, which can be normal or hyperthrophic, is then removed and the dural sac exposed. Partial facetectomy is carried out to free the emerging nerve root which may be compressed by the superior and/or inferior facet joint. The extension of facetectomy varies depending on the severity of stenosis. Usually, in the presence of moderate-severe central stenosis both the inferior and superior facets should be extensively resected (approximately the medial two thirds of the facet joints), whereas a less extensive facetectomy may be performed in patients with moderate isolated lateral stenosis. The orientation of facet joints in the horizontal plane also affects the extension of facetectomy. When facet joints show a coronal, or slight sagittal, orientation, stenosis is often caused by the anteromedial portion of the superior and inferior facets. In this case, partial facetectomy may be accomplished by removing initially the medial one half or two thirds of the inferior facet with a small osteotome, and then the medial one half or two thirds of the superior facet with a pituitary rounger. When facet joints show a marked sagittal orientation, stenosis is often caused by the anterior slipping of the inferior facet, whereby its anterior portion needs to be excised.

Once the emerging nerve root and the thecal sac are decompressed at the disc level—that is, where stenosis is usually more severe—laminotomy should be extended somewhat distally in the radicular canal until the point where the nerve root reaches the intervertebral foramen. However, foraminotomy should be avoided since DS causes stenosis of the lateral, or central, portion of the spinal canal but not foraminal stenosis.

If total facetectomy is performed, spinal fusion should be carried out.

The postoperative course includes standing and walking from the first operative day as tolerated by the patient. We encourage six walks of 5 minutes from the second postoperative day and as long as possible from the fourth day after the operation. Hospital discharge usually occurs the second or third day after surgery.

RESULTS

Although degenerative spondylolisthesis is probably one of the spinal conditions that require surgery more frequently, few studies have analyzed in detail the results of the surgical treatment in DS. Feffer et al. (2) analyzed the surgical outcome in 19 patients with DS treated in two different hospitals. Eight patients underwent decompression and fusion, and 11 decompression alone. All patients had leg pain equal to or greater than their back pain and radiologic investigations showing a compression of the nervous structures. Length of follow-up ranged from 12 months to 72 months. In the fused group, the clinical result was rated as good in 5 patients and fair in 3. In the decompressed group, the clinical result was rated as good in 5, fair in 3, and poor in 3 patients. Lombardi et al. (5) analyzed the surgical outcome in 47 patients with DS treated with wide decompression (bilateral total facetectomy) in 6 patients, standard decompression (partial facetectomy) in 20 patients, and decompression with partial facetectomy plus posterolateral fusion in 21 patients. The follow-up ranged from 24 months to 7 years. The surgical outcome was rated as excellent or good in 30% of the patients who had wide decompression, in 80% of those who had standard decompression, and in 90% of those who had decompression plus fusion. Herron and Trippi (8) reported on 24 patients submitted to simple decompression and evaluated 18 to 71 months after surgery. They found that 83% of the patients reported good results.

A meta-analysis of literature on DS patients treated with laminectomy alone or laminectomy and instrumented or noninstrumented fusion revealed satisfactory results in 69% of those who had laminectomy alone, and 90% and 86% of those who had laminectomy with noninstrumented and instrumented fusion, respectively (6).

An unpublished series of selected patients with DS treated with simple decompression was recently reported (19). The series included 35 patients, 24 women and 11 men, with a mean age of 67 years (range 52 to 79 years). Inclusion criteria to undergo simple decompression were: (a) presence of radicular pain as the only or predominant symptom; (b) no evidence of marked hypermobility of the olisthetic vertebra on flexion-extension radiographs; (c) lateral stenosis or mild central stenosis, which could be treated with unilateral or bilateral laminotomy. Patients were evaluated after a minimum follow-up of 8 years using validated spinal questionnaires. The results showed that 32 patients (91%) reported satisfactory outcomes (21 excellent and 11 good results) and 3 (9%) reported fair results. None of the patients needed spinal fusion during the follow-up period due to spinal instability at the operated or adjacent level.

CONCLUSIONS

Data on the surgical outcome in patients with DS are largely incomplete due to methodologic limitations of the studies. Most of the series are retrospective, did not analyze the functional outcome, did not address possible causes of failures, and are based on short-term follow-ups. Nevertheless, most of the studies show that DS is one of the spinal conditions in which the result of surgical treatment is predictable and successful in most of the patients. Overall, patients with DS who underwent decompression and fusion report better outcomes than those undergoing simple decompression. However, by selecting patients with DS showing no evidence of spinal instability on clinical and radiologic evaluation, simple decompression may be highly successful and, possibly, by avoiding the long-term complications related to spinal fusion, even more successful than fusion in the long term.

REFERENCES

1. Bridwell KH, Sedgewick TA, O'Brien MF, et al. The role of fusion and instrumentation in the treatment of degenerative spondylolisthesis with spinal stenosis. *J Spinal Disord* 1993;6:461–472.
2. Feffer HL, Wiesel SW, Cuckler JM, et al. Degenerative spondylolisthesis: to fuse or not to fuse. *Spine* 1985;10:287–289.
3. Fox MW, Onofrio BM, Hanssen AD. Clinical outcomes and radiological instability following decompressive lumbar laminectomy for degenerative spinal stenosis: a comparison of patients undergoing concomitant arthrodesis versus decompression alone. *J Neurosurg* 1996;85:793–802.
4. Herkowitz HN, Kurz LT. Degenerative lumbar spondylolisthesis with spinal stenosis: a prospective study comparing decompression and intertransverse process arthrodesis. *J Bone Joint Surg Am* 1991;73:802–808.
5. Lombardi JS, Wiltse LL, Reynolds J, et al. Treatment of degenerative spondylolisthesis. *Spine* 1985;10:821–827.
6. Mardjetko SM, Connolly PJ, Shott S. Degenerative lumbar spondylolisthesis: a meta-analysis of literature 1970–1993. *Spine* 1994;19:S2256–S2265.
7. Epstein NE. Decompression in the surgical management of degenerative spondylolisthesis: advantages of a conservative approach in 2290 patients. *J Spinal Disord* 1998;11(2)116–122.
8. Herron LD, Trippi AC. L4–L5 degenerative spondylolisthesis: the results of treatment by decompressive laminectomy without fusion. *Spine* 1989;14:534–538.
9. Fischgrund JS, Mackay M, Herkowitz HN, et al. Degenerative lumbar spondylolisthesis with spinal stenosis: a prospective, randomized study comparing arthrodesis with and without instrumentation. *Spine* 1997;22:2807–2812.

10. Banwart JC, Asher MA, Hassanein RS. Iliac crest bone graft harvest donor site morbidity: a statistical evaluation. *Spine* 1995;20:1055–1060.
11. Colterjohn NR, Bednar DA. Procurement of bone graft from the iliac crest: an operative approach with decreased morbidity. *J Bone Joint Surg Am* 1997;79:756–759.
12. Cinotti G, Postacchini F, Fassari F, et al. Predisposing factors in degenerative spondylolisthesis: a radiographic and ct study. *Intern Orthop* 1997;21:337–342.
13. Johnsson KE, Uden A, Jonsson K. Postoperative instability after decompression for lumbar spinal stenosis. *Spine* 1996;1:92–-98.
14. Jonsson B, Akesson M, Jonsson K, et al. Low risk for vertebral slipping after decompression with facet joint preserving technique for lumbar spinal stenosis. *Eur Spine J* 1992;1:90–94.
15. Kinoshita T, Ohki I, Roth KR, et al. Results of degenerative spondylolisthesis treated with posterior decompression alone via a new surgical approach. *J Neurosurg* 2001;95:11–16.
16. Kleeman TJ, Hiscoce AC, Berg EE. Patient outcome after minimally destabilizing lumbar stenosis decompression: the "port-hole" technique. *Spine* 2000;25:865–870.
17. Abumi K, Panjabi MM, Kramer KM, et al. Biomechanical evaluation of lumbar spine stability after graded facetectomies. *Spine* 1990;15:1142–1147.
18. Postacchini F, Cinotti G, Perugia D, et al. The surgical treatment of central lumbar stenosis: multiple laminotomy compared with total laminectomy. *J Bone Joint Surg Br* 1993;75:386–392.
19. Cinotti G. Simple decompression without fusion. 11th Brussels International Spine Symposium: Spondylolysis, Spondylolisthesis and Degenerative Spondylolisthesis. Brussels, 2004.

28

Pedicle Navigation in Spondylolisthesis

C. Bolger and M. Bourlion

Pedicle screw fixation has been widely used for stabilization of the spine for conditions such as trauma, deformity, tumors, and the degenerative spine since its introduction in the late 1950s (1–6). One of the main problems facing the surgeon during pedicle screw placement is the inability to visualize the actual pedicle during both preparation of the pedicle and the actual screw placement, a situation that makes perforation of the vertebral wall a surgical risk. Numerous published studies have looked at the rate of both cortical breaches and screw misplacement, concluding that between 15% and 55% of screws breach some aspect of the pedicle. Complications of such breaches include but are not limited to dysesthesia, paraparesis, or paraplegia (7–13).

To achieve optimal placement of pedicle screws and to avoid the complications described above, surgeons have increasingly used computer-assisted and spinal-monitoring devices. Such techniques include, but are not limited to, mechanical probing, electromyography (EMG), somatosensory evoked potentials (SEEP), and spinal cord monitoring, along with image guidance. However, these methods all have their drawbacks. Probing is an inconsistent method, the results of which depend on the operator. The use of intraoperative EMG and monitoring is complex and requires the participation of trained personnel for the duration of the surgery (14–16).

Postoperative solutions for detection of accurate pedicle screw placement include computed tomography (CT), fluoroscopy, and roentgenography, as well as feedback from the patient. However, these are carried out after the screw placement and are therefore too late to avoid neurologic deficit.

SURGICAL NAVIGATION

Surgical navigation techniques offer many benefits to the surgeon for the accurate placement of pedicle screws. Preoperative CT scanning loaded into the system allows the surgeon to plan preoperatively for the best trajectory for optimal placement of the screws. The option to measure all dimensions of the pedicle, which is normally not visible to the surgeon, avoids the risk of breaches as a direct result of the actual screw. For more complex and deformed spines, the three-dimensional (3D) image generated by the computer is beneficial in defining complex and disrupted anatomy, allowing the surgeon to operate in confidence and increasing the accuracy of the placement of the pedicle screws (11,17–21).

However, surgical navigation also has its drawbacks insofar as it is an expensive system and requires preoperative CT scanning and time for the surgeon to load the scanning and plan the exams preoperatively. To gain the best advantage from the system there is a rather long learning curve for the user, which can lead to the risk of overreliance on technology for completion of the surgery. Moreover, when using image guidance for

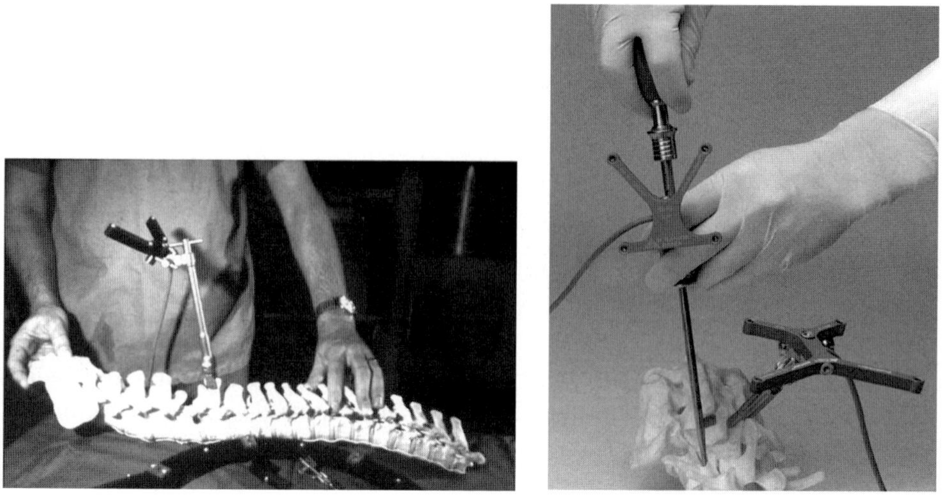

FIG. 28.1. Reference arc is attached to the spinous process for registration purposes.

multiple-level spinal fusions, the actual registration tends to lose its accuracy over the multilevel procedure and may require the surgeon to reregister the system to another anatomical landmark in the spine, thus lengthening the actual surgical procedure.

IMAGE GUIDANCE IN SPONDYLOLISTHESIS

In order to use image guidance, the spine needs to be both orientated and registered to the computer-generated 3D model that has been obtained from preoperative CT. A reference arc is clasped onto one of the exposed spinous process, and this is registered onto the 3D model (Fig 28.1). The remainder of the registration is generated around this point.

However, in spondylolisthesis, a stress fracture of the pars interarticularis (Fig. 28.2) causes detachment of the stabilizing elements posterior to the motion segments. This

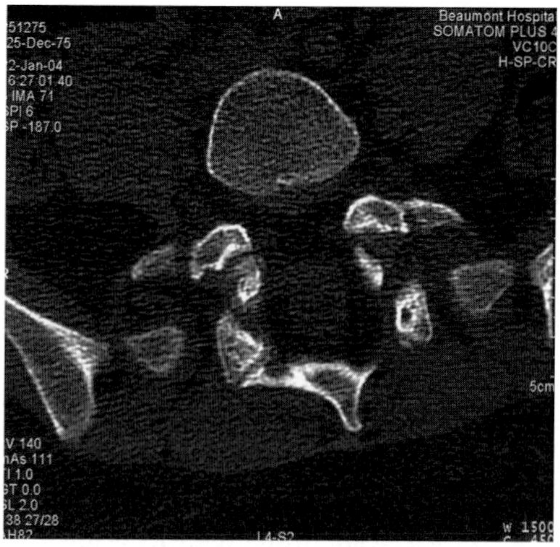

FIG. 28.2. Pars fracture in a patient with spondylolisthesis.

detachment causes a biomechanical imbalance resulting in a shearing and eventual failure of the disc annulus, which results in displacement of the vertebral body. Therefore, because there is no stable anatomy for placement of the reference frame for image guidance, this method of navigational surgery is not suitable for accurate navigation in patients with spondylolisthesis. Hence, there is a need for an efficient and cost-effective device that will assist the surgeon to navigate the pedicle in relative safety that is adaptable to be used in most spinal conditions, including spondylolisthesis.

ELECTRICAL IMPEDANCE IN SPINE SURGERY

In biologic tissues, electrical conductivity depends on tissue structure and blood content. The basic idea is that by assessing electrical conductivity, one can distinguish cortical bone from cancellous bone and both from soft tissue. Electrical impedance measurements have been used previously in spinal surgery. Although some authors have suggested that impedance is not effective for detecting screw fractures (22,23), this conclusion was biased by several technical artifacts, as described below.

Probing versus Drilling Instrument

When an instrument is used to probe the pilot hole measuring electrical impedance, the pilot-hole is often full of blood, leading to shunting or partial shunting. In this case, there is no way to know whether there is a breach or not in the pedicle wall. No significant impedance difference can be measured between a breached pedicle wall and an intact pedicle wall in this case. This observation is also confirmed and well explained by Toleikis (24).

Monopolar Probe

Previous authors have used a monopolar probe. This means that the active and return electrodes are far away (a few centimeters) from each other, and there is no way to be sure that the current will flow through a breach if there is a breach. The current will flow through the pathway of least resistance. And this pathway may be out of the pedicle hole. Further, with a monopolar probe, the distance between electrodes changes with the depth of insertion, thus leading to an unstable measured electrical impedance.

Absolute Measurement

Trying to correlate absolute electrical impedance measurements with detection of pedicle wall breaches does not provide statistically significant outcome. There is a large difference of absolute electrical impedance between subjects.

Impedance Measuring Tool

For analyzing these limitations, an impedance measuring tool (PediGuard, SpineVision, France) was designed as a freehand drilling bipolar instrument that measures electrical impedance at the tip. The measured impedance is translated into a visible and audible signal to inform the surgeon, in real time, when a change in resistance occurs at the tip. This measurement tool features bipolar electrodes that avoid any shunting effect and keep the

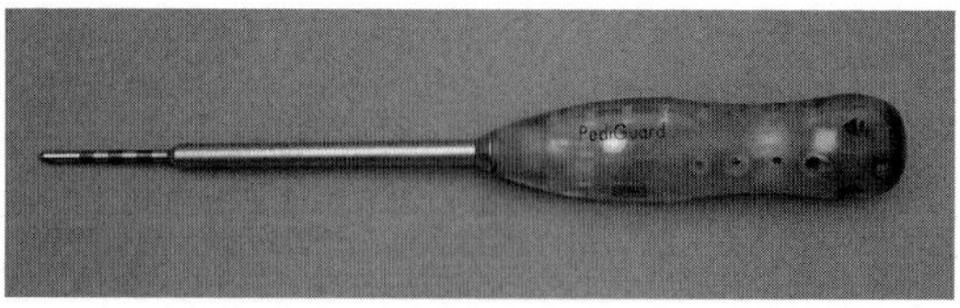

FIG. 28.3. General view of impedance-measuring tool with built-in electronic printed circuit board.

measured electrical impedance independent of the insertion depth. In a constant medium, the electrical impedance remains constant while the instrument is advanced into the vertebral pedicle and variation occurs when the instrument passes through a boundary between two different media.

As shown in Figure 28.3, this tool consists of an awl instrument with a hollow handle that accepts a built-in electronic printed circuit board. The electronic components allow performing impedance measurement and translation to audible signal and colored light emitting diodes (LEDs) to be used as feedback to the surgeon. In addition, this impedance measuring tool features a neurostimulator that can used in conjunction with a standard EMG.

NUMERICAL MODELING

A numerical model was developed by means of a finite-element computation in two-dimensional axisymmetric geometry to measure the impedance when the instrument is moving along a line that is perpendicular to the planes of the different layers, as shown in Figure 28.4.

The geometry of the tool representation being axisymmetric, of axis OZ, we have to solve Poisson's equation ($\Delta V = 0$, where V stands for the electrostatic potential), which is written as follows in these conditions:

$$\frac{\partial^2 V}{\partial r^2} + \frac{1}{r}\frac{\partial V}{\partial r} + \frac{\partial^2 V}{\partial z^2} = 0$$

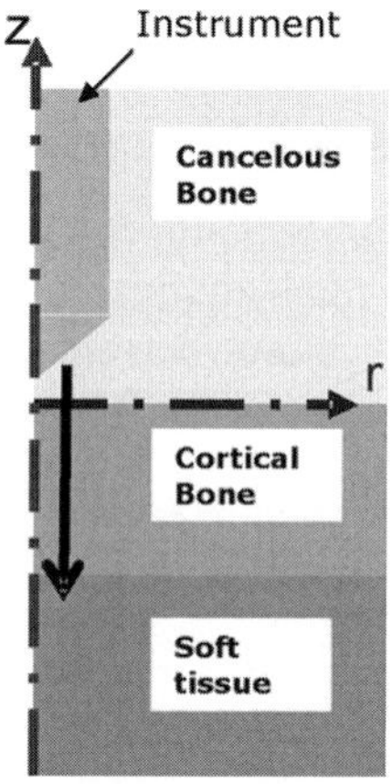

FIG. 28.4. Studied bidimensional geometrical model.

TABLE 28.1. *Instrument tip geometrical parameters*

	Conical 1	Conical 2
Diameter	3.2 mm	4 mm
Tip angle	120°	120°
	Ellipsoidal 1	Ellipsoidal 2
Diameter	3.2 mm	4 mm
Major radius	3.2	4
Minor radius	1.6	2
Eccentricity	0,866	0,866

The parameters of the problem are the geometrical dimensions as well as the electrical resistivities ρi of the different layers. The only variable is the distance between the tip of the tool and the interface between the cancellous bone and the cortical bone. The lateral extension of the domain is taken large to avoid any limit influence regarding current lines.

The different areas are meshed with a refining of the meshing near the critical interfaces (for each calculation, the number of nodes ranges between 5,000 and 8,000 depending on the value of d).

We have chosen to impose the potentials at the tip on the electrode and to compute the resulting current. Injected current at the tip of the instrument, null potential at the periphery, and null lateral leakage current $\partial V/\partial n = 0$ (where n is the normal axis at the surface) are selected as boundary conditions.

The solution consists in the values of $V(r,z)$ at each node, and the value of $R(d)$, resistance as a function of d is then deduced from the computation of the intensity of the current flowing into the inner electrode.

Geometry and Parameters

Electrical resistivity ρi of the three layers are $5\Omega.m$, $= 10\Omega.m$, and $= 2.5\Omega.m$ for cancellous bone, cortical bone, and soft tissue respectively. These values are consistent with those reported in literature (23), and their computed resistance values are the same as those measured experimentally with the actual tool during an animal study (25). The thickness of the cortical layer is 3 mm.

The tip of the instrument is either conical (with a 120 degree angle at the top) or ellipsoidal. Two diameters for both shapes were selected—4 mm and 3.2 mm. Geometrical tip parameters are given in Table 28.1.

Results

Figure 28.5 shows the curves representing the computed values of $R(d)$ for the four proposed geometries. The origin of d is taken at the interface between the cancellous bone and the cortical bone. The values of d between -3 mm and 0 mm correspond to the drilling into the cortical, and values of d smaller than -3 mm to the ones in the soft tissue. Rather than representing the value of the resistance, we preferred to represent the relative value (the reference value is taken in the cancellous bone, far from the interfaces), which gives a better view of the ability to detect when the tool is getting into the "dangerous zone."

From a quantitative point of view, the amplitude difference of the measured value of R is higher when the perforation instrument passes from cortical bone to soft tissue than

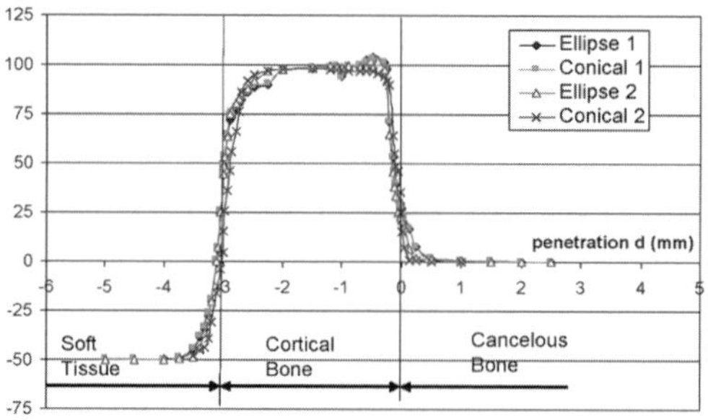

FIG. 28.5. Relative variation of the resistance "seen" by the surgical instrument as it goes through the different media. (On this graph, the instrument is moving forward from the right to the left.)

when it passes from cancellous bone through cortical bone. From a qualitative point of view, the curves are similar to the different optimized tip shapes. We can also plot the evolution of the electromagnetic field while the instrument is progressing through the different types of layers. In Figure 28.6 we provide two pictures of this computed field. On the left side, the instrument is in the cortical bone just before creating a breach. One can see that when in the cortical the electromagnetic field is constrained due to weak electrical conductivity of the medium. And on the right side, the instrument is creating a breach leading to high current leakage due to electrical conductivity decrease and spreading electromagnetic field.

Animal Studies

To confirm the results of the modeling, an animal study was performed. Using standard operative techniques, 168 pedicle drillings were performed on the lumbar and thoracic spines of 11 young pigs under general anesthetic. All drillings were performed by a surgeon trained in the use of an impedance measurement tool (PediGuard, SpineVision). Record of breaches was taken from both the surgeon and the instrument.

Following pedicle drillings and pedicle screw placement, the pigs were sacrificed and the pedicles were anatomically assessed for signs of breaches. These breaches were compared to the recording taken from both the surgeon and the electrical impedance measuring instrument.

Using this protocol, the device demonstrated a 100% positive predictive value, 96% negative predictive value, 100% specificity, and 97% sensitivity when computed with the actual necroscopically confirmed breaches.

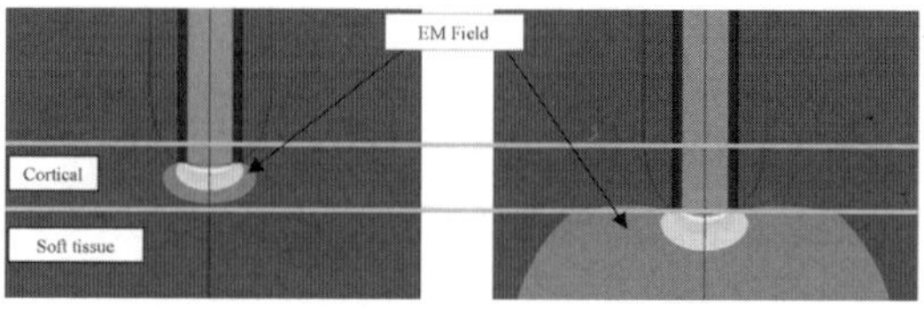

FIG. 28.6. Electromagnetic field shape. In the cortical bone prior to a breach (*left*); immediately after the breach in soft tissue (*right*).

Of the 18 drillings, there were:

- Two false negatives, leading to a minor effraction, cranially in the intervertebral discs
- Nine screw threads breaching the vertebral cortex when inserting screws, although preparation of the holes did not indicate any perforation
- Twenty-three percent of breaches detected by the device and not detected by the surgeon
- Twenty-seven drillings were in the growth cartridge, consistency similar to soft tissue, and these were all detected by the instrument.

CLINICAL STUDIES

First Human Trials

Eleven senior surgeons at nine hospitals throughout Europe were given an electrical impedance device (PediGuard, SpineVision) to be used in conjunction with their normal methods of pedicle preparation. Data were collected twofold; initially comparison was made between the impedance measurement tool's ability to detect a breach and the surgeon's own detection of a breach, as measured by independent postoperative CT scanning. However, since the surgeons were not blinded to the information from the instrument, a second set of data was collected looking at the accuracy of the impedance measurement in detecting a breach in isolation.

A total of 521 pedicle perforations were carried out on 97 patients, 147 drillings were recorded in the initial study, and the subsequent 374 drillings occurred in the second phase of the study.

Outcome Measures

A comparison was made between impedance measurement and the other detection possibilities (surgeon's tactile feeling, mechanical probing, fluoroscopy, CT scans, EMG, SEEP, surgical navigation, depending on their availability, peri- and/or postoperatively). Thus were registered and compared the detections of vertebral cortex fractures indicated:

- By the measurement of electrical impedance
- By any other available method

Results

Of 147 drillings, 23 vertebral cortex fractures (16%) were confirmed. Of these 23 fractures, 22 were identified preoperatively by impedance measurement. Fifty-two percent (12 of 23) of these breaches were detected by the impedance instrument but not by the surgeon. In one case, the neurostimulator integrated to the device induced visible leg twitches, simultaneously with an audio signal rise of the drilling instrument. There was one false positive, where there was a rise in the bleep but no fracture was confirmed postoperatively: positive predictive value 96%.

On the 374 drillings, 41 (11%) breaches were confirmed, with the device detecting 100% of these breaches; these also being detected by the surgeon. There were three false negatives, where there was a rise in the bleep but no fracture was confirmed either by the surgeon intraoperatively or on CT scanning postoperatively: positive predictive value 93%.

A total of 521 drillings were performed while measuring impedance; 64 (12.3%) breaches were confirmed. The device offers the surgeon 98% sensitivity on the detection of a breach during pedicle preparation with 99% specificity.

CONCLUSION: BENEFITS IN SPINAL SURGERY, ESPECIALLY SPONDYLOLISTHESIS SURGERY

As previous studies have shown, this electrical impedance measurement has a sensitivity of >98% in the detection of breaches. Over and above this, impedance measurement detected between 36% and 52% more breaches than the actual surgeon performing the surgeries.

By its very nature, as a hand-held wireless tool that is used not only for navigation but also for perforation, the tool gives real-time feedback to the surgeon, without the surgeon having to change instruments and without causing the surgeon to lose momentum during pedicle preparation. The fact that there is no need for preoperative CT scanning or preoperative planning saves time for the surgical team. Because this tool does not require computer registration or vertebral tracking, it can be used in all aspects of spinal fixation, inclusive of fractures and spondylolisthesis cases, regardless of the degree of pars fracture and dislocation.

REFERENCES

1. Montesano PX, McLain RF, Benson DR. Spinal instrumentation in the management of vertebral column tumours. *Semin Orthop* 1991;6:237–246.
2. Punjabi MM, Oda T, Wang J. The effects of pedicle adjustments on neural spaces in burst fracture surgery. *Spine* 2000;25:1637–1643.
3. Roy-Camille R, Saillant G, Mazel C. Internal fixation of the lumbar spine with pedicle screw plating. *Clin Orthop* 1986;7–17.
4. Roy-Camille R, Saillant G, Mazel C: Plating of thoracic, thoracolumbar, and lumbar injuries with pedicle screw plates. *Orthop Clin North Am* 1986;17: 147–159.
5. Vaccaro R, Conant RF, Hilibrand AS, et al. A plate-rod device for treatment of cervicothoracic disorders: comparison of mechanical testing with established cervical spine in vitro load testing data. *J Spinal Disord* 2000;13:350–355.
6. Xu R, Ebraheim NA, Ou Y, et al. Anatomic considerations of pedicle screw placement in the thoracic spine: Roy-Camille technique versus open-lamina technique. *Spine* 1998;23:1065–1068.
7. Davne, SH, Myers DL. Complications of lumbar spine fusion with transpedicular instrumentation. *Spine* 1992;17:184–189.
8. Esses SI, Sachs BL, Dreyzin V. Complication associated with technique of pedicle screw fixation. *Spine* 1993;18:2231–2239.
9. Gertzbein SD, Robbins SE. Accuracy of pedicular screw placement in vivo. *Spine* 1990;15:11–14.
10. Lonstein JE, Denis F, Perra JH. Complications associated with pedicle screws. *J Bone Joint Surg Am* 1999;81:1519–1528.
11. Xu R, Ebraheim NA, Ou Y, et al. Anatomic considerations of pedicle screw placement in the thoracic spine. *Spine* 1998;23:1065–1068.
12. Vaccaro A, Rizzolo SJ, Balderston RA, et al. Placement of pedicle screws in the thoracic spine. Part II: an anatomical and radiographic assessment. *J Bone Joint Surg Am* 1995;77:1200–1206.
13. West JL, Ogilvie JW, Bradford DS. Complications of the variable screw plate pedicle screw fixation. *Spine* 1991;16:576–579.
14. Calancie B, Madsen P, Lebwohl N. Stimulus-evoked EMG monitoring during transpedicular lumbosacral spine instrumentation. Initial clinical results. *Spine* 1994;19(24):2780–2786.
15. Gundanna M, Eskenazi M, Bendo J, et al. Somatosensory evoked potential monitoring of lumbar pedicle screw placement for in situ posterior spinal fusion. *Spine* 2003;5:370–376.
16. Welch WC, Rose RD, Balzer JR, et al. Evaluation with evoked and spontaneous electromyography during lumbar instrumentation: a prospective study. *J Neurosurg* 1997;87:397–402.
17. Amiot LP, Lang K, Putzier M, et al. Comparative results between conventional and computer-assisted pedicle screw installation in the thoracic, lumbar and sacral spine. *Spine* 2000; 25(5):606–614.
18. Bolger C, Wigfield C. Image-guided surgery: application to the cervical and thoracic spine and a review of the first 120 procedures. *J Neur Spine* 2000;92:175–180.

19. Laine T, Lund T, Ylikoski M, et al. Accuracy of pedicle screw insertion with and without computer assistance: a randomised controlled clinical study in 100 consecutive patients. *Eur Spine J* 2000;9(3):235–240.
20. Rampersaud Y, Simon DA, Foley KT. Accuracy requirements for image-guided spinal pedicle screw placement. *Spine* 2000;26(4):352–359.
21. Youkilis AS, Quint DJ, McGillicuddy JE, et al. Stereotactic navigation for placement of pedicle screws in the thoracic spine. *Neurosurgery* 2001;48:771–778; discussion 778–779.
22. Darden BV, Owen JH, Hatley MK, et al. A comparison of impedance and electromyogram measurements in detecting the presence of pedicle wall breakthrough. *Spine* 1998;23:256–262.
23. Myers BS, Hasty CC, Floberg DR, et al. Measurement of vertebral cortical integrity during pedicle exploration for intrapedicular fixation. *Spine* 1995;20;2:144–148.
24. Toleikis JR. Neurophysiological monitoring during pedicle screw placement. In: Deletis V, Shils J, ed. *Neurophysiology in Neurosurgery: A Modern Intraoperative Approach*. New York: Academic Press; 2002:231–234.
25. Carozzo C, Bourlion M, Vanquaethem A, et al. A new device to detect iatrogenic initial pedicle perforation: a preliminary study of reliability in the porcine model. *Eur Spine J* 2002;11(1).

29

Bone Graft Alternatives in Spinal Surgery

Alberto Di Martino, Jeff S. Silber, and Alexander R. Vaccaro

The accomplishment of a successful spinal fusion depends on the stability of the fusion bed, the viability of the local blood supply, and the responsiveness of the cellular environment to osteoinductive and osteoconductive elements. The prospect of a successful fusion depends on four distinct processes: osteogenesis, osteoinduction, osteoconduction, and stability, or lack of motion. Osteogenesis describes the process of new bone formation occurring at a cellular level and implies the recruitment of osteoprogenitor stem cells. Osteoinduction is the cytokine-mediated recruitment and differentiation of various cell types essential for new bone formation; an osteoinductive material must contain one or more growth factors that can induce de novo ectopic bone formation through differentiation of progenitor cells into osteoblasts. Osteoconduction is defined as the apposition of growing bone to the three-dimensional surface of the graft structural scaffold with the graft providing the framework for the ingrowth of the tissue.

Autogenous bone graft, due to its intrinsic osteogenic, osteoinductive, and osteoconductive properties, is an optimal graft source for a spinal fusion. In addition, modern surgical techniques provide early stability through the use of spinal instrumentation; nonetheless, long-term stability is dependent on the development of a solid biologic fusion.

PRINCIPLES OF BONE GRAFTING IN SPINAL FUSION

The local host environment is of critical importance in obtaining a solid spinal fusion. The presence of an adequate blood supply is essential. Disruption of the blood supply can be minimized during surgery through careful surgical manipulation of the surrounding bony and soft tissue elements. Experimental models of posterolateral intertransverse fusions demonstrate that blood supply to the graft arises from the decorticated transverse processes; inadequate decortication leads to failure of the graft to incorporate and achieve fusion (1). Preserving an intact blood supply maintains oxygen tension as well as the nutrient levels; these are necessary to preserve cellular synthetic activity, promote neovascularization, and allow migration of cells into the developing fusion mass.

Systemic illnesses such as diabetes or chronic renal failure can also have an adverse impact on fusion rates; this mechanism is supposed to be related mostly to the impairment in vascular ingrowth. Additionally, cigarette smoking, most likely as a result of the effect of nicotine on vascular supply (2), and malnutrition are associated with a general impairment of wound healing and may also have an adverse effect on fusion healing.

Local biomechanical factors are dependent on the type and position of the bone graft applied to the spine. Anterior interbody structural grafts are exposed to local compressive forces. Precise contouring and fit may affect ultimate fusion success or failure. On the contrary, a posterior applied bone graft is placed along the tension side of the spinal column.

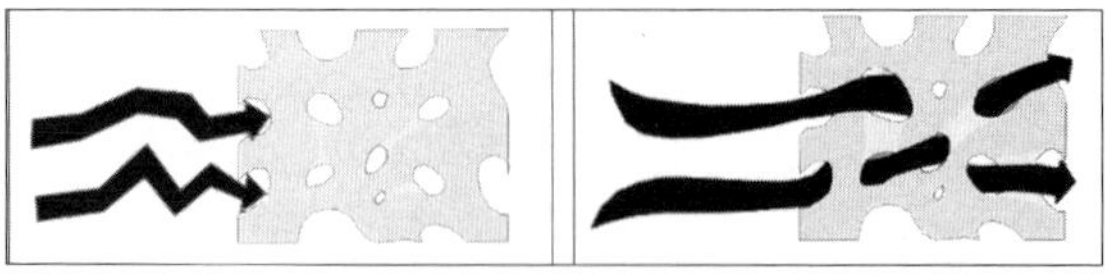

FIG. 29.1. Osteoconduction: scheme of impeded (**A**) and complete (**B**) bone ingrowth through a porous structure. Reprinted, with permission, from Interpore Cross International, Irvine, CA.

Because there are no local compressive stimuli, bone graft incorporation is not as directly affected by local biomechanical factors. The lack of stability of this grafting technique and the presence of excessive strain may lead to inadequate neovascularization into the graft and ultimately failure to attain a successful arthrodesis.

Osteogenic cells responsible for new bone formation are an absolute requirement for a successful fusion. Autograft bone directly provides viable progenitor stem cells and mature osteoblasts. The bone extracellular matrix provided by the autograft as well as the local wound hematoma at the fusion site are sources of osteoinductive factors such as bone morphogenetic proteins (BMPs). These play a critical role in the formation and maturation of new bone and stimulate the recruitment of additional osteogenic cells. Many growth factors (GFs) are involved in the process of osteogenesis; these include platelet-derived growth factor (PDGF), transforming growth factor beta (TGF-β), and vascular endothelial growth factor (VEGF), but BMPs are the only known factors able to induce the entire process of new bone formation (3).

Osteoconductive substitutes may be used as scaffolds to deliver bone growth factors. These materials facilitate bone formation but do not contain natural growth factors that can attract osteoblast precursor cells and initiate osteoblast differentiation. They include collagen, ceramics, polymers, coral, and allograft bone, and they function similarly to the native collagen and hydroxyapatite of autograft bone, providing a lattice within the developing fusion mass for new blood vessels and migrating stem cells (4). Osteoconductivity of a graft material is a function of its geometric and biomechanical properties and of the similarity of the graft to the native bone. In particular, pore size and three-dimensional interconnectivity of the host and donor tissue must be closely matched; this allows the migration of osteoblastic precursor cells and the ingrowth of new bone (Fig. 29.1) (4). The graft also has to be biocompatible to minimize interference with bone induction from an autoimmune inflammatory reaction (5).

AUTOGRAFT AND ALLOGRAFT BONE

The term *autograft* implies that a piece of bone is harvested from one donor anatomical site and then transplanted to a receptor site in the same individual. Autograft sources include the fibula, ribs, posterior spinal elements, and tibia, although the gold standard for the majority of spinal procedures is autograft taken from the iliac crest. The latter contains osteoblasts and mesenchymal osteogenic precursor cells with osteogenic potential; moreover, it has osteoconductive and osteoinductive properties. A bone allograft is defined as a piece of bone transferred between individuals of the same species.

As demonstrated by Goldberg and Stevenson (6), the incorporation of a bone graft occurs in five distinct stages. Initially, autograft and allograft evoke an acute inflammatory response followed, in 2 weeks, by granulation tissue deposition and activation of osteoblastic activity due to osteoinduction. Vascularization and continued osteoinduction

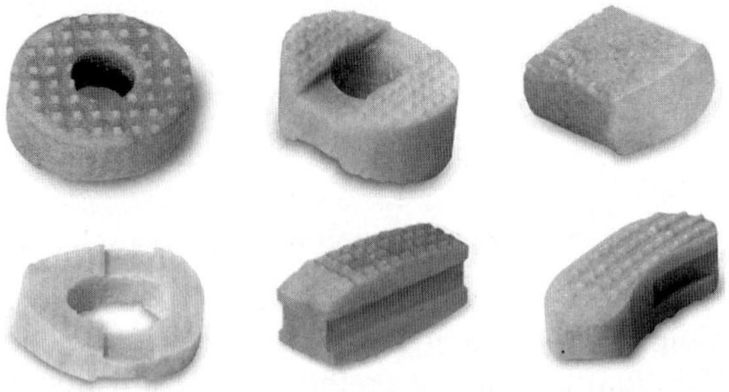

FIG. 29.2. Allograft bone wedges and spacers designed to provide anterior support column support for spinal procedures. Reprinted, with permission, from Musculoskeletal Transplant Foundation, Edison, NJ.

then occurs; it is during these stages of incorporation that the host's immune system becomes sensitized to donor antigens if allograft is used. After this stage, the graft's three-dimensional lattice acts through osteoconduction to promote infiltration of osteoprogenitor cells within its boundaries. This phase lasts from several months for trabecular grafts to years for cortical grafts. Over time, the voids between the graft and host bone are bridged by new bone. Concurrently, remodeling of the graft occurs through local mechanical stimuli (6). Lastly, segmental stiffness increases as new bone is deposited and remodeled onto the osteoconductive matrix of the graft.

In general, as compared to autograft, allograft bone incorporates more slowly and less completely, which may be a manifestation of the host's immune response to Class I and II major histocompatibility complex antigens (HLA) contained in the allograft. Experimental allograft bone grafting studies have demonstrated that HLA-matched allografts incorporate in a fashion closely resembling incorporation of autograft bone (7).

The use of allograft bone in spine surgery has increased greatly as a result of improved procurement, preparation, and storage methods. Allograft bone is available in different forms to match the surgeon's needs in spinal applications (Fig. 29.2). It is both osteoconductive and weakly osteoinductive, the degree of osteoinductivity being directly related to the method of preparation and sterilization of the allograft bone. The processing consists of removal of cells and extraneous debris from the allograft bone, thus minimizing the risk of infection as well as the immunogenicity (8). The downside of this process is a dampening of the osteogenic potential of the allograft tissue.

Allograft preparations are available clinically as either fresh frozen or freeze dried. Both processes start with graft cooling to –70°C. Freeze-dried specimens undergo an additional lyophilization step that destroys any remaining viral DNA. Unfortunately, this process often denatures contained BMPs. Manufacturers of particular demineralized bone matrix (DBM) products that use freeze-dry processing have noted preservation of osteoinductive capabilities resulting from the presence of active BMPs. The most commonly expressed concern among patients who are intended to receive an allograft is the potential that the bone graft will transmit infection to them. Studies suggest the risk of human immunodeficiency virus (HIV) infection to be about 1 per 1.6 million procedures of all allograft bone grafting. The risk of hepatitis B or C transmission is less with freeze-dried than with fresh-frozen allografts (9).

Healing of allograft bone to native bone is partially dependent upon its anatomical placement within the spine. Compared to autograft used in anterior column applications, allograft bone used in posterior or posterolateral position is associated with reduced fusion rates. In this position, allograft is associated with more extensive resorption, slower incorporation rates, and increased infection risk compared with autologous bone graft (10–12).

A recent literature review on spinal fusion trends for the treatment of lumbar degenerative disk disease over the last 20 years revealed that iliac crest autograft was the most common graft source utilized, with reported fusion rates of 87%. Allograft fusion alone was successful in 86% of cases, being more frequently used as an interbody graft compared to autograft. Combined autogenous/allogenous grafts resulted in overall fusion rates of 86% (13). Therefore, depending on the clinical situation, an acceptable fusion rate may be achieved using an allograft source alone such as, in a nonsmoker, a single-level anterior cervical discectomy and fusion followed by anterior cervical plating. In this clinical scenario, the morbidity of autograft harvest can often be avoided without compromising outcomes (7,14–17).

The principal disadvantage of using autograft bone remains the morbidity associated with graft harvest. In fact, in anterior cervical discectomy and fusion procedures, complications related to the graft harvesting site occur more commonly than complications related to the anterior cervical fusion. Incidence of donor-site complication ranges from 4% to 49%, the major complications associated with graft harvest procedures being chronic pain and infection, wound drainage, hematoma formation, pelvic ring destabilization, formation of enterocutaneous fistula, neurosensory loss, gait disturbance, and bowel herniation (8).

The morbidities associated with bone graft harvest have led to the development of numerous biologic and synthetic graft alternatives, including allograft machined implants, demineralized bone matrix, recombinant bone growth factors, and ceramics. These alternatives can be used alone, in combination with one another, with autologous bone marrow, or together with autologous bone graft as bone graft extenders.

BONE MARROW ASPIRATE AND GROWTH FACTORS

Bone marrow aspirate represents an important source of a population of pluripotential progenitor cells, referred to as mesenchymal stem cells, capable of differentiation into cells able to produce bone, cartilage, tendon, and muscle. The percentage of stem cells among nucleated cells varies according to age, decreasing in the bone marrow of elderly patients (18). Stem cell concentration is 1 in 50,000 nucleated cells in young patients and becomes 1 in 2 million in the elderly. Centrifugation of the marrow aspirate allows increasing the relative concentration of stem cells (19).

The procedure of bone marrow aspiration (BMA) from the iliac crest is associated with minimal morbidity; once harvested, the bone marrow can be used as an adjunct to grafting procedures for spinal fusion (Fig. 29.3). Adding bone extracts containing BMPs to the BMA enhances its potential usefulness. Currently, BMA is used clinically as an adjunct to various autograft alternatives, thus providing the osteogenic potential to the osteoinductive and osteoconductive properties of the grafting material.

As noted above, the use of autologous marrow is limited by the relatively low osteoprogenitor cell frequency and number in the starting marrow population. However, a number of groups have shown that human adipose tissue is also a source of osteoprogenitor cells (20–24). Unlike marrow, adipose tissue can be obtained in relatively large quantities with minimal morbidity. In a recent study, Cowan et al. demonstrated the ability of cells derived from murine adipose tissue seeded onto an apatite-coated scaffold to

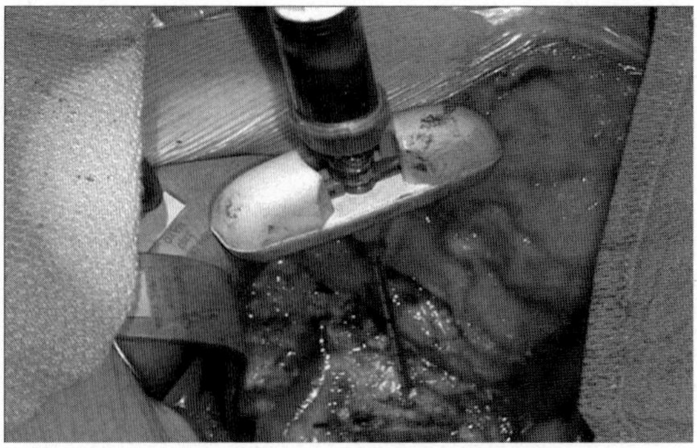

FIG. 29.3. Intraoperative bone marrow aspiration from the iliac crest. Reprinted, with permission, from Orthovita, Malvern, PA.

promote healing in a critical-size (4-mm) calvarial defect in mice (25). The authors also noted that the cells derived from adipose tissue reached confluence approximately 7 times faster than marrow-derived cells (2–3 days compared to 2–3 weeks). Further, De Ugarte et al. (26) compared adipose-derived and marrow-derived stem cells and showed that adipose cells grew approximately 20-fold more effectively than those from marrow of the same donor. Thus, adipose tissue may represent a superior source of osteoprogenitor cells for orthopedic applications.

Another fusion enhancement strategy is the addition of growth factors as a bone graft promoter. Following injury, white blood cells and platelets collect at the site of insult and form a clot while attracting reparative growth factors. The osteopromotive nature of this clot has been studied extensively by Muschler et al. (27). Using a canine posterior spinal fusion model, they compared fusion rates of cancellous bone matrix (mineralized or demineralized) combined with bone marrow–derived cells containing osteoblastic progenitor cells with and without a bone marrow clot. They found that adding the bone marrow clot to an enriched cell-matrix composite graft resulted in a significant increase in bone graft healing. At present, several commercial products are available that assist in separating out and concentrating specific blood components such as platelets, growth factors, and the leukocyte-rich buffy coat at the time of surgery. These blood products are prepared in the form of a gel and combined with bone grafting materials to be used as a bone graft extender during a fusion procedure.

The local application of platelet-rich plasma (PRP) to promote or enhance the maturation of bone fusion is based on the release of the growth factors present in platelets, such as PDGF, TGF-β (28), and insulin growth factor-I (IGF-I), which have been shown to be involved in the process of osteogenesis. One commercially available service, Autologous Growth Factor (AGF, Biomet, Warsaw, IN, USA), collects a unit of blood through a cell saver and separates it into three parts: red cells, plasma, and a buffy coat. The buffy coat is then removed and ultraconcentrated. This concentrate is then added to thrombin to form a soft or hard gel, which then is added to an osteoconductive carrier or delivered directly to the fusion site (29). Schlegel et al. (30), in a skull defect model in adult pigs, found that animals treated with a combination of PRP and bovine collagen demonstrated new bone growth similar to that found with the use of autologous bone alone. In contrast, Jensen et al. (31) found no benefit in using PRP combined with allograft in a canine proximal humerus defect model. Walsh et al. (32)

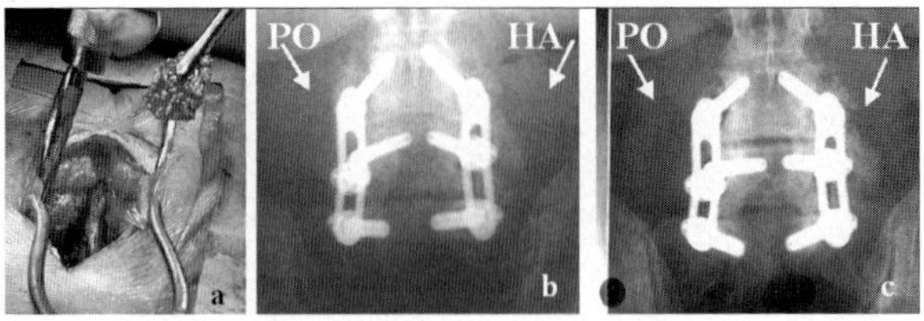

FIG. 29.4. Intraoperative picture of Pro-Osteon 500R granules mixed with Autologous Bone Graft (ABG) and autologous platelet gel in instrumented posterolateral lumbosacral fusion (**A**). Radiographic results at 6 weeks (**B**) and 6 months (**C**) postoperatively. This study compared the resorption rates of Pro Osteon 500R to Pro Osteon 500HA granules. Reprinted, with permission, from Interpore Cross International, Irvine, CA.

recently reported that the combination of autologous bone marrow, buffy coat derived growth factors, and a porous ceramic (Pro-Osteon 500R) used as a graft substitute in an instrumented posterolateral fusion model resulted in a fusion rate similar to autograft bone alone (Fig. 29.4). At present, blood-derived growth factors have found useful applications in maxillofacial and spinal fusion procedures. Further studies are needed to analyze the potential benefits of these techniques in bone healing in the appendicular skeleton.

DEMINERALIZED BONE MATRIX

Demineralized bone matrix (DBM) is generally a weakly osteoinductive allograft bone graft extender. The osteoinductive potential of DBM is partly dependent on how it is processed, with some proving experimentally to be more osteoinductive than others (33). DBM is produced via removal of the mineral content of bone through mild acid extraction; this process leaves an organic product made predominantly by BMPs, collagen, and various noncollagenous proteins (18). The trabecular structure of the original tissue is retained and can serve as a biologic scaffold; however, the original structural strength contributed by the bone mineral is no longer present. The naturally occurring BMPs present in DBM stimulate mesenchymal stem cells to differentiate into chondrocytes and osteoblasts, thus exerting their osteoinductive effect (29). Extensive processing makes DBM the least immunogenic of all currently available allograft bone products. DBM has reported excellent results in stable and well-supported skeletal defects in animal studies, as well as in the treatment of giant cell tumors of bone in humans (34,35). In addition, Glowacki and Mulliken (36) found that DBM and bone marrow composite grafts were comparable to autogenous iliac crest bone graft in some arthrodesis procedures.

A variety of DBM products are commercially available. One of the most intensively studied and used product is Grafton Demineralized Bone Matrix (Osteotech, Eatontown, NJ, USA). This allograft material is considered banked human tissue by US regulatory authorities: it consists of DBM in a glycerol carrier (18). Grafton DBM is available in five different forms (Fig. 29.5): Gel, which consists of particulate DBM; Grafton DBM Putty, which contains DBM in fiber form (fibers have been shown to be more osteoconductive than particles (37); Grafton DBM Flex, which is made of nonwoven sheets of DBM fibers; Grafton DBM Matrix, a preformed fiber material designed for specific spinal applications; and Grafton Plus DBM, a paste product designed to be moldable and irrigable. Grafton has proven to be osteoinductive in animal models, and preclinical studies have

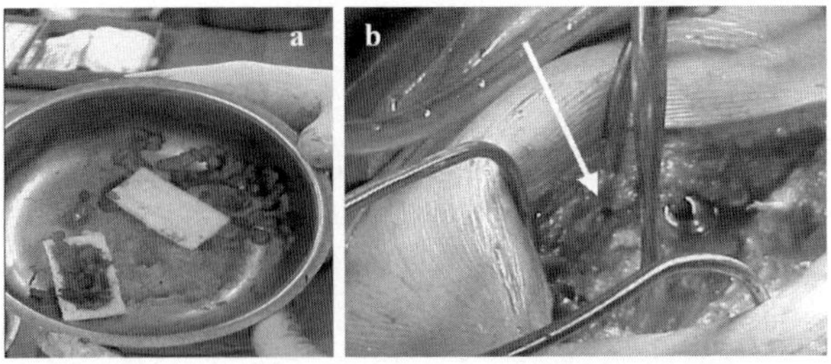

FIG. 29.5. The Grafton DBM product consists of demineralized bone matrix in a glycerol carrier and is available in gel, putty, paste, crunches, flex, and matrix forms. A picture of Grafton Matrix combined with autologous bone graft (**A**) and intraoperatively implanted in lumbar instrumented posterolateral fusion (**B**). Reprinted, with permission, from Osteotech, Inc., Eatontown, NJ.

yielded favorable results when Grafton was used either alone or as an autograft extender. A recently reported clinical trial of 120 patients who underwent a posterolateral instrumented lumbar spine fusion using autograft alone on one side and Grafton DBM Gel as an autograft extender on the other side found similar fusion results for both sides (38,39).

Other commercially available DBM preparations use a variety of carriers such as calcium sulfate (Allomatrix, Wright Medical Technology, Memphis, TN, USA); hyaluronic acid (DBX, Synthes, Paoli, PA, USA); porcine collagen (Osteofil, Regeneration Technologies Inc., Alachua, FL, USA) (40); cortical bone chips (Opteform, Regeneration Technologies, Inc., Alachua, FL, USA); and poloxamer excipient (Dynagraft, GenSci Regeneration Sciences, Inc., Irvine, CA, USA).

CERAMICS

Ceramics are synthetic bone graft alternatives. The biggest advantages of their use are their limitless availability and the absence of disease transmission. Ceramics are not derived from bone and are purely osteoconductive without possessing osteogenic or osteoinductive properties. The two-dimensional surface of ceramics provides the scaffold for adherence and migration of bone-forming cells, but it is their three-dimensional microarchitecture (pore diameter and void interconnectedness) that is the major determinant of the rate of graft incorporation and remodeling. The optimal pore size for osteoconduction ranges from 150 μm to 500 μm (41). These highly porous, low-density implants offer a large surface area for nutrient access, neovascularization, and bony ingrowth (9).

Depending on their method of manufacture, ceramics are divided into sintered, replamiform, or collagen mesh. Sintered ceramics are porous forms of hydroxyapatite or calcium phosphate that may contain interconnectivity between pores resulting from the use of poragen, which is removed during high-temperature processing. Replamiform ceramic is derived from sea coral and possesses a microarchitecture closely resembling bone. Collagen mesh and injected molded ceramics are newer forms of synthetic ceramics still under development. It is postulated that this form of ceramic, when combined with bone marrow aspirate or recombinant BMPs as a composite graft, will possess a biologic efficacy similar to that of autograft (42). The major disadvantage of coralline hydroxyapatite ceramics is their relatively poor mechanical properties. They are quite brittle, providing little fracture resistance or tensile strength. Implants using this material when designed as structural grafts must be shielded from loading until substantial bone ingrowth occurs (43).

Popular ceramics used in clinical application for spinal fusion include calcium phosphate biomaterials and their composites, such as hydroxyapatite (HA) combined with tricalcium phosphate (TCP) (18). These compounds have been used alone or in combination with autologous bone graft or bone graft extenders and appear to elicit little immunologic reaction in surrounding tissues, presumably due to their biochemical resemblance to normal bone. The advantage of the mixture of hydroxyapatite and tricalcium phosphate combined in optimal proportions is that the end product can benefit from the unique characteristics of both. Tricalcium phosphate dissolves readily in vivo via osteoclastic activity, allowing new bone to form along its osteoconductive framework, while deriving its strength from a combination of its geometric structure and the low solubility of hydroxyapatite, making the graft composite stable over the long term. The compressive strength of ceramic significantly increases after implantation following successful incorporation into the fusion mass (44,45).

Synthetic ceramics have proven efficacy in spinal fusion performed for deformity and trauma. In a large prospective, randomized study on 341 adolescents undergoing posterior spinal fusion for idiopathic scoliosis, the efficacy of synthetic porous ceramic blocks (macroporous biphasic calcium phosphate [MBCP]) (Triosite, Zimmer, Inc., Warsaw, IN, USA) was compared with autograft (46). Fusion rates were comparable between the two groups; but the rate of wound complications was significantly decreased in the group receiving the ceramic. Another study demonstrated the ability of MBCP Triosite granules to act effectively as a graft extender in patients undergoing surgery for scoliosis when combined with local decorticated bone graft, thus eliminating the necessity for harvesting autologous bone graft from the iliac crest (44). Another prospective study evaluated 106 patients with degenerative scoliosis and/or spondylolisthesis who underwent a posterior lumbar fusion procedure; in this study, MBCP Triosite granules were used in combination with corticocancellous allograft bone chips and bone marrow aspirate (47). Radiographic fusion was achieved in all but six patients, demonstrating that MBCP can function as an adequate substitute to autograft in this patient population.

Pro Osteon (Biomet, Warsaw, IN, USA) is a ceramic derived from sea coral. The production of Pro Osteon involves the high-temperature chemical transformation of calcium carbonate (constituent of the sea coral) into hydroxyapatite. Different pore sizes can be created, yielding a three-dimensional structure resembling either cortical or cancellous bone. The initial commercial available formulation of Pro Osteon demonstrated extremely slow resorption rates in clinical follow-up studies with complete resorption occurring only after 15 to 20 years.

Several clinical studies have demonstrated successful use of structural anterior column coralline implants when protected by load-sharing internal fixation. Thalgott et al. (48) used Pro Osteon 200 (pore diameter of 200 microns) in combination with rigid anterior plating in 26 patients undergoing anterior cervical decompression and fusion procedures. After a 2-year minimum follow-up, the reported fusion rate was 100%, with a mean decrease in overall pain of 76%. McConnell et al. reported the outcome of anterior cervical interbody fusion using Pro-Osteon 200 as an anterior structural graft followed by anterior plate fixation. They noted clinical improvement comparable to autologous iliac crest bone graft at follow-up (49). In a clinical study of 20 patients undergoing a combined anterior-posterior lumbar fusion, Pro Osteon 200 was utilized as an anterior lumbar interbody graft (50). With a minimum 37-month follow-up, fusion rates were 93.7%, and pain decreased by an average of 61.8% with an overall patient satisfaction rate of

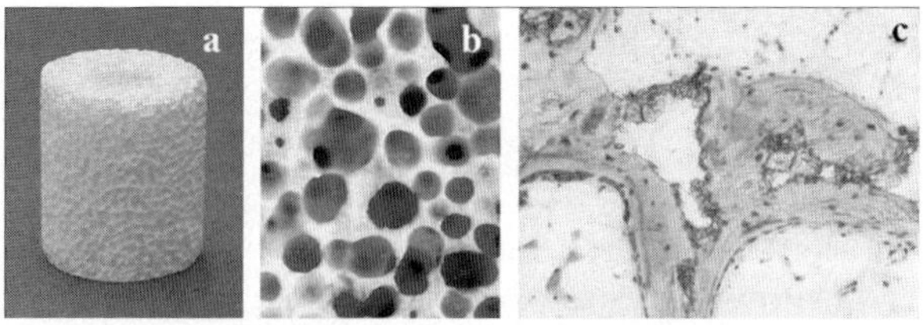

FIG. 29.6. Pictures of nonimplanted Norian ChronOs, showing its high porosity (**A**,**B**). Once implanted, the ceramic is replaced by normal bone (**C**) in 6 to 18 months. Reprinted, with permission, from Synthes Inc., West Chester, PA.

90%. The authors concluded that Pro Osteon 200 represented a reasonable bone graft substitute as an anterior lumbar interbody graft because of its structure resembling cortical bone and its good resistance to compressive loadings. Pro-Osteon 500 (porous diameter of 500 microns) has a structure resembling cancellous bone. It has 25% of the compressive resistance compared to Pro Osteon 200, and has been shown to be effective as a bone graft extender in instrumented posterolateral lumbar fusion procedures (51).

ChronOS (Synthes Inc., West Chester, PA, USA) is a ceramic made up of pure (β-tricalcium phosphate. Its strength is similar to that of cancellous bone (7.5 ± 1 MPa), and its three-dimensional scaffold provides an ideal structure for osteoconductivity. ChronOs features pore sizes in the range of 100–550 μm and has a 60% to 80% porous structure that mimics trabecular bone (Fig. 29.6) (45). It is gradually resorbed and replaced by new bone, with remodeling occurring over 6 to 18 months. ChronOs has been developed to be used in spinal applications such as posterolateral fusions mixed with autologous bone graft to improve graft volume. The substance can also serve as filler for structural grafts. Muschik demonstrated the efficacy of ChronOS compared to allograft as a bone graft extender in posterolateral spinal fusion surgery in adolescents with idiopathic scoliosis (52).

VITOSS (Orthovita, Malvern, PA) is a commercially available, highly porous (β-tricalcium phosphate bone void filler (53). The material contains 90% interconnected void space, resembling the trabecular structure of cancellous bone (8). Pore sizes range from 1 μm to 1,000 μm; the smaller pores induce capillary wicking of phagocytic cells for implant resorption and bone-forming cells, nutrients, and cytokines for new bone formation, while the larger pores encourage neovascularization and structural bone ingrowth (9).

Because of its interconnected microporosity, VITOSS represents an excellent carrier for bone marrow aspirate or recombinant BMPs as a composite implant (Fig. 29.7). The hydrophilic properties of the scaffold encourage retention of both seeded marrow cells and growth factors. The range in pore size may also allow greater penetration of bone-forming cells and phagocytic cells as well as enhanced diffusion of cytokines and nutrients from adjacent bone (9). Because of the low mechanical properties of the porous substance, VITOSS cannot be used in situations in which immediate structural strength is required. In a prospective study of 50 patients undergoing a posterolateral lumbar spinal fusion and decompressive laminectomy, VITOSS was used as an autograft extender with either local bone or iliac crest autograft (54). Both noninstrumented and instrumented fusions were performed; some patients were also subjected to a posterior lumbar interbody fusion (PLIF) using interbody cages and autograft. One hundred percent of the 32 patients examined at 5- to 7-month follow-up demonstrated radiographic evidence of progressive bone graft consolidation. Iliac crest bone graft was avoided in 7 (14%) patients, and an average of 30% less autograft was required when iliac crest autograft was used.

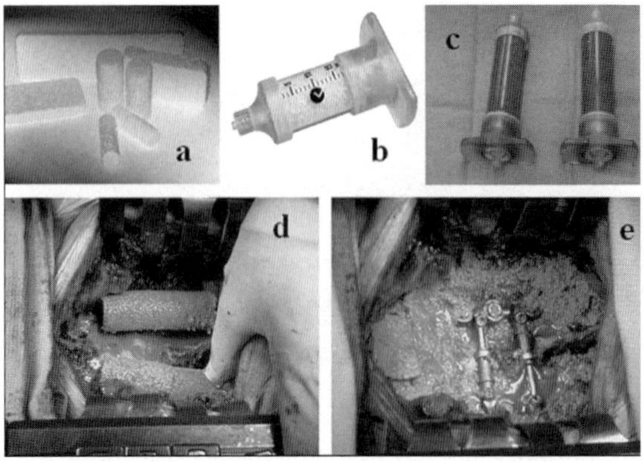

FIG. 29.7. VITOSS Scaffold (**A**) is composed of nanometer-sized (β-tricalcium phosphate particles with 90% interconnecting porosity and is available as a scaffold matrix in both morsel and block forms. A picture of the VITOSS Scaffold canister (**B**): bone marrow aspirate (**C**) is added to the VITOSS Scaffold to obtain a composite. Two pictures of the VITOSS/BMA composite in an instrumented posterolateral fusion patient: the compound is first applied (**D**) and then spread over the fusion surfaces (**E**) (Dr. Joe Ellis Wheeler, Neurosurgeon, Fort Worth, TX). Reprinted, with permission, from Orthovita, Malvern, PA.

In a small study, 7 patients underwent either an anterior (ALIF) or posterior (PLIF) lumbar interbody fusion for a total of 12 levels fused using femoral-ring allograft combined with VITOSS and venous blood without autograft (55). At both the 3- and 6-month follow-up, progressive radiographic fusion was present in 100% of patients; there was no evidence of allograft subsidence, extrusion, fracture, or resorption.

INJECTABLE CERAMIC CEMENTS

Injectable ceramic cements combine the utility of cement with the biomechanical properties of a synthetic bone graft (41). Norian (Norian SRS, Synthes Inc., West Chester, PA, USA) is injectable calcium phosphate cement containing α-TCP, calcium carbonate, and monocalcium phosphate monohydrate in a solution of sodium phosphate. The resulting ceramic is an injectable, fast setting paste that cures in vivo at a physiologic pH and temperature to form an osteoconductive carbonate apatite with chemical and physical properties similar to bone mineral. It can be injected by syringe into a bone defect or fracture site. It is biocompatible, and in vivo it hardens into a material that has an initial compressive strength comparable to cancellous bone. Within a few weeks of introduction, vascular channels invade the implant, osteoclastic activity appears, and new bone formation occurs in direct contact with the ceramic. Over time, the implant undergoes remodeling and is ultimately replaced by host bone with minimal foreign body reaction (56).

Norian SRS has been used successfully in the treatment of distal radial fractures (57), symptomatic vertebral compression fractures, and in the reinforcement of pedicle screw fixation (58). It has been suggested that this material could be used prophylactically to improve the compressive strength of osteoporotic vertebral bodies to help prevent future fractures. In a vertebral body burst fracture model, Norian SRS has been shown to enhance the strength of pedicle screw fixation, which might eliminate the need for supplemental anterior reconstruction in certain fracture patterns (59). A potential concern of

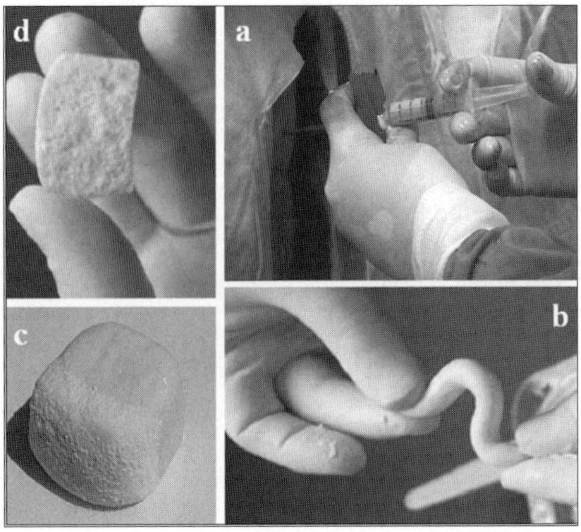

FIG. 29.8. Kryptonite is a self-setting, calcified polyurethane cement. When in liquid form, it can be injected for vertebroplasty (**A**). During the curing process, the material morphs from a liquid to a putty (**B**), and then to a paste (**C**); it acquires a bonelike consistency (**D**) in 48 hours. Reprinted, with permission, from Doctor Research Group, Inc., Plymouth, CT.

liquid injectable cement is extraosseus extrusion. Fortunately, Norian cures and hardens without significant production of heat, decreasing the potential risk of thermal injury to surrounding neural elements and other tissues (41).

Other injectable calcium phosphate cements are currently under evaluation for augmentation of vertebral body/pedicle screw fixation and for vertebral body augmentation procedures such as vertebroplasty and kyphoplasty (60–62). A silica-based ceramic cement (Cortoss Synthetic cortical Bone Void Filler, Orthovita, Inc.) has been approved by the US Food and Drug Administration (FDA) for dental applications; it is used in Europe to reinforce pedicle screw fixation in osteopenic bone, and as a polymethylmethacrylate substitute for vertebroplasty techniques (63,64). A newer compound, Kryptonite (Doctor Research Group, Inc., Plymouth, CT, USA) is a self-setting, polyurethane cement (Fig. 29.8). It is made of a bioabsorbable-calcified triglyceride, which is extremely adhesive and has bonelike mechanical properties. During the curing process, the material changes from a liquid to a putty, and then to a bonelike consistence through a low exothermic curing reaction (45°C). The unique property of this material resides in its osteoconductivity secondary to its porous structure that develops once hardened; moreover, it is reabsorbed over time and is replaced with bone. It is currently pending FDA approval as a bone void filler and for augmentation of internal fixation in patients with poor bone quality. Biomechanical strength and stiffness testing of Kryptonite is underway in a three-level vertebral augmentation cadaver model, as well as a posterolateral fusion model in athymic rats comparing it to autograft and DBM.

BONE MORPHOGENETIC PROTEINS

Bone morphogenetic proteins consist of at least 15 structurally related osteoinductive growth factors, which make up part of the transforming growth factor-β (TGF-β) superfamily. These were first identified in 1976 as the active osteoinductive fraction of DBM and then characterized by molecular cloning in 1988. Similar to other members of the TGF-β superfamily, BMPs are multifunctional and regulate several critical functions ranging from skeletal morphogenesis and development, to angiogenesis and tissue homeostasis. Moreover, BMPs promote the differentiation and proliferation of mesenchymal stem cells into osteochondrogenic cells lineage; they enhance matrix synthesis and apoptosis of osteoblasts, osteoclasts, and vascular endothelial cells. The property of BMPs that has generated the most interest is their ability to initiate and conduct new bone formation. Utilizing recombinant gene technology, BMPs can be produced in an essentially unlimited supply. Recombinant human bone morphogenetic protein-2 (rhBMP-2, Genetics Institute, Cambridge, MA, USA) and rhBMP-7 (Creative Biomolecules, Hopkinton, MA, USA) are the first two products undergoing extensive evaluation and clinical application (55).

A new bone-derived mixture of BMPs, Ne-Osteo, has recently been evaluated in a nonhuman primate model and a human posterolateral lumbar spine fusion pilot clinical trial assessing the optimal quantity needed for humans for induction of new bone formation for an adequate fusion (65).

Both rhBMP-2 and rhBMP-7, also known as osteogenic protein-1 (OP-1), are approved by the FDA for both trauma and spine applications. In 2002, rhBMP-2 was approved in spine using a type I collagen sponge carrier (InFuse bone graft, Medtronic Sofamor Danek, Memphis TN) for use within a cylindrical cage (LT-Medtronic Sofamor Danek) for the surgical management of symptomatic degenerative lumbar disk disease (Fig. 29.9). rhBMP-2 is also approved for use in fresh fractures. rhBMP-7 (OP-1), was approved by the FDA in 2001 for human use for the treatment of recalcitrant tibial nonunions (OP-1 Implant, Stryker Biotech, Hopkinton, MA, USA) (66), and in April 2004 received an additional approval for revision posterolateral fusions utilizing its putty formulation (OP-1 Putty, Stryker Biotech, Hopkinton, MA, USA) (Fig. 29.10). Off-label usage of BMP has been studied extensively. In a recent study, 45 patients undergoing anterior cervical discectomy and fusion with anterior iliac crest autograft were examined (67). Various concentrations of rhBMP-2 were combined with a collagen sponge in order to repair the defect in the iliac crest resulting from graft procurement. Preliminary results are promising and the authors are awaiting long-term follow-up.

rhBMP-7 has been studied extensively in animal spinal fusion models, and presently human clinical trials are underway. An investigational study evaluated the safety and efficacy of rhBMP-7 in patients with single-level degenerative spondylolisthesis (Grade 1 and 2) and spinal stenosis undergoing a posterolateral noninstrumented fusion (68). In this study, iliac crest autograft combined with rhOP-1 in a collagen and carboxymethilcellulose (CMC) carrier was used. Results from 12 patients with 1-year follow-up

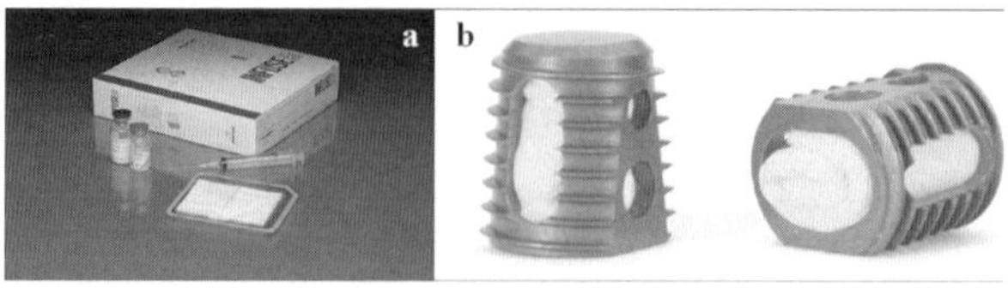

FIG. 29.9. Infuse consists of rhBMP-2 carried by a type I collagen sponge (**A**) is used in anterior interbody procedures in combination with the LT (**B**) cage for treatment of degenerative lumbar disc disease (incorporates technology developed by Gary K. Michelson, MD). Reprinted, with permission, from Medtronic Sofamor Danek, Memphis, TN.

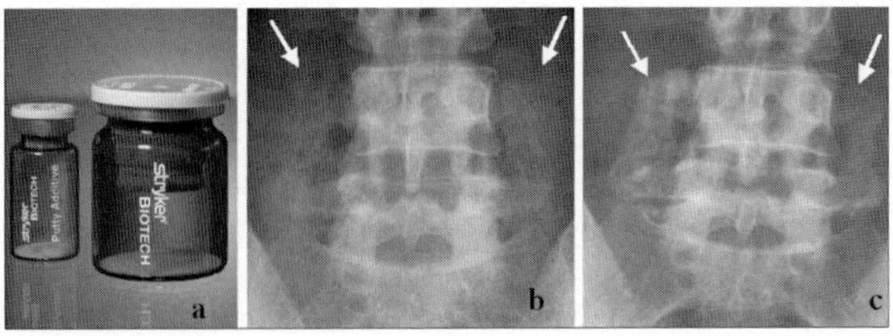

FIG. 29.10. The OP-1 putty implant contains 3.5 mg of lyophilized rhOP-1 mixed with 230 mg carboxymethylcellulose (CMC). At the time of surgery, the powdered mixture (**A**) is reconstituted by adding saline solution to form putty. Six-month (**B**) and 24-month (**C**) follow-up anteroposterior radiograph of OP-1/autograft patient showing the formation of a solid bridge bone (*arrows*) between the transverse processes after noninstumented posterolateral fusion. Reprinted, with permission, from Stryker Biotech, Hopkinton, MA.

revealed 92% of patients demonstrating new bone formation in the intertransverse region (69). Currently, an FDA-approved clinical study is underway evaluating posterolateral uninstrumented fusions randomized to either iliac crest autograft or rhOP-1 in a collagen and CMC carrier.

GENE THERAPY

Gene therapy is the newest method of osteoindutive protein delivery, and therefore relatively few published studies exist. Local gene therapy to achieve a spinal fusion is a multistep procedure designed to deliver a gene with a complementary deoxyribonucleic acid (cDNA) sequence coding for an osteoinductive factor in order to produce specific osteoinductive proteins. This is in place of the actual physical delivery of the protein itself (70). Once an osteoinductive gene is selected, there are several critical decisions to consider when formulating a potential gene therapy program to achieve a fusion. These include the choice of delivery vector, gene, the establishment of the transduction conditions necessary to produce a desired protein or proteins, the selection of carrier matrix, and the establishment of adequate in vivo and in vitro testing models (71).

Vectors may be viral or nonviral. When using viruses for therapeutic gene transfer, they must be modified so that the viral component allowing for protein replication is eliminated from the genome and not reproduced as well. At present, the main recombinant viral vectors used are retroviruses, adenovirus, and adeno-associated viruses. Nonviral vectors include plasmids, cationic liposomes, and DNA-ligand complexes that are capable of transferring genetic material into cell genomes.

Use of gene therapy to obtain a spinal fusion may have several advantages over the local introduction of recombinant BMPs. Modified genetic material may be more physiologically useful than an osteoconductive matrix, providing a more prolonged delivery of the desired signal with continued protein production. More recently, the discovery of LIM mineralization protein-1 (LMP-1), a protein with the ability to initiate membranous bone formation in vivo and in vitro, has provided the opportunity to develop a spinal fusion gene therapy approach through an intracellular activator of the osteoinductive cascade (72). There is now compelling evidence that LMP-1 induces the expression of several BMPs (mostly BMP-4 and BMP-7, less BMP-2, BMP-6 and TGF- β 1 protein). In vivo studies have shown that most of the implanted buffy-coat cells expressing LMP-1 survive for less than 1 week in vivo, but there is indirect evidence of an influx of host cells that differentiate into bone-forming cells. Lastly, LMP-1 appears to induce membranous bone formation without a clear cartilage interphase common with many of the BMPs (73).

COMPOSITE AND BIODEGRADABLE POLYMERIC GRAFTS

A composite graft is defined as combinations of organic and synthetic materials that are designed to provide osteoconductive, osteoinductive, and possibly osteogenic potential. HEALOS (DePuy Spine, Raynham, MA, USA) is an osteoconductive matrix composed of cross-linked type I collagen fibers that are fully coated with 30% hydroxyapatite through a proprietary 360° accretion process (Fig. 29.11). When combined with autogenous bone marrow aspirate, HEALOS provides an environment for osteoprogenitor cell attachment, proliferation, and differentiation. The hydroxyapatite-coated collagen microfibers in HEALOS are similar in structure and composition to bone, thereby recreating the natural human response. The matrix can be saturated with BMA (63), and remodels into new bone at the graft site.

HEALOS has unique graft handling characteristics due to its three-dimensional architecture, which imparts unique tensile strength and "shape memory"; in fact, it retains structural integrity and porosity despite extensive handling. In addition, the flexible, spongelike strips expand and can be molded for graft site coverage, even in irregular spaces. In a rabbit posterolateral intertransverse lumbar fusion model, Tay et al. (74) observed that HEALOS augmented with whole bone marrow produced fusion rates comparable to those of autologous bone graft. HEALOS has also been combined with recombinant human growth/differentiation factor-5 (MP52) in an endoscopic sheep posterolateral fusion model and has demonstrated similar results as autograft in terms of fusion healing (75).

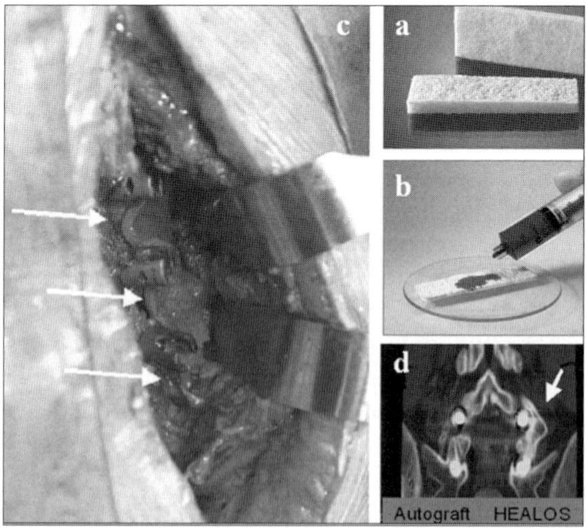

FIG. 29.11. HEALOS is an osteoconductive matrix of cross-linked type I collagen fibers coated with hydroxyapatite (**A**). It is combined with autogenous bone marrow aspirate and molded for complete graft site coverage (**B**). An intraoperative picture of HEALOS plus BMA (*arrows*) versus autograft in instrumented posterolateral fusion (**C**); 12-month follow-up CT reconstruction in the coronal plane showing solid bridge bone between the transverse processes (*arrow*) (Courtesy S. Kitchel, Eugene, OR). Reprinted, with permission, from DePuy Spine, Raynham, MA.

Recently, porous ceramic granules coated with cultured mesenchymal stem cells have been shown to be useful as an alternative to autogenous graft in critical-size defects of long bone, and now are being evaluated as grafting material in experimental posterolateral spinal fusion models. Results demonstrate fusion success comparable to autograft and superior to porous ceramic alone (76). Van Gaalen et al. (77) attached osteoprogenitor cells derived from cultured marrow onto porous HA granules and subcultured them for a week. The granules were then implanted paravertebrally, intramuscularly, and in the subcutaneous tissue in an athymic nude rat model. In all three anatomical sites, new bone formation was observed at the 6- to 9-week postmortem evaluation (78).

Collagraft (Collagraft, Warsaw, IN, USA) is a composite of collagen gel and granules of a biphasic ceramic consisting of 60% HA and 40% TCP. Its structural microarchitecture is designed to resemble the composition of natural bone. This composite has been studied primarily in animal models and was found to be effective as an autograft extender in a canine anterior spinal fusion model, but demonstrated poorer results in a posterior spinal fusion model. In studies of long bone fracture treatment, the use of Collagraft and autologous marrow was compared with iliac crest autograft alone. The researchers found no significant differences in radiographic healing rates or functional outcomes, and its use decreased surgical time and autograft harvesting morbidity (79,80).

Considerable research is being directed toward identifying the optimal carrier to deliver recombinant BMPs. An absorbable collagen sponge (ACS) derived from bovine tendons and a collagen matrix derived from demineralized/guanidine-extracted bovine bone have been used successfully in the delivery of rhBMP-2 and rhBMP-7, respectively. An important advantage of collagen as a carrier material is that it is an endogenous protein, readily metabolized by the body following implantation (81). The disadvantage of its use in its native form is the lack of biomechanical rigidity; thus it can't be used as a structural graft; however, this limitation may be overcome by the addition of hydroxyapatite (82–84). The immunologic potential of collagen derived from allogeneic or xenogeneic sources is also a concern (85).

Biodegradable polymers offer the possibility of replacing collagen as a delivery agent for BMPs or cells, thus eliminating the use of xenogeneic material (86). Two categories of polymeric membranes being investigated for containing or guiding bone growth in bone grafting procedures are the nonbiodegradable polytetrafluoroethylene (PTFE) and biodegradable poly α-hydroxy acids (PHAs), including polylactic acid (PLA) and polyglycolic acid (PGA) (87,88). Biodegradable polymers (PLA and PGA) are already in clinical use as absorbable sutures, fixation pins and screws, and spinal graft buttress implants. In the form of a solid device, PLA spinal cages filled with rhBMP-2-soaked collagen sponge resulted in bridging bone in 100% of the patients as early as 3 months in the cervical region (89) and 98% solid fusion at 6 months in the lumbar region (90). Early studies on these materials as potential growth factor carriers in their porous form have shown promising results. Poly [D,L lactide-co-glycolide)] (PLGA) porous scaffolds have been evaluated in a canine spinal fusion model combined with rhBMP-2 (87), and compared directly to both autograft bone and PLGA alone. No differences were identified in terms of fusion rates or biomechanical properties between the rhBMP-2/PLGA composite and the autograft alone groups, and both treatments were superior to the use of PLGA alone. A more recent canine study showed faster spinal fusion in the rhBMP-2/PLA scaffold group compared to the autograft or scaffold alone (91). Porous PHAs demonstrated their potential as carriers for bone marrow–derived osteoprogenitor cells in the late 1990s (92), and this combination of osteogenic cells and porous PLGA scaffold displayed osteoinductive properties by inducing ectopic bone formation. As mentioned earlier, osteoprogenitor cells derived from adipose tissue also promoted healing in a critical-size murine calvarial defect when delivered using an apatite-coated PLGA scaffold (25). Recently, PLGA has been combined with a calcium-phosphate cement composite for the delivery of rhBMP-2. This model demonstrated that the release of rhBMP-2 was dependent on composite composition and nanostructure as well as the pH of the release medium (93). A copolymer of PLA and polyethylene glycol (PLA-PEG) has recently been developed. Advantage of this material is that plasticity, stiffness, and biodegradability of the polymer can be controlled by altering the PLA to PEG ratio (94,95). These composites have demonstrated good osteoinductivity and osteoconductivity when combined with BMPs in preliminary studies.

CONCLUSIONS

Obtaining a successful spinal fusion can be extremely challenging. Careful patient selection and surgical technique are paramount and remain the most important variables in obtaining satisfactory outcomes in a majority of patients. Unfortunately, a failed spinal fusion continues to represent a considerable source of unsatisfactory clinical outcomes. Utilizing a generous amount of autograft bone has previously provided the most reliable means of achieving a rapid and robust fusion mass, but results have nevertheless remained unpredictable, and the morbidity associated with graft harvest has often overshadowed positive clinical results from the primary operation. Numerous alternatives to autograft bone have been developed, none of which possess all the crucial properties of autograft, including being osteoconductive, osteoinductive, and osteogenic. Recombinant BMPs and advances in gene therapy may provide fusion-enhancing capacity that matches or even exceeds the performance of autograft. The recent development of newer and more effective composite grafts has developed a new and exciting field of research in regard to biomaterials and biotechnology, promising a more effective treatment for patients requiring spinal fusion.

REFERENCES

1. Boden SD. Biology of lumbar spine fusion and use of bone graft substitutes: present, future, and next generation. *Tissue Eng* 2000;6(4):383–399.
2. Boden SD, Schimandle JH. Biology of lumbar spine fusion and bone graft materials. In: International Society for Study of the Lumbar Spine Editorial Committee, ed. *The Lumbar Spine*. 2nd edition. Philadelphia: WB Saunders, 1996:1284–1306.
3. Boden SD. Overview of the biology of lumbar spine fusion and principles for selecting a bone graft substitute. *Spine* 2002;27(16 suppl);S26–S31.
4. Simon SR, ed. *Orthopaedic Basic Science*. 2nd edition. Rosemont, IL: American Academy of Orthopaedic Surgeons; 1994:284–293.
5. Vaccaro AR. The role of the osteoconductive scaffold in synthetic bone graft. *Orthopedics* 2002;25(5 suppl):S571–S578.
6. Goldberg VM, Stevenson S. Natural history of autografts and allografts. *Clin Orthop* 1987;225:7–16.
7. Malloy KM, Hilibrand AS. Autograft versus allograft in degenerative cervical disease. *Clin Orthop* 2002;394:27–38.
8. Erbe EM, Marx JG, Clineff TD, et al. Potential of an ultraporous β-tricalcium phosphate synthetic cancellous bone void filler and bone marrow aspirate composite graft. *Eur Spine J* 2001;10:S141–S146.
9. Betz RR. Limitations of autograft and allograft: new synthetic solutions. *Orthopedics* 2002;25(5 suppl):S561–S570.
10. Jorgenson SS, Lowe TG, France J, et al. A prospective analysis of autograft vs. allograft in posterolateral fusion in the same patient: a minimum one year follow-up in 144 patients. *Spine* 1994;19:2048–2053.
11. Malinen TI, Brown MD. Bone allografts in spine surgery. *Clin Orthop* 1981;154:68–73.
12. May VR Jr, Mauck WR. Exploration of the spine for pseudoarthrosis following spinal fusion in the treatment of scoliosis. *Clin Orthop* 1967;53:115–122.

13. Bono CM, Lee CK. Critical analysis of trends in fusion for degenerative disc disease over the past 20 years: influence of technique on fusion rate and clinical outcome. *Spine* 2004;29:455–463.
14. Arrington ED, Smith WJ, Chambers HG, et al. Complications of iliac crest bone graft harvesting. *Clin Orthop* 1996;329:300–309.
15. Banwart JA, Asher MA, Hassanein RS. Iliac crest bone graft harvest donor site morbidity: a statistical evaluation. *Spine* 1995;20:1055–1060.
16. Enneking WF, Early JL, Burchardt H. Autologous cortical bone grafts in the reconstruction of segmental skeletal defects. *J Bone Joint Surg Am* 1975;57:237–252.
17. Younger EM, Chapman MW. Morbidity at bone graft donor sites. *J Orthop Trauma* 1989;3:192–195.
18. Khan SN, Tomin E, Lane JM. Clinical applications of bone graft substitutes. *Orthop Clin North Am* 2000;31:389–398.
19. Connolly JF, Guse R, Tiedman J, et al. Autologous marrow injection as a substitute for operative grafting of tibial nonunions. *Clin Orthop* 1991;266:259–270.
20. Dragoo JL, Choi JY, Lieberman JR, et al. Bone induction by BMP-2 transduced stem cells derived from human fat. *J Orthop Res* 2003;21:622–629.
21. Dragoo JL, Samimi B, Zhu M, et al. Tissue-engineered cartilage and bone using stem cells from human infrapatellar fat pads. *J Bone Joint Surg Br* 2003;85:740–747.
22. Halvorsen YD, Franklin D, Bond AL, et al. Extracellular matrix mineralization and osteoblast gene expression by human adipose tissue-derived stromal cells. *Tissue Eng* 2001;7:729–741.
23. Zuk PA, Zhu M, Mizuno H, et al. Multilineage cells from human adipose tissue: implications for cell-based therapies. *Tissue Eng* 2001;7:211–228.
24. Zuk PA, Zhu M, Ashjian P, et al. Human adipose tissue is a source of multipotent stem cells. *Mol Biol Cell* 2002;13:4279–4295.
25. Cowan CM, Shi YY, Aalami OO, et al. Adipose-derived adult stromal cells heal critical-size mouse calvarial defects. *Nat Biotechnol* 2004;22:560–567.
26. De Ugarte DA, Morizono K, Elbarbary A, et al. Comparison of multi-lineage cells from human adipose tissue and bone marrow. *Cells Tissues Organs* 2003;174:101–109.
27. Muschler GF, Nitto H, Matsukura Y, et al. Spine fusion using cell matrix composites enriched in bone marrow–derived cells. *Clin Orthop* 2003;407:102–118.
28. Weiner BK, Walker, M. Efficacy of autologous growth factors in lumbar intertransverse fusions. *Spine* 2003;28:1968–1971.
29. Vaccaro AR, Sharan AD, Tuan RS, et al. The use of biologic materials in spinal fusion. *Orthopedics* 2001;24:191–197.
30. Schlegel KA, Donath K, Rupprecht S, et al. De novo bone formation using bovine collagen and platelet-rich plasma. *Biomaterials* 2004;25(23):5387–5393.
31. Jensen TB, Rahbek O, Overgaard S, et al. Platelet rich plasma and fresh frozen bone allograft as enhancement of implant fixation: an experimental study in dogs. *J Orthop Res* 2004;22:653–658.
32. Walsh WR, Loefler A, Nicklin S, et al. Spinal fusion using an autologous growth factor gel and a porous resorbable ceramic. *Eur Spine J* 2004 Mar 18 [Epub ahead of print].
33. Bauer T. A comparative evaluation of the osteoinductivity of two formulations of human demineralized bone matrix. Presented at the 69th meeting of the American Academy of Orthopaedic Surgeons. February 13–17, 2002, Dallas, TX.
34. Oikarinen J. Experimental spinal fusion with decalcified bone matrix and deep frozen allogenic bone in rabbits. *Clin Orthop* 1982;162:210–218.
35. Pals SD, Wilkins RM. Giant cell tumor treated by curettage, cementation, and bone grafting. *Orthopedics* 1992;15:703–708.
36. Glowacki J, Mulliken JB. Demineralized bone implants. *Clin Plast Surg* 1985;12:233.
37. Martin GJ, Boden SD, Titus L, et al. New formulations of demineralized bone matrix as a more effective alternative in experimental posterolateral lumbar spine arthtrodesis. *Spine* 1999;24:637–645.
38. Cammisa FP Jr, Lowery G, Garfin SR, et al. Two-year fusion rate equivalency between Grafton DBM gel and autograft in posterolateral spine fusion: a prospective controlled trial employing a side-by-side comparison in the same patient. *Spine* 2004;29:660–666.
39. Louis-Ugbo J, Murakami H, Kim HS, et al. Evidence of osteoinduction by Grafton demineralized bone matrix in nonhuman primate spinal fusion. *Spine* 2004;29:360–366.
40. Iwata H, Sakano S, Itoh T, et al. Demineralized bone matrix and native bone morphogenetic protein in orthopaedic surgery. *Clin Orthop* 2002;395:99–109.
41. Kim DH, Jenis L, Berta SC, et al. Bone graft alternatives in spinal fusion surgery. *Curr Opin Orthop* 2003;14: 127–137.
42. Vaccaro AR, Chiba K, Heller JG, et al. Bone grafting alternatives in spinal surgery. *Spine J* 2002;2:206–215.
43. Constantz BR, Ison IC, Fulmer MT, et al. Skeletal repair by in situ formation of the mineral phase of bone. *Science* 1995;267:1796–1799.
44. Delecrin J, Takahashi S, Gouin F, et al. A synthetic porous ceramic as a bone graft substitute in the surgical management of scoliosis: a prospective, randomized study. *Spine* 2000;25(5):563–569.
45. Gazdag AR, Lane JM, Glaser D, et al. Alternatives to autogenous bone graft: efficacy and indications. *J Am Acad Orthop Surg* 1995;3:1–8.

46. Ransford AO, Morley T, Edgar MA, et al. Synthetic porous ceramic compared with autograft in scoliosis surgery: a prospective, randomized study of 341 patients. *J Bone Joint Surg Br* 1998;80:13–18.
47. Cavagna R. Daculsi G. Bouler JM. Macroporous calcium phosphate ceramic: a prospective study of 106 cases in lumbar spinal fusion. *J Long Term Eff Med Implants* 1999;9(4):403–412.
48. Thalgott JS, Fritts K, Giuffre JM, et al. Anterior interbody fusion of the cervical spine with coralline hydroxyapatite. *Spine* 1999;24:1295–1299.
49. McConnell JR, Freeman BJ, Debnath UK, et al. A prospective randomized comparison of coralline hydroxyapatite with autograft in cervical interbody fusion. *Spine* 2003;28:317–323.
50. Thalgott JS, Fritts K, Giuffre JM, et al. The use of coralline hydroxyapatite for interbody spinal fusions. *Spine* 1997;11:325–340.
51. Thalgott JS, Klezl Z, Timlin M, et al. Anterior lumbar interbody fusion with processed sea coral (coralline hydroxyapatite) as part of a circumferential fusion. *Spine* 2002;27:E518–E525.
52. Muschik M, Ludwig R, Halbhubner S, et al. Beta-tricalcium phosphate as a bone substitute for dorsal spinal fusion in adolescent idiopathic scoliosis: preliminary results of a prospective clinical study. *Eur Spine J* 2001;10(suppl 2):S178–S184.
53. Resnick DK. Vitoss bone substitute. *Neurosurgery* 2002;50:1162–1164.
54. Meadows GR. Adjunctive use of ultraporous β-tricalcium phosphate bone void filler in spinal arthrodesis. *Orthopedics* 2002;25(5 suppl):S579–S584.
55. Ludwig SC, Boden SD. Osteoinductive bone graft substitutes for spinal fusion: a basic science summary. *Orthop Clin North Am* 1999;30:635–644.
56. Cornell CN. Osteoconductive materials and their role as substitutes for autogenous bone grafts. *Orthop Clin North Am* 1999;30:591–598.
57. Cassidy C, Jupiter JB, Cohen M, et al. Norian SRS cement compared with conventional fixation in distal radial fractures: a randomized study. *J Bone Joint Surg Am* 2003;85:2127–2137.
58. Wuisman PI, Van Dijk M, Staal H, et al. Augmentation of (pedicle) screws with calcium apatite cement in patients with severe progressive osteoporotic spinal deformities: an innovative technique. *Eur Spine J* 2000;9:528–533.
59. Keating JF, McQueen MM. Substitutes for autologous bone graft in orthopaedic trauma: substitutes for autologous bone graft in orthopaedic trauma. *J Bone Joint Surg Br* 2001;83:3–8.
60. Bai B, Kummer FJ, Spivak J. Augmentation of anterior vertebral body screw fixation by an injectable, biodegradable calcium phosphate bone substitute. *Spine* 2001;26:2679–2683.
61. Blattert TR, Delling G, Weckbach A. Evaluation of an injectable calcium phosphate cement as an autograft substitute for transpedicular lumbar interbody fusion: a controlled, prospective study in the sheep model. *Eur Spine J* 2003;12(2):216–223.
62. Lim TH, Brebach GT, Renner SM, et al. Biomechanical evaluation of an injectable calcium phosphate cement for vertebroplasty. *Spine* 2002;27:1297–1302.
63. Bauer TW, Smith ST. Bioactive materials in orthopaedic surgery: overview and regulatory considerations. *Clin Orthop* 2002 395:11–22.
64. Heini PF, Berlemann U. Bone substitutes in vertebroplasty. *Eur Spine J* 2001;10(suppl 2):S205–S213.
65. Boden SD, Grob D, Damien C. Ne-osteo bone growth factor for posterolateral lumbar spine fusion: results from a nonhuman primate study and a prospective human clinical pilot study. *Spine* 2004;29:504–514.
66. Sandhu HS. Bone morphogenetic proteins and spinal surgery. *Spine* 2003;28(15 suppl):S64–S73.
67. Sandhu HS, Grewal HS, Parvataneni H. Bone grafting for spinal fusion. *Orthop Clin North Am* 1999;30(4):685–698.
68. Vaccaro AR, Patel T, Fischgrund J, et al. A pilot safety and efficacy study of OP-1 putty (rhBMP-7) as an adjunct to iliac crest autograft in posterolateral lumbar fusions. *Eur Spine J* 2003;12:495–500.
69. Patel TCh, Hopkinton MA, Vaccaro AR, et al. Two-year follow up of a safety and efficacy study of op-1 (rhbmp-7) as an adjunct to posterolateral lumber fusion. Presented at 16th Annual Meeting of the North American Spine Society. October 31–November 3, 2001, Seattle, WA.
70. Yoon ST, Boden SD, Titus L, Hair G, et al. Lumbar spine fusion by local gene therapy with a cDNA encoding a novel osteoinductive protein (LMP-1). *Spine* 1998;23:2486–2492.
71. Boden SD. Spine fusion by gene therapy. *Gene Ther* 2004;11:360–367.
72. Cha CW, Boden SD. Gene therapy applications for spine fusion. *Spine* 2003;28(15 suppl):S74–S84.
73. Minamide A, Boden SD, Viggeswarapu M, et al. Mechanism of bone formation with gene transfer of the cDNA encoding for the intracellular protein LMP-1. *J Bone Joint Surg Am* 2003;85:1030–1039.
74. Tay BK, Le AX, Heilman M, et al. Use of a collagen-hydroxyapatite matrix in spinal fusion: a rabbit model. *Spine* 1998;23:2276–2281.
75. Jahng TA, Fu TS, Cunningham BW, et al. Endoscopic instrumented posterolateral lumbar fusion with Healos and recombinant human growth/differentiation factor-5. *Neurosurgery* 2004;54:171–180.
76. Cinotti G, Patti AM, Vulcano A, et al. Experimental posterolateral spinal fusion with porous ceramics and mesenchymal stem cells. *J Bone Joint Surg Br* 2004;86:135–142.
77. van Gaalen SM, Dhert WJ, van den Muysenberg A, et al. Bone tissue engineering for spine fusion: an experimental study on ectopic and orthotopic implants in rats. *Tissue Eng* 2004;10:231–239.
78. Cui Q, Ming Xiao Z, Balian G, et al. Comparison of lumbar spine fusion using mixed and cloned marrow cells. *Spine* 2001;26:2305–2310.

79. Chapman MW, Bucholz R, Cornell C. Treatment of acute fractures with a collagen-calcium phosphate graft material: a randomized clinical trial. *J Bone Joint Surg Am* 1997;79:495–502.
80. Cornell CN, Lane JM, Chapman M, et al. Multicenter trial of collagraft as bone graft substitute. *J Orthop Trauma* 1991;5:1–8.
81. Uludag H, Gao T, Porter TJ, et al. Delivery systems for BMPs: factors contributing to protein retention at an application site. *J Bone Joint Surg Am* 2001;83:S1128–S1135.
82. Nakashima, M. Induction of dentine in amputated pulp of dogs by recombinant human bone morphogenetic protein-2 and -4 with collagen matrix. *Arch Oral Biol* 1994;39:1085–1099.
83. Takaoka K, Koezuka M, Nakahara H. Telopeptide-depleted bovine skin collagen as a carrier for bone morphogenetic protein. *J Orthop Res* 1991;9:902–907.
84. Takaoka K, Nakahara H, Yoshikawa H, et al. Ectopic bone induction on and in porous hydroxyapatite combined with collagen and bone morphogenetic protein. *Clin Orthop* 1988;234:250–254.
85. DeLustro F, Dasch J, Keefe J, et al. Immune responses to allogeneic and xenogeneic implants of collagen and collagen derivatives. *Clin Orthop* 1990;260:263–279.
86. Saito N, Takaoka K. New synthetic biodegradable polymers as BMP carriers for bone tissue engineering. *Biomaterials* 2003;24:2287–2293.
87. Muschler GF, Hyodo A, Manning T, et al. Evaluation of Human Bone Morphogenetic Protein 2 in a Canine Spinal Fusion Model. *Clin Orthop* 1994;35:279–284.
88. Peter SJ, Miller MJ, Yasko AW, et al. Polymer concepts in tissue engineering. *J Biomed Mater R*es 1998;43:422–427.
89. Lanman TH, Hopkins TJ. Lumbar interbody fusion after treatment with recombinant human bone morphogenetic protein-2 added to poly(L-lactide-co-D,L-lactide) bioresorbable implants. *Neurosurg Focus* 2004; 16(3):E9.
90. Lanman TH, Hopkins TJ. Early findings in a pilot study of anterior cervical interbody fusion in which recombinant human bone morphogenetic protein-2 was used with poly(L-lactide-co-D,L-lactide) bioabsorbable implants. *Neurosurg Focus* 2004;16(3):E6.
91. Sandhu HS, Kanim LE, Kabo JM, et al. Evaluation of rhBMP-2 with an OPLA carrier in a canine posterolateral (transverse process) spinal fusion model. *Spine* 1995;20(24):2669–2682.
92. Ishaug-Riley SL, Crane GM, Gurlek A, et al. Ectopic bone formation by marrow stromal osteoblast transplantation using poly(DL-lactic-co-glycolic acid) foams implanted into the rat mesentery. *J Biomed Mater Res* 1997;36:1–8.
93. Ruhe PQ, Hedberg EL, Padron NT, et al. rhBMP-2 release from injectable poly(DL-lactic-co-glycolic acid)/calcium-phosphate cement composites. *J Bone Joint Surg Am* 2003;85(suppl 3):75–81.
94. Miyamoto S, Takaoka K, Okada T, et al. Polyactic acid-polyethylene glycol block copolymer. a new biodegradable synthetic carrier for bone morphogenetic protein. *Clin Orthop* 1993;294:333–343.
95. Saito N, Okada T, Toba S, et al. New synthetic absorbable polymers as BMP carriers: plastic properties of poly-D,L-lactic acid-polyethylene glycol block copolymers. *J Biomed Mater R*es 1999;47:104–110.

30

The Place of Vertebrectomy in the Treatment of Spondylolisthesis/ Spondyloptosis

Helton Defino

DEFINITION

Spondyloptosis represents the most advanced and severe degree of spondylolisthesis, when the L5 body is located below the top of S1. The slip angle and the tilt angle vary considerably among different patients. The rarity of this deformity has not permitted the collection of large clinical series, so that rational decisions about treatment have been difficult.

PHYSIOPATHOLOGY

The stability of the lumbosacral junction depends on static factors (spatial orientation of L5 to sacrum, lumbosacral angle, sacral slope, and osteodiscoligamentous complex) and dynamic factors (interaction of neuromuscular system with osteodiscoligamentous complex). The compression forces are supported by the vertebral body and disc; the shear forces are supported by the disc and by posterior bone elements. The pars articularis acts as a bone bridge and is the apparent link between these two regions (1,2).

The progression of spondylolisthesis to a high-grade slip or spondyloptosis is related to the degree of dysplasia of the vertebra and to external factors such as age, growth, weight bearing, and muscle imbalance. The degree of developmental dysplasia associated with lumbosacral kyphosis results in the different types of spondylolisthesis. Spondyloptosis is the final result of developmental high-dysplastic spondylolisthesis associated with ventral translation and lumbosacral kyphosis that was untreated or mismanaged (1–3).

The majority of slips do not progress significantly, but some patients progress to high-grade slips and spondyloptosis. Some factors predicting the risk for progression have been identified: i.e., female gender, great growth potential, increased slip angle, trapezoidal L5, domed and vertical sacrum, and sagittal rotation. High-grade slips and younger age are the most significant risk factors for progression (1,3–6).

The sagittal balance and spinopelvic relationship associated with the degree of vertebral slip are related to progression of the slip. Kyphosis and increased slip angle occur late, and they are as much a result as a cause of progressive high-grade slips. They can be considered to be markers of the risk for spondyloptosis (4–7).

The increase in lumbar lordosis is present from the early phases as a response compensating for the increased translation and slip angle. Lordosis also increases in the more delayed forms to compensate for sagittal imbalance. Sagittal balance can be achieved by only hyperlordosis, perhaps to anatomic extremes. In situations in which further compensation to maintain sagittal balance is necessary in addition to lordosis, verticalization of the sacrum occurs. Verticalization of the sacrum is accompanied by contraction of the hamstrings, which promotes caudal rotation of the ischium and anterior rotation of the pelvis in a cephalic direction. These actions occur at the level of the coxofemoral joint and therefore affect posture (hyperlordosis) and gait (crouched or waddling gait), in a manner that characterizes patients with high-degree slip or spondyloptosis (1,4,6,8).

Not all patients with dysplastic posterior elements develop a high-grade spondylolisthesis or ptosis. The morphology of the spine and of the pelvis (inclination of the sacrum, distance between the femoral head and the sacrum) contributes to the cascade of events and is a determinant factor in progression to slip and lumbosacral kyphosis.

The natural history of spondyloptosis is unknown, and its clinical manifestations are not uniform, with different clinical characteristics being observed in different patients.

CLINICAL PICTURE

The clinical picture of patients with spondyloptosis is not uniform: some patients are almost asymptomatic and others present intense symptoms accompanied by a marked degree of functional disability. The symptoms are related to mechanical changes in the lumbosacral region (pain), compression of nervous structures (weakness, numbness, changes in sphincter function), and sagittal imbalance (thoracolumbar fatigue, muscle weakness, gait abnormality) (3–5).

INDICATIONS

The indication of surgical treatment should take into account the age of the patient. For children, surgical treatment should be indicated in the presence of slips over 50% or documented progression regardless of symptoms. All efforts should be made to prevent the occurrence of a significant slip angle (6,8–10).

For adults, the indication of surgical treatment is related to the importance of symptoms, persistent leg pain, neurologic deficit, cauda equina syndrome, and major sagittal imbalance (walking, standing, or visual difficulties)(3,6,11,12).

Surgical indication for pain relief is still a matter of debate since the exact source of nociception is unclear and a full resolution of pain by surgical treatment is not certain.

Vertebrectomy has also been indicated as a salvage reconstruction procedure for failed primary surgery on Grades 4 and 5 spondylolisthesis when the patients present pain, progressive deformity, or bowel and bladder dysfunction (3,10,13,14)

OBJECTIVES AND OPTIONS OF TREATMENT

In general, the purpose of treatment is to fuse as few segments as possible, restore or maintain spinal balance, preserve neurologic status, obtain a solid arthrodesis, and treat patient's clinical symptoms.

In cases of spondylolisthesis with a high degree of deviation, surgical treatment, in general, should consist of in situ arthrodesis of the deformity, or a reduction (close, open, vertebral resection) should be attempted. The final decision is still subjective and depends on the treatment philosophy of the surgeon. The treatment of high-grade spondylolisthesis and ptosis has not been specifically reported as a large series. However, complication rates are higher, especially if reduction is attempted and the deformity is rigid (3,6,9,11,15).

There is considerable controversy about the treatment of spondyloptosis and high-grade spondylolisthesis due to the lack of understanding of the biomechanical causes and sequelae of these disorders.

VERTEBRECTOMY

L5 vertebrectomy for the treatment of spondyloptosis was developed by Gaines in 1979 (13), and the description of the technique with the results for the first patients was published in 1985 (14). The technique was elaborated due to the fact that the techniques available at the time did not permit improved alignment along the sagittal plane and caused iatrogenic lesions of cauda equina nerves in situations in which Harrington rods were used for reduction.

The surgical procedure described by Gaines and Nichols (14) is performed in two stages (anterior and posterior approach), which may be part of the same surgical act or may be separated by a 1-week interval. In the first stage, the intervertebral L4–L5-S1 discs are removed and the L5 vertebral body is fully resected by means of a retroperitoneal approach using a transverse abdominal incision that transects one rectus abdominis muscle completely and at least half of the contralateral rectus abdominis muscle. The L5 vertebral body must be resected up to the pedicles, which represent the posterior margin of the anterior stage resection. No attempt at reduction is made during this treatment stage and epidural bleeding can be controlled with Gelfoam. In the second stage, the L4-S1 vertebral segment is exposed through a posterior approach, the posterior elements of L5 (lamina, pedicles, and transverse process) are resected; the L5 root is identified and exposed bilaterally; and reduction, fixation, and arthrodesis of L4 over S1 are performed. L4-S1 fixation is performed with pedicular screws, and cancellous bone from the L5 vertebrectomy is used as a posterolateral graft. Modification of the Gaines technique has been observed in sporadic clinical case reports in which treatment is started by approach to, and removal of the posterior elements of L5, by anterior approach to and resection of the L4–L5-S1 discs and the L5 vertebral body, followed by skeletal traction. Treatment is finalized with the second posterior approach for L4-S1 reduction, fixation, and arthrodesis.

RESULTS

The largest series and the longest follow-up of patients submitted to these techniques belong to the author of the procedure himself, Robert W. Gaines, who, at the 2003 Scoliosis Research Society Meeting, presented a review of 24 years of experience with the use of L5 vertebrectomy for the surgical treatment of spondyloptosis. Twenty-seven patients have been operated since 1979, 20 of them aged 12 to 25 years and three aged 30 to 50 years. The latter three patients had already undergone surgical treatment. One had had two previous procedures; another had had four, and one had six previous procedures (13).

The independent evaluation of patients carried out in 1994 (16) showed that they were satisfied with the treatment, felt better, and were not taking narcotics, and that each would recommend the procedure to other patients. However, one patient operated upon after the revision performed in 1994 has been presenting pain despite the good radiologic result.

When he first started to use the technique, Gaines recommended routine re-exploration of the fusion mass and removal of implants 4 to 6 months following the reconstruction.

This re-exploration is no longer recommended; breaking of the pedicular screws due to fibrous union was observed in two patients over the last 3 years, and the problem was solved by reinstrumentation and a bone graft (3).

No junctional problem was observed in any of the patients over the 24 years of follow-up, and it was possible to improve lumbopelvic alignment and spinal posture, although the restoration of the C7 plumb line is unpredictable.

General complications such as death, pulmonary emboli or other serious medical problems, or bowel, bladder, or sexual dysfunction were not observed. Lesion of the vena cava occurred in one patient and was repaired during the primary procedure.

Temporary L5 neuropraxis was the neurologic complication most frequently observed in the 27 patients of the series reported by Gaines (13), occurring unilaterally or bilaterally in 20 of the 27 patients operated upon. In view of the frequent occurrence of this complication, counseling about it has been recommended as a standard preoperative procedure. All but two of the 20 patients with L5 deficit totally recovered their motor function. A few patients had lingering numbness in the L5 distribution, which is a nuisance grade annoyance that causes no functional limitation for any of the patients who have it.

No neuropraxis in any other nerve root except L5 was observed in the series reported by Gaines (13).

CONCLUSIONS

L5 vertebrectomy is an alternative for the treatment of spondyloptosis associated with severe lumbopelvic deformity and sagittal plane imbalance, and can also be used as a salvage reconstruction procedure for patients with high-grade spondylolisthesis who have already been operated upon. This procedure permits the alignment of the spine on the sagittal plane; because of the shortening of the spine that occurs due to vertebral resection, the adjacent nervous elements are protected, with their stretching being prevented during reduction. However, neuropraxis of the L5 root has frequently been observed in patients submitted to this procedure and, even though many patients present motor recovery of this root, the occurrence of this event should be considered during treatment planning. Prevention of spondyloptosis by early and adequate treatment of spondylolisthesis still seems to be the most effective way to avoid the need for surgical treatment of a severe deformity such as spondyloptosis, whose treatment is not free from the risk of lesion of the L5 root.

REFERENCES

1. Österman K, Schlenzka D, Poussa M, et al. Isthmic spondylolisthesis in symptomatic and asymptomatic subjects: epidemiology and natural history with special reference to disk abnormality and mode of treatment. *Clin Orthop* 1993;297:65–70.
2. Saraste H. Spondylolysis and spondylolisthesis. *Acta Orthop Scand* 1993;251(suppl):84–86.
3. Gaines RW. The L5 vertebrectomy approach for the treatment of spondyloptosis. In: Bridwell KH, DeWald RL, ed. *The Textbook of Spinal Surgery.* 2nd edition. Philadelphia: Lippincott–Raven; 1999:1357–1370.
4. Curylo LJ, Edwards C, de Wald RW. Radiographic markers in spondyloptosis: implications for spondylolisthesis progression. *Spine* 2002;27(18):1–5.
5. Huang RP, Bohlman HH, Thompson GH, et al. Predictive value of pelvic incidence in progression of spondylolisthesis. *Spine* 2003;28(20):2381–2385.
6. Szpalski M, Gunzburg R. Surgery for high-grade spondylolisthesis. In: Herkowitz HN, Dvořák J, Bell JR, Nordin M, et al. *The Lumbar Spine*. 3rd edition. Philadelphia: Lippincott Williams & Wilkins; 2004:59–597.
7. Schwab F, Farcy JP, Roye DP. The sagittal pelvic index as a criterion in the evaluation of spondylolisthesis: preliminary observations. *Spine* 1997;22(14):1661–1677.
8. Poussa M, Schlenzka, Seitsalo S, et al. Surgical treatment of severe isthmic spondylolisthesis in adolescents: reduction or fusion in situ. *Spine* 1993;18:894–901.

9. DeWald RL, Faut MM, Taddonio RF, et al. Severe lumbosacral spondylolisthesis in adolescents and children. *J Bone Joint Surg Am* 1981;63:619–626.
10. Wild A, Jager M, Werner A, et al. Treatment of congenital spondyloptosis in an 18-months-old patient with a 10-year follow-up. *Spine* 2001;26(21):502–505.
11. Dimar JR, Hoffman G. Grade 4 spondylolisthesis: two-stage therapeutic approach of anterior vertebrectomy and anterior-posterior fusion. *Orthop Rev* 1986;15:504–509.
12. Verbiest H. The treatment of lumbar spondyloptosis or impending lumbar spondyloptosis accompanied by neurologic deficit and/or neurogenic intermittent claudication. *Spine* 1979;4(1):68–77.
13. Gaines R. Treatment by L5 spondylectomy. Scoliosis Research Society CME Course. Quebec City, Quebec, Canada, September 10, 2003.
14. Gaines RW, Nichols WK. Treatment of spondyloptosis by two-stage L5 vertebrectomy and reduction of L4 onto S1. *Spine* 1985;10:680–686.
15. Molinari RW, Bridwell KH, Lenke LG, et al. Complications in the surgical treatment of pediatric high-grade, isthmic dysplastic spondylolisthesis: a comparison of three surgical approaches. *Spine* 1999;24(16):1701.
16. Lehmer S, Steffe AD, Gaines RW. Treatment of L5-S1 spondyloptosis by staged L5 resection with reduction and fusion of L4 onto S1. *Spine* 1994;19:1916–1925.

31

Surgery for Spondylolisthesis: RCT Evidence from the Cochrane Review

J. N. Alastair Gibson and Gordon Waddell

Ideally, any surgical intervention should be evidence based, and surgery for spondylolisthesis is no exception. The first, clinical demand is that surgery should be effective, but in these days of finite health care funding, it should also be cost effective. Indeed, a marginally less effective, yet safer or cheaper intervention may be the treatment of choice in some situations. This may be especially relevant to the choice of intervention for spondylolisthesis.

We have recently collated all randomized controlled trials (RCTs) on surgical interventions for the latest update of the Cochrane Review of Degenerative Lumbar Spondylosis (1). From that review, it was possible to extract data pertaining to the treatment of spondylolysis and the various types of spondylolisthesis for this chapter. Critical analysis allows important questions to be addressed with respect to the type of surgery, timing of surgery, and cost.

METHODS

Selection of Trials

All trials published as full articles or abstracts were collected from computer searches of Medline, PubMed, and the Cochrane Controlled Trials Register. *Spine*, the *Journal of Spinal Disorders*, and other specialized periodicals were hand-searched and, in addition, surgical colleagues around the world forwarded RCTs known to them. All RCTs were checked by both authors for details of the trial methodology and quality rated. Those RCTs with any reference to spondylolysis or spondylolisthesis were then extracted and all relevant data analyzed for this paper.

Outcome Analysis

Outcome data presented in the trials varied considerably in its content and substance, but most trials contained some relevant results that could be analyzed using the Cochrane review manager PC software (Revman®). Where appropriate, meta-analysis was performed and odds ratios (OR) with 95% confidence limits (CI) calculated. Patient or surgeon ratings of outcome were treated by pooling the data, classifying excellent or good outcomes as "success" and fair or poor as "failure."

TRIALS

In the 2005 update of the Cochrane Review on lumbar spondylosis, 31 published RCTs are included. Eleven contain data relating to patients with spondylolisthesis. Two of these analyzed outcomes following treatment of an isthmic type spondylolisthesis, while the remainder assessed some aspect of treatment of spinal stenosis in conjunction with degenerative spondylolisthesis. The characteristics of these trials are presented in Table 31.1.

TABLE 31.1. *Characteristics of trials*

Trial	Methods	Interventions	Participants	Outcomes
Laminotomy versus laminectomy				
Postacchini et al. (6)	Alternate assignment Blinding: nil Rating: C	Experiment: Multiple laminotomy Control: Laminectomy	70 patients: • 34 male, 36 female • Age 43–79 years	Outcomes at 3.7 years: Patient's rating Surgeon's rating Spondylolisthesis progression Operating time Blood loss
Arthrodesis versus decompression alone				
Herkowitz and Kurz (8)	Alternate assignment Blinding: nil Rating: C	Experiment: Posterolateral arthrodesis and decompression Control: Decompression	50 patients: • 14 male, 36 female • Age 52–84 years • Loss to follow-up: 0/50	Outcomes at 3 years: Back pain Leg pain Surgeon's rating Fusion Spondylolisthesis progression
Bridwell et al. (7)	Randomization method unknown Blinding: nil Rating: B	Experiment: a. Posterolateral fusion b. Instrumented posterolateral fusion (Steffee system mostly) Control: Decompression	44 patients: • 10 male, 34 female • Age 44–79 years • Loss to follow-up: 1/44	Outcomes at 2 years: Spondylolisthesis progression Secondary surgery Walking distance
Fischgrund et al. (10)	Closed envelope allocation Assessor blinded Rating: A	Experiment: Instrumented posterolateral fusion (Steffee system) Control: Posterolateral fusion	76 patients: • 17 male, 59 female • Age 52–86 years • Loss to follow-up: 8/76	Outcomes at 2 years: Back pain score Leg pain score Surgeon's rating Fusion Progression of spondylolisthesis
Kitchel and Matteri (11)	Randomization method unknown Blinding: nil Rating: B	Experiment: Instrumented posterolateral (system unknown) and posterior interbody fusion (autogenous graft) Control: Instrumented posterolateral fusion (system unknown)	62 patients: no details	Outcomes at 2 years: Fusion Change in Oswestry Disability Index
Isthmic spondylolisthesis				
Carragee (2)	Closed envelope randomization Blinding: nil Rating: A	Experiment: a. Smokers with instrumented arthrodesis (Texas Scottish Rite Hospital System) b. Nonsmokers with graft alone Control: Same groups with no laminectomy	42 patients: • 26 male, 16 female • Age 19–51 years • Loss to follow-up: 2/42	Outcomes at 3 years: Fusion Patient's rating

TABLE 31.1. *Continued*

Moller and Hedlund (29,30)	Blindly selected choice of three Blinding: nil Rating: A	Experiment: a. Instrumented posterolateral fusion (Cotrel–Dubousset system) b. Posterolateral fusion Control: Exercise program	111 patients: • 57 male, 54 female • Age 18–55 years • Loss to follow-up: 8/114 randomized	Outcomes at 2 years: Disability rating index Pain score Assessor rating Patient rating Fusion Return to work
Spondylolisthesis instrumentation				
Zdeblick (16)	Random number generation Blinding: nil Rating: A	Experiment: a. Instrumented posterolateral fusion (Texas Scottish Rite Hospital System) b. Semirigid instrumented posterolateral fusion (Luque II system) Control: Posterolateral fusion	124 patients: • Age 20–80 years • Loss to follow-up: 1/124	Outcomes at 16 months: Surgeon's rating Second procedure
Thomsen et al. (15)	Closed envelope randomization Assessor blinded Rating: A	Experiment: Instrumented posterolateral fusion (Cotrel–Dubousset system) Control: Posterolateral fusion	130 patients: • 60 male, 69 female • Age 20–67 years • Loss to follow-up: 3/129	Outcomes at 2 years: Functional scale Patient's rating Fusion Second procedure
France et al. (14)	Randomization method unknown Blinding: nil Rating: B	Experiment: Instrumented posterolateral fusion (Steffee system) Control: Posterolateral fusion	83 patients: • 58 male, 25 female • Age 19–76 years • Loss to follow-up: 12/83	Outcomes at 2 years: Back pain scale Patient's rating Fusion
Christensen et al. (17)	Closed envelope randomization Independent radiologist Rating: A	Experiment: Circumferential fusion with anterior interbody fusion (Brantigan cage) and posterior instrumentation (Cotrel–Dubousset system or transarticular screws) Control: Instrumented posterolateral fusion (Cotrel–Dubousset system)	148 patients: • 88 male, 58 female • Age 20–65 years • Loss to follow-up: 9/146	Outcomes at 2 years: Dallas pain score Low back rating Work status

Note: Allocation concealment was rated into three grades: (A) clearly yes, some form of centralized randomization scheme or assignment; (B) unclear, assignment envelopes, a list, or table, evidence of possible randomization failure, or those trials stated to be random but with no description of the method; (C) clearly no, including quasi-randomization where patients were allocated by alternation, case number, or date of birth in which the method of allocation was transparent before assignment to a given group.

Isthmic Spondylolisthesis

Spondylolisthesis of isthmic type generally presents clinically in early adulthood and this was reflected in both included trials (2,3). Moller (3) compared posterolateral fusion with an exercise program in 111 patients, 62% of whom reported low back pain and sciatica, 31% low back pain only, and 7% sciatica only. Fusion was performed either with or without supplementary transpedicular fixation. The patients performed strength training exercises three times per week for 6 months, then twice a week for a further 6 months. Posterolateral fusion produced significantly less pain and disability and better patient- and observer-rated outcomes at 2 years ($p = 0.002$), although instrumentation had no effect. Exercises had limited effect on pain relief or observer ratings. No treatment had any significant effect on occupational outcomes.

Recently, long-term outcomes from this trial have been presented (4). The earlier differences noted between the two groups have not been maintained; only the "global self-assessment" rating showed any significant difference at a mean of 9 years. Following fusion, 76% of patients felt better or much better, compared with 50% in the exercise group. There was no significant difference in Oswestry Disability Score.

Preliminary results from a parallel Swedish study were also recently reported at the SpineWeek 2004 meeting (5). This trial compared disability outcomes in patients with adult isthmic spondylolisthesis treated by posterolateral lumbar interbody fusion (PLIF) with the data from the intervention groups of the earlier study by Moller et al. (3) There was no evidence of a positive effect from interbody fusion.

A separate RCT by Caragee analyzed the effect on back pain of supplementary spinal decompression in patients who had a primary posterolateral arthrodesis for isthmic spondylolisthesis. Adding the decompression seemed to make no material difference to the end result, although group numbers were small. The result was similar whether or not instrumentation was used to facilitate fusion (in smokers only).

Spinal Stenosis and Degenerative Spondylolisthesis

Most surgeons advocate spinal decompression for severe, symptomatic spinal stenosis, but techniques vary widely. In patients with degenerative spondylolisthesis, Postacchini et al. (6) attempted to address this issue by comparing outcomes following multiple laminotomies with those following a traditional laminectomy. At three years, no differences were noted between the two groups of patients, although several confounding factors have to be considered. Some patients were "group changers" for technical reasons from laminotomy to laminectomy, and a few in both groups had a lateral mass fusion.

If laminectomy is required to relieve stenosis, then there is some evidence from two RCTs that patients fare better after supplementing decompression with an intertransverse arthrodesis (7,8). Outcomes improved (OR 4.41 [range 1.09 to 17.8]) and less spondylolisthesis progression probably occurred (though that was not quite statistically significant). However, both these trials had small numbers. An increase in vertebral slip and "instability" at the operative level was associated with a poor clinical result, a finding contrasting with that reported in the case series of Jonsson et al. (9).

Two other trials compared instrumented fusion with posterolateral arthrodesis alone (10,11). In one, the intervention group were stabilized using the Steffee pedicular instrumentation system (10), and in the other posterior lumbar interbody cages were inserted (11). No additional benefit was gained from instrumentation in either RCT. This conclusion is broadly in line with our previous meta-analysis of all available evidence (from heterogeneous patient groups) that instrumenting an intertransverse arthrodesis with a rigid fixation system increases fusion rate but has no effect on clinical outcome (12). It is also well recognized that complication rate increases with the complexity of the surgery (13).

Four further RCTs included some data from patients with degenerative spondylolisthesis. Three of these were comparisons of an instrumented arthrodesis with some form of pedicle screw system versus posterolateral arthrodesis only (14–16). The other compared results from a circumferential fusion (anterior interbody cage plus posterior instrumentation) with those following an instrumented posterolateral fusion alone (17). In the latter study, the chance of reoperation within 2 years of spinal fusion was lower for those who had received a 360 degree fusion. Unfortunately, all three of these trials include heterogeneous groups of patients and it is not possible to extract separate data about spondylolisthesis.

DISCUSSION

Isthmic spondylolisthesis is a distinct condition from degenerative spondylolisthesis, and most authors have separated the two entities. Progression of spondylolysis to spondylolisthesis in adults, although recognized, is very uncommon (15,18).

Pain in the presence of a spondylolysis may arise either from micromovement at the pars defect or from irritation of the nerve root exiting at that site due to tissue overgrowth. Theoretically, the only treatment required is some form of stabilization of the defect to restore segmental rigidity, although the benefits of this procedure are probably limited to patients less than 30 years of age (19,20). The two trials of isthmic spondylolisthesis included in this review analyzed a subcategory of older individuals who presumably had all developed some associated degenerative changes. In this patient group, there is limited evidence supporting spinal fusion over an exercise program, at least for a few years (3). However, no separate data were presented in Moller's trial for back pain, and it is not clear how much of the success reported was attributable to relief of sciatica from foraminal stenosis. Stabilization of the spine alone may be sufficient to adequately relieve symptoms, as suggested by Caragee, rather than any formal decompression (2). There are no RCTs dealing with high-grade spondylolisthesis in the absence of spinal stenosis, but evidence from nonrandomized trials suggests that fusion in children, and in adults with greater than Grade 3 slippage, usually also yields good clinical outcomes (21).

In degenerative spondylolisthesis, facet arthritis, loss of disc height, and ligamentum flavum hypertrophy are the main pathologic features, and decompression is the primary goal of surgery. This procedure may, however, lead to incremental instability, and the majority of the clinical trials have considered whether stabilization by arthrodesis will prevent this and provide better patient outcomes. The trials included in the Cochrane review probably show some benefit from adjunctive noninstrumented fusion, but the level of evidence is weak (7,8). Indeed, Herkowitz and Kurz studied only 50 patients, and 9 of the 25 who had an arthrodesis probably developed a pseudarthrosis. The conclusion that the development of a pseudarthrosis did not preclude a successful result casts some doubt on the trial's overall findings. Similarly, the conclusions drawn from Bridwell's trial are weak. In this study, the control group consisted of only nine patients and there was inadequate data for intention to treat analysis to demonstrate any significant effect of performing fusion per se versus decompression alone. The place of arthrodesis is supported by long-term evidence from one arm of the trial published Fischgrund et al. in 1997 (10). Analysis of data from 47 of 58 patients treated by decompression and arthrodesis without instrumentation showed that symptom severity and physical function were better in those with a solid arthrodesis than in those considered to have a pseudarthrosis ($p = 0.01$) although patient satisfaction was similar (22).

A secondary issue is whether instrumentation adds any value to fusion. A recent survey of the North American Spine Society membership found that 67% of respondents would recommend an instrumented arthrodesis, compared with only 9% recommending noninstrumented arthrodesis (23). Although this approach is underwritten by the meta-analysis by Mardjetko et al. in 1994 (24), of nine small, mainly nonrandomized trials (84 patients noninstrumented, 101 patients instrumented) and a retrospective cohort study of 2,684 patients with degenerative spondylolisthesis, in which the authors show higher fusion rates with instrumentation (25), there is some equivocal evidence. In a much larger analysis of 84 trials (randomized and nonrandomized) in degenerative disc disease published between 1979 and 2000, Bono and Lee (26) found that although instrumentation seemingly led to a higher fusion rate than graft alone, the rate of fusion did not actually alter between the 1980s and 1990s (88% vs. 87%) despite increased use of instrumentation. As in this present review, a positive effect on clinical outcome was not detected.

Instrumentation of the spine clearly has significant cost implications, and no trial has dealt adequately with cost effectiveness. It is estimated that compared with decompression alone, a noninstrumented fusion increases hospital costs by 50% and an instrumented fusion by 100% (27). Kuntz in 2000 calculated that the latter would lead to an additional $8,700 per person over 10 years compared with a noninstrumented fusion that resulted in one additional quality-adjusted day, with a cost-effectiveness ratio of just over $3 million per quality-adjusted year of life (28). It is of course difficult to calculate cost without information on complications. In none of the currently presented trials were complications adequately addressed despite rates up to 10% quoted by Mardjetko et al. in their review (24).

All the data available at present is from RCTs of “rigid” instrumentation. There is no RCT evidence at present on the value of tension band systems, such as the Graf ligament, and only one on any form of anterior stabilization. The reader should also recognize that any instrumentation system used is likely to be outdated and replaced by a second or third generation implant by the date that a trial is published (although there is no clear evidence whether that makes any difference to outcomes [26]).

CONCLUSIONS

- There is limited evidence (Level C—direct from one low-quality RCT, and indirect evidence from two other RCTs) that patients with symptomatic isthmic spondylolisthesis who are candidates for surgery have better clinical outcomes from arthrodesis than from an intensive exercise program (at least in the medium term).
- Degenerative spondylolisthesis is a common accompaniment of spinal stenosis. In general, the displacement is stable and it is only after a wide decompression that progression can occur. There is limited evidence (Level C—from multiple low-quality RCTs) that the benefits of routine intertransverse arthrodesis are marginal and that supplementary posterior lumbar interbody fusion provides no additional benefit.
- There is strong evidence (Level A—from two RCTs, and multiple RCTs in degenerative spondylosis) that instrumentation of an intertransverse arthrodesis increases fusion rates but has marginal if any affect on clinical outcomes.
- Further RCTs are required to improve our confidence in these conclusions.

REFERENCES

1. Gibson JNA, Waddell G. Surgery for degenerative lumbar spondylosis. In: The Cochrane Library, Issue 2, 2005. Oxford, Update Software. (www.cochrane.org).
2. Carragee EJ. Single-level posterolateral arthrodesis, with or without posterior decompression, for the treatment of isthmic spondylolisthesis in adults. *J Bone Joint Surg Am* 1997;79:1175–1180.
3. Moller H. Isthmic spondylolisthesis in adults: a randomized controlled trial [Thesis]. Stockholm: Karolinska Institute; 1999.
4. Ekman P, Moller H, Hedlund R. The long-term effect of fusion in adult isthmic spondylolisthesis: a prospective randomized study. Proceedings of SpineWeek 2004.Porto, Portugal.
5. Ekman P, Hedlund R, Moller H, et al. PLIF vs. posterolateral fusion in adult isthmic spondylolisthesis: a preliminary report. Proceedings of SpineWeek 2004. Porto, Portugal.
6. Postacchini F, Cinotti G, Perugia D, et al. The surgical treatment of central lumbar stenosis. *J Bone Joint Surg Br* 1993;75:386–392.
7. Bridwell KH, Sedgewick TA, O'Brien MF, et al. The role for fusion and instrumentation in the treatment of degenerative spondylolisthesis with spinal stenosis. *J Spinal Disord* 1993;6:461–472.
8. Herkowitz HN, Kurz LT. Degenerative lumbar spondylolisthesis with spinal stenosis: a prospective study comparing decompression with decompression and intertransverse process arthrodesis. *J Bone Joint Surg Am* 1991;73:802–808.
9. Jonsson B, Annertz M, Sjoberg C, et al. A prospective and consecutive study of surgically treated lumbar spinal stenosis, part 2: five-year follow-up by an independent observer. *Spine* 1997;22:2938–2944.
10. Fischgrund JS, Mackay M, Herkowitz HN, et al. Degenerative lumbar spondylolisthesis with spinal stenosis: a prospective randomized study comparing decompressive laminectomy and arthrodesis with and without spinal instrumentation. *Spine* 1997;22:2807–2812.
11. Kitchel SH, Matteri RE. Prospective randomized evaluation of PLIF in degenerative spondylolisthesis patients over 60 years old. *Curr Concepts Rev* 2002.
12. Gibson JNA, Waddell G. Rationale for the surgical treatment of degenerative disc disease from the Cochrane Review. In: Gunzburg R, Szpalski M, Andersson GBJ ed. *Degenerative Disc Disease*. Philadelphia: Lippincott Williams & Wilkins; 2004:291–301.
13. Christensen FB. Lumbar spinal fusion: outcome in relation to surgical methods, choice of implant and postoperative rehabilitation. *Acta Orthop Scand* 2004;75(313):1–43.
14. France JC, Yaszemski MJ, Lauerman WC, et al. A randomized prospective study of posterolateral lumbar fusion. *Spine* 1999;24:553–560.
15. Thomsen K, Christensen FB, Eiskjaer SP, et al. The effect of pedicle screw instrumentation on functional outcome and fusion rates in posterolateral lumbar spinal fusion: a prospective randomized clinical study. *Spine* 1997; 22:2813–2822.
16. Zdeblick TA. A prospective, randomized study of lumbar fusion: preliminary results. *Spine* 1993;18(8): 983–991.
17. Christensen FB, Hansen ES, Eiskjaer SP, et al. Circumferential lumbar spinal fusion with Brantigan cage versus posterolateral fusion with titanium Cotrel–Dubousset instrumentation: a prospective, randomized clinical study of 146 patients. *Spine* 2002;27:2674–2683.
18. Fredrickson BE, Baker D, McHolick WJ, et al. The natural history of spondylolysis and spondylolisthesis. *J Bone Joint Surg Am* 1984;66:699–707.
19. Buck JE. Direct repair of the defect in spondylolisthesis. *J Bone Joint Surg Br* 1970;52:432–437.
20. Nicol RO, Scott JHS. Lytic spondylolysis: repair by wiring. *Spine* 1986;11:1027–1030.
21. Butterman GR, Garvey TA, Hunt AF, et al. Lumbar fusion results related to diagnosis. *Spine* 1998;18:23:116–127.
22. Kornblum MB, Fischgrund JS, Herkowitz HN, et al. Degenerative lumbar spondylolisthesis with spinal stenosis: a prospective long-term study comparing fusion with pseudarthrosis. *Spine* 2004;29:726–733.
23. Phillips FM. The argument for noninstrumented posterolateral fusion for patients with spinal stenosis and degenerative spondylolisthesis. *Spine* 2004;29:170–172.
24. Mardjetko SM, Connoly PJ, Shott S. Degenerative lumbar spondylolisthesis: a meta-analysis of the literature 1970–1993. *Spine* 1994;10:S2256–S2265.
25. Yuan HA, Garfin SR, Dickman CA, et al. A historical cohort study of pedicle screw fixation in thoracic, lumbar and sacral spinal fusions. *Spine* 1994;19(suppl):S2279–S2296.
26. Bono CM, Lee CK. Critical analysis of trends in fusion for degenerative disc disease over the past 20 years: influence of technique on fusion rate and clinical outcome. *Spine* 2004;29:455–463.
27. Katz JN, Lipson SJ, Lew RA, et al. Lumbar laminectomy alone or with instrumented or noninstrumented arthrodesis in degenerative lumbar spinal stenosis. Patient selection, costs and surgical outcomes. *Spine* 1997;22:1123–1131.
28. Kuntz KM, Snider RK, Weinstein JN, Pope MH, Katz JN. Cost-effectiveness of fusion with and without instrumentation for patients with degenerative spondylolisthesis and spinal stenosis. *Spine* 2000;25(9):1132–1139.
29. Moller H, Hedlund R. Surgery versus conservative management in adult isthmic spondylolisthesis: a prospective randomized study: part 1. *Spine* 2000;25:1711–1715.
30. Moller H, Hedlund R. Instrumented and non-instrumented posterolateral fusion in adult spondylolisthesis: a prospective randomized study: part 2. *Spine* 2000;25:1716–1721.

32

The Use of Outcome Scales in the Management of Spondylolysis

Finn Bjarke Christensen and Thomas Andersen

Why should outcome measurement of spinal patients' health and treatment be less accurate than corresponding measurements in other fields such as evaluation of educational achievements? There truly is no reasonable justification for this discrepancy; individual outcome assessment of patients receiving spinal treatment is essential in today's health care environment. In the construction of a spinal health index, a fundamental issue is how to select among the virtually unlimited number of questions that could potentially be included. The vast numbers of assessment techniques reported in the literature complicates the choice of appropriate tools for the assessment of clinical results. Thus, it is difficult to recommend the "best questionnaire buy" without knowledge of the study in which the user intends to use the method. The user must decide exactly what is required of the measurement. For example, will it be used to evaluate a program of care, or to study individual patients? What type of patient will be assessed (what diagnosis, age group, level of disability)? What time frame must the assessment cover: acute or long-term conditions?

Patient-oriented outcome measurements should include categories pertaining to health-related quality of life (symptoms and pain, activities of daily living, social, psychological, role status/employment), satisfaction, and costs.

Clearly, no single variable adequately describes health; rather, its measurement relies on compilation of a number of variables as indicators of outcome or health, each of which represents an element of the overall concept. Although there is a broad range of available tools, only a limited number of measurement instruments are frequently used.

The impact of low back pain can generally be described and measured on three different levels:

a. Physical impairment (decreased range of motion, reduced muscle strength, neurologic deficiency, etc.)
b. Physical disability (reduced walking ability; impaired lifting capacity; decreased ability to sit, stand, and perform other physical functions)
c. Social handicap (the resulting limitations in social, vocational, and recreational life as well as life satisfaction).

In the selection of outcome questionnaires, the following aspects should be considered:

1. Is the questionnaire validated? (Does it measure what it claims to measure?)
2. Is it reliable? (Is it consistent and reproducible?)
3. Is it responsive? (Is it capable of detecting subtle change?)
4. Is the questionnaire available in the target language?
5. Is the questionnaire sensible? (Is it relevant, and easy to complete and score?)

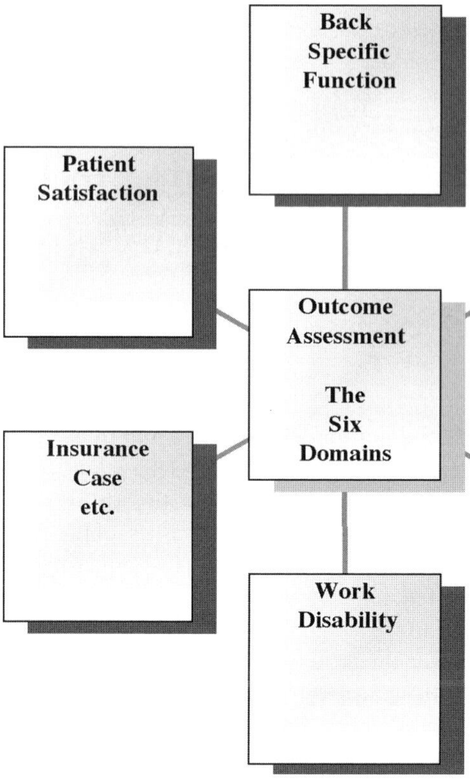

FIG. 32.1. The six recommended outcome assessment domains.

For outcome assessment, we recommend the six domains shown in Figure 32.1. However, if there is a risk of burdening the patient, which may result in loss of compliance, fewer domains might be relevant.

Some of the most commonly used questionnaires in relation to management of spondylolysis are reviewed in this chapter, and the pertinent area of dysfunction covered by each of them is indicated.

FUNCTIONAL OUTCOME

Oswestry Disability Index

The Oswestry Disability Index (ODI) (1,2) is a multiple-choice questionnaire filled out by the patient. It consists of 10 sections related to different activities of daily living. Each section describes six different levels of disability, which are scored by the sections answered and multiplied by 100. The first section rates pain intensity, while the remaining nine cover the disabling effects of pain on typical daily activities: personal care, lifting, walking, sitting, standing, sleeping, sex life, social life, and traveling. This allows potentially irrelevant sections, such as sex life, to be omitted. The Oswestry Disability Index is available in many languages.

Dallas Pain Questionnaire

The Dallas Pain Questionnaire (DPQ) (3) is disease-specific questionnaire in the form of a 16-item visual analogue scale. It was developed by Lawlis et al. to assess the amount of chronic spinal pain that affects four aspects of the patients' lives: daily activities, work–leisure activities, anxiety–depression, and social concerns. At our institution, it has been used as the main outcome instrument in several randomized and prospective studies as well as several other studies on the treatment of low back pain (4–9). Ozguler et al. (10) recently published a new way of scoring this questionnaire. In a population still in the work force despite low back pain, the authors were able to classify the individuals into one of four groups based on their degree of disability and the presence of emotional distress. We have demonstrated that this classification is of use in relation to spinal fusion patients.

Roland-Morris Disability Questionnaire

Roland-Morris Disability Questionnaire (RDQ) (2,11,12) is a back-specific scale that is completed by selecting 24 items from the Sickness Impact Profile (e.g., "I avoid heavy jobs around the house," "I sleep less well") and adding the phrase "because of my back." Patients completing the RDQ are asked to place a check mark beside a statement if it applies to them that day. The RDQ score is calculated by adding up the number of items checked. Items are not weighted. The scores therefore range from 0 (no disability) to 24 (maximum disability). The scale has become popular among back pain researchers and has been translated into several languages.

GENERIC OUTCOME

SF-36

The SF-36 (Short-Form Health Survey) (13) was designed as a multipurpose generic questionnaire containing 36 questions on various aspects of the person's general health. Health status is measured in eight dimensions: physical functioning, role-physical, bodily pain, general health, vitality, social functioning, role-emotional, mental health. These eight scales are summarized in two summary measures: a physical health component score and a mental health component score. In addition, the SF-36 contains a health transition item that evaluates the average change in health during the year prior to administration of the questionnaire.

In general, most studies of patients with back problems have found back-specific questionnaires to be more responsive to change in the patient's condition than SF-36. However, some have advocated the use of SF-36 because the pain and functions scales of the SF-36 have been nearly as responsive to change as some back-specific questionnaires and the SF-36 affords the possibility of requiring less time for the respondent than when several questionnaires are administered. Recently a low-back-specific version of the physical functioning scale has been developed. By adding four questions, the scale has been made more back-specific. This version will require further investigation.

One study has shown that spinal pain patients fall into three SF-36-based categories: highly functional (relatively high health status), dysfunctional (relatively low health status), or emotional adapters (low scores on the physical scales, relatively high scores on the mental scales). The distribution of patients in these three clusters was diagnosis-dependent, with 33% of spondylolysis patients being dysfunctional, 40% being emotional adapters, and 27% being highly functional (14).

PAIN ASSESSMENT

The Low Back Pain Rating Scale (LBPRS) (15) is a measurement that consists of three scales: pain (leg and back pain), disability, and physical impairment. Impairment is measured by testing endurance and flexibility. (If the scale is self-administered, this part is omitted.)

Disability measurement is based on 15 questions relating to specific daily activities. Pain intensity is measured using an 11-point numerical rating scale divided into "back pain" and "leg pain." Within each category, the patients are asked to quantitate both their current pain and their worst and average pain within the previous 14 days. While we have used this scale in a single study regarding rehabilitation after spinal surgery (16), the numerical rating scale has been of great value in several other studies performed at our institution. It has the advantages of differentiating between back and leg pain and being easy to understand and answer. Furthermore, this type of scale makes available data on the magnitude of clinically important change (16,17).

WORK DISABILITY

Health-related work outcomes have not received much attention in the literature, despite the fact that production loss (due to absenteeism and disability) associated with back pain is the greatest economic burden to the society. At a minimum, work status should be measured at the first and final visits. We recommend the following to be included: employment at usual job, on light duty or some restricted work assignment, paid leave/sick leave, unpaid leave, unemployed because of health problems, unemployed because of other reasons, student, keeping house/homemaker, retired, on disability. We believe, however, that it is difficult to use work status as a measure of treatment success due to the fact that both socioeconomic and psychologic factors may influence work status.

INSURANCE CASES, ETC.

In accordance with previously published studies (18,19), we found that patients with ongoing litigation due to work injury, patient insurance, or other indemnity were at high risk for an inferior functional outcome (17,20) (Fig. 32.2). We therefore recommend that the following questions be asked:

- Are you currently being trained for another job?
- Are you applying for pension due to back pain or other reason?
- Are you awaiting the outcome of a work injury case, patient insurance case, indemnity case, or complaints case?

PATIENT SATISFACTION

There are many approaches to the measurement of patient satisfaction. Some ask a few global questions, while others consist of multidimensional questionnaires. The heterogeneity of patient satisfaction measurements confuses the choice of measure. It is noteworthy that the word "satisfaction" does not even appear in many measures that otherwise implicitly reflect this concept. The association between care and outcome is complex and not well understood; there is, however, evidence to indicate that many patients evaluate care and outcome separately (21). An example of an outcome and a care question: "How satisfied are you with the overall result of your back surgery?" (17,22,23) and "In an overall, general sense, how satisfied are you with the service you received?"

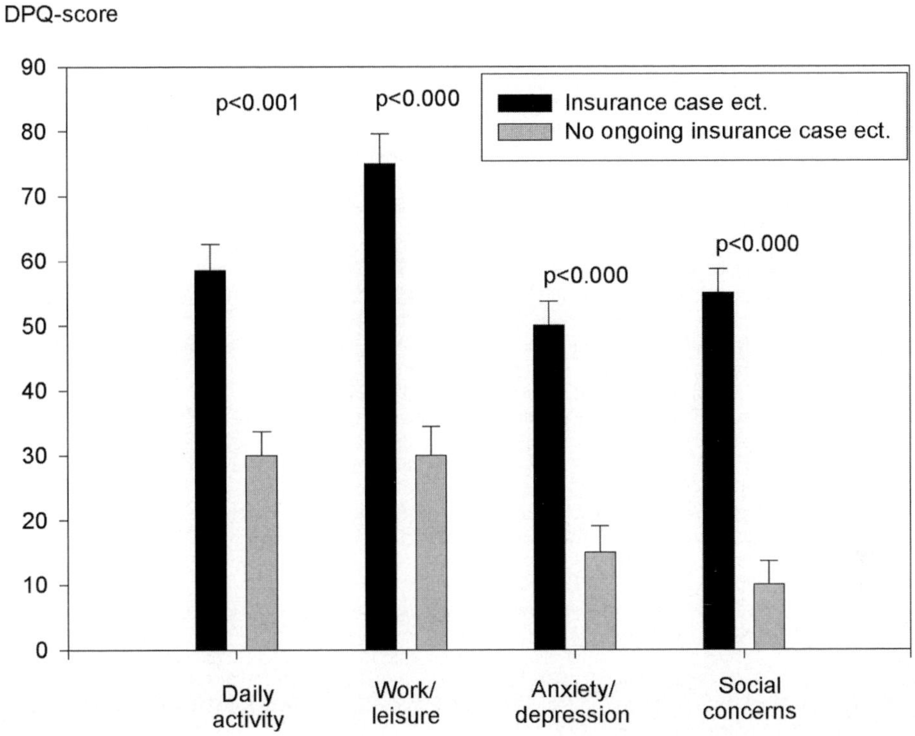

FIG. 32.2. Dallas Pain Questionnaire scores 5 years after posterolateral spinal fusion for patients with and without involvement in a work injury case, patient insurance case, indemnity case, or complaints case. Mean values and standard error of the mean for the categories daily activity, work–leisure activities, anxiety–depression, and social function. High scores indicate poor condition (NS = not significant).

CONCLUSIONS

Outcome assessment of patients receiving spinal treatment is essential in a contemporary health care environment. Quality results are complex, highly personal, and difficult to determine without standardized and validated instruments. Outcome evaluation seeks to answer questions regarding relief from pain, recovery of function, return to work, patient satisfaction, and costs of resources used to attain such result. Outcome data are necessary in guiding the direction of future treatment.

REFERENCES

1. Fairbank JC, Couper J, Davies JB, et al. The Oswestry low back pain disability questionnaire. *Physiotherapy* 1980;66:271–273.
2. Roland M, Fairbank J. The Roland-Morris Disability Questionnaire and the Oswestry Disability Questionnaire. *Spine* 2000;25:3115–3124.
3. Lawlis GF, Cuencas R, Selby D, et al. The development of the Dallas Pain Questionnaire: an assessment of the impact of spinal pain on behavior. *Spine* 1989;14:511–516.
4. Andersen T, Christensen FB, Hansen ES, et al. Pain 5 years after instrumented and non-instrumented posterolateral lumbar spinal fusion. *Eur Spine J* 2003;12:393–399.
5. Andersen T, Christensen FB, Laursen M, et al. Smoking as a predictor of negative outcome in lumbar spinal fusion. *Spine* 2001;26:2623–2628.

6. Christensen FB, Hansen E, Laursen M, et al. Long-term functional outcome of pedicle screw instrumentation as a support for posterolateral spinal fusion: randomized clinical study with a 5-year follow-up. *Spine* 2002;27: 1269-1277.
7. Christensen FB, Bunger CE. Retrograde ejaculation after retroperitoneal lower lumbar interbody fusion. *Int Orthop* 1997;21:176–180.
8. Christensen FB, Hansen ES, Eiskjaer SP, et al. Circumferential lumbar spinal fusion with Brantigan cage versus posterolateral fusion with titanium Cotrel–Dubousset instrumentation: a prospective, randomized clinical study of 146 patients. *Spine* 2002;27:2674–2683.
9. Christensen FB, Karlsmose B, Hansen ES, et al. Radiological and functional outcome after anterior lumbar interbody spinal fusion. *Eur Spine J* 1996;5:293–298.
10. Ozguler A, Gueguen A, Leclerc A, et al. Using the Dallas Pain Questionnaire to classify individuals with low back pain in a working population. *Spine* 2002;27:1783–1789.
11. Roland M, Morris R. A study of the natural history of back pain. Part I: development of a reliable and sensitive measure of disability in low-back pain. *Spine* 1983;8:141–144.
12. Roland M, Morris R. A study of the natural history of low-back pain. Part II: development of guidelines for trials of treatment in primary care. *Spine* 1983;8:145–150.
13. Ware JE, Jr. SF-36 health survey update. *Spine* 2000;25:3130–3139.
14. Fanciullo GJ, Hanscom B, Weinstein JN, et al. Cluster analysis classification of SF-36 profiles for patients with spinal pain. *Spine* 2003;28:2276–2282.
15. Manniche C, Asmussen K, Lauritsen B, et al. Low back pain rating scale: validation of a tool for assessment of low back pain. *Pain* 1994;57:317–326.
16. Christensen FB, Laurberg I, Bunger CE. Importance of the back-cafe concept to rehabilitation after lumbar spinal fusion: a randomized clinical study with a 2-year follow-up. *Spine* 2003;28:2561–2569.
17. Christensen FB. Lumbar spinal fusion. Outcome in relation to surgical methods, choice of implant and postoperative rehabilitation. *Acta Orthop Scand* 2004;75:2–43.
18. Frymoyer JW, Cats-Baril W. Predictors of low back pain disability. *Clin Orthop* 1987;89–98.
19. Greenough CG. Recovery from low back injury. *J Bone Joint Surg Br* 1994;76:859–861.
20. Christensen FB, Bunger C. Stabilisation surgery for chronic low back pain: indications, surgical procedures, and outcome. *Scand J Rheum* 2004;33:210–217.
21. Fitzpatrick R, Hopkins A. Problems in the conceptual framework of patient satisfaction research: an empirical exploration. *Sociol Health Illn* 1983;5:297–311.
22. Fritzell P, Hägg O, Wessberg P, et al. The Swedish spine study: lumbar fusion for chronic low back pain: a multicenter RCT comparing surgery with physiotherapy. EuroSpine 2000. October 2000.
23. Moller H, Hedlund R. Surgery versus conservative management in adult isthmic spondylolisthesis—a prospective randomized study: part 1. *Spine* 2000;25:1711–1715.

33

The Problems of Instrumentation in Poorer Countries

Helton Defino

The implants used for surgeries of the spine are the segment of highest growth on the orthopedic market. This growth is directly related to the changes that have occurred in the treatment of spinal diseases. Originally, instrumentation was used only in the correction of spinal deformities such as scoliosis. Over the past 10 to 15 years, however, the application of internal fixation has also been used for other conditions such as degenerative, traumatic, tumoral, and infectious diseases. Other devices used in spine surgery such as bone graft substitutes, growth factors technologies, and spinal arthroplasty devices have also contributed to the growth of this market, side by side with the increasing population of elderly patients, favorable changes regarding reimbursement, and the development of minimally invasive surgical techniques. The global spine market was valued at $2.4 billion in 2003, with a 14.9% increase compared to 2002, and by 2008 it is expected to be over $3.7 billion.

The problems related to the application of modern technologies in the health area are complex and are intimately linked to the economic and cultural characteristics of each country or region. The analysis of these problems cannot be generalized but must focus on a region of interest. The Latin American spine market represents a small part of the global spine market and was valued at $56 million in 2003. This figure reflects the influence of the economic situation and of the organization and funding of the health systems on the spinal implant market. For the purpose of analysis of the spinal implant market, Latin America is considered here to consist of Brazil, Mexico, Colombia, Argentina, Venezuela, and Chile.

Despite the low absolute value of the Latin American implant market in relation to the world market, growth is predicted to occur over the next few years, influenced by recovery of the market as a function of the improved economic situation of the countries, reforms to improve the health care system in several countries, increased training of surgeons in the use of orthopedic devices, and an aging population likely to have a greater incidence of degenerative disc disease, arthritis, and osteoporosis. Unemployment and a high level of poverty continue to be limiting factors regarding the growth of the orthopedic implant market in Latin America.

The orthopedic implant market was estimated at $200 million (US dollars) in 2003, with reconstructive implants ($90.0 million) and trauma implants ($69.1 million) accounting for the leading shares of this market, followed by spinal implants ($56.93 million) (Fig. 33.1). The vertebral implant market has been negatively affected by the devaluation of some currencies (real, bolivar, and Argentine peso) in Latin America, by the bankruptcy of the Venezuelan health care system, and by the lack of training of surgeons in the use of new techniques. Driving the market over the forecast period, however, is an increase incidence of degenerative disc disease stemming from an aging population and improvement in various health care systems, notably in Chile and Mexico.

	Reconstructive Implants (US$M)	Trauma Devices (US$M)	Spinal Implants (US$M)
2002	87.6	62.1	53.5
2003	90.4	69.1	56.9
2004	97.3	77.2	64.2

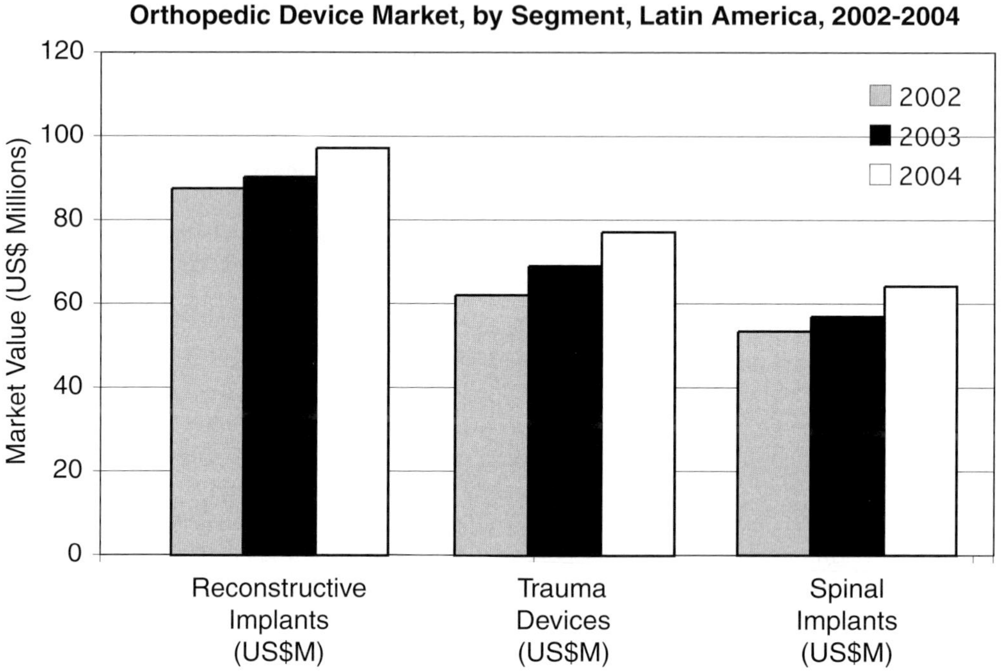

Source: Millenium Research Group

FIG. 33.1. Orthopedic device market, by segment, Latin America, 2002–2004.

In Latin America, the implant market is directly related to population size (Figs. 33.2,33.3). Thus, Brazil, the country with the largest population (fifth in the world), represents, in general, the largest orthopedic implant market, estimated at $70 million in 2003. The Brazilian market is price sensitive and has the highest number of strong domestic manufacturers of reconstructive, trauma, and spinal implants, with five manufacturers being among the top 20 competitors in the Latin American orthopedic market. Argentina also has various domestic manufacturers, whereas few are available in Mexico and Colombia, which rely primarily on imported products. Similarly, Venezuela and Chile import most of their products and have the smallest number of domestic implant manufacturers.

CHARACTERISTICS OF THE DIFFERENT COUNTRIES

Argentina

Argentina was the second smallest market in Latin America in 2003, valued at $5.1 million. The limiting factors for the growth of the vertebral implant market in Argentina are the high price of imported implants; the recession and the devaluation of the Argentine peso;

Brazil	Mexico	Colombia	Argentina	Chile	Venezuela
73	61	31	28	15	15

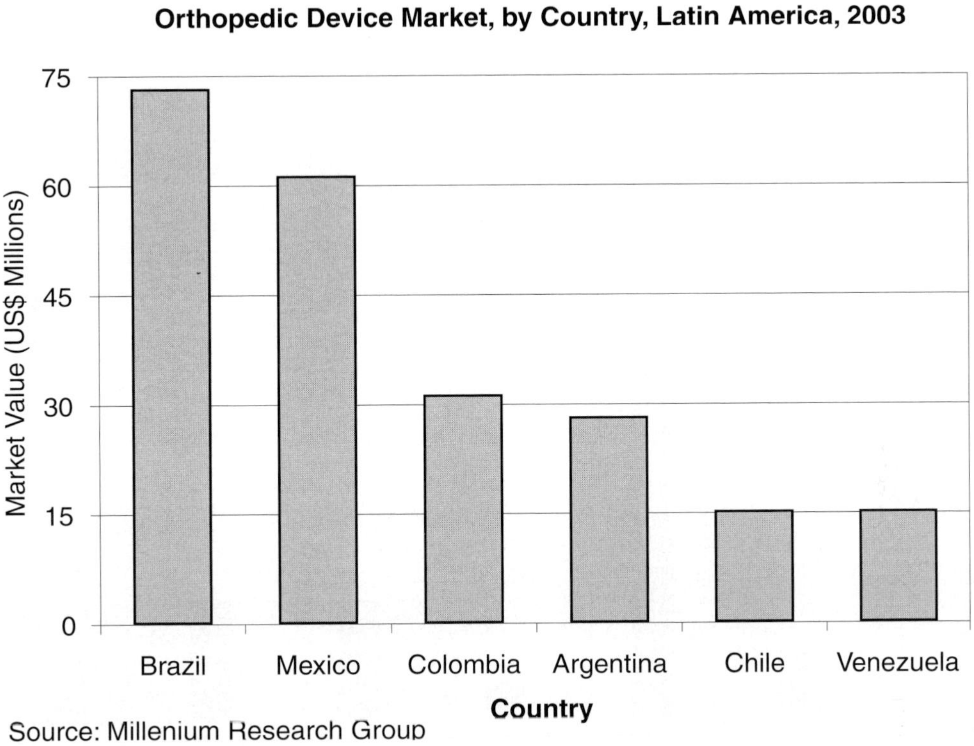

FIG. 33.2. Orthopedic device market, by country, Latin America, 2003.

a deficit in the number of dedicated surgeons; and a narrow selection of spinal implant products relative to other Latin American markets. Nevertheless, an expansion of the market is expected, driven primarily by an increase of the population and especially of the elderly segment. Thoracolumbar implants are the devices most frequently used on the Argentinian market (78.1%), whereas the cervical implant and interbody fusion device markets are limited by the number of qualified surgeons available to perform these surgeries.

Brazil

The spinal implant market in Brazil has considerably increased over the last few years as the result of increased access to public health care and the decentralization of health care to municipal levels, together with the reimbursement of spinal surgery in the public sector by Sistema Unico de Saude (SUS). SUS has not taken into consideration the devaluation of Brazilian currency for the payment of implants, a fact that has been particularly beneficial to local manufacturers, who are better positioned to accommodate the price ceilings set by SUS through lower-priced offerings. As a consequence, more than half the implants commercially sold in Brazil for spinal surgery come from domestic manufacturers, and they are the lowest priced devices in Latin America.

In 2003, thoracolumbar implants represented 69.5% of the market and cervical implants 10.6%. The number of interbody fusion procedures exceeds the number of cervical

	Argentina (US$M)	Brazil (US$M)	Chile (US$M)	Colombia (US$M)	Mexico (US$M)	Venezuela (US$M)
2002	5.1	22	2.4	7.9	7.5	8.5
2003	5.1	25.5	2.8	8.7	8.8	6
2004	5.2	29.7	3.3	9.8	10.3	6

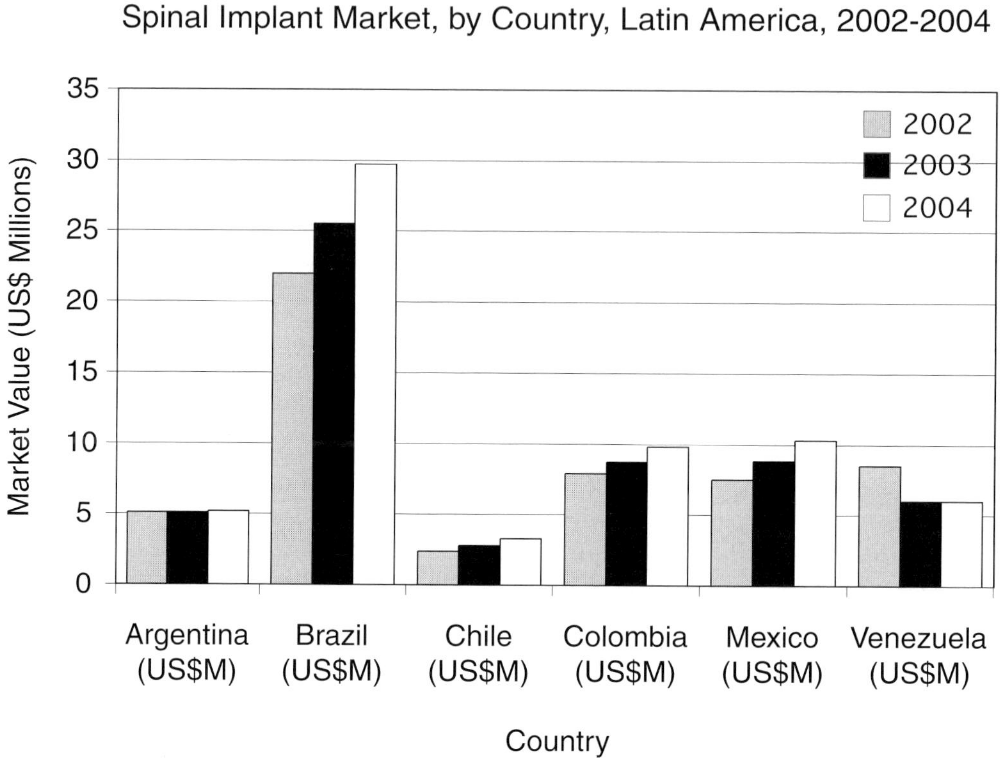

Source: Millenium Research Group

FIG. 33.3. Spinal implant market, by country, Latin America, 2002–2004.

implant procedures, and the popularity of interbody fusion devices is related to the increased use of mesh in tumor surgery, the increased use and instruction of interbody fusion techniques in medical schools, and the patient perception of these devices as new and innovative technologies. The use of thoracolumbar implants was directly related to the use of pedicular screws for the treatment of degenerative disease and deformity disorders.

Chile

The spinal implant market in Chile was valued at $2.8 million in 2003, and this small amount is related in part to the size of the population. Thoracolumbar implants represented 58.9% of total spinal devices in 2003, and cervical implants represented 22.8%. Only 215 interbody fusion devices were implanted in 2003, but an increased use of this type of device is expected to occur.

Colombia

The spinal implant market in Columbia was valued at $8.7 million in 2003, with 72.4% of the devices being represented by thoracolumbar implants. The market has been limited by the high prices of spinal implants as a result of the almost complete absence of domestic manufacturers. In Colombia, the mean sale price of spinal implants is the highest in Latin America. There is a significant range in prices among products manufactured in South America ($850 to $2,500) and products shipped abroad ($4,000 and $5,000). Cervical and interbody fusion implants are lower-priced than thoracolumbar implants, but the procedures are more complicated and a large number of alternatives are available. Both of these markets are still in an initial phase.

Mexico

Mexico is the third largest market for spinal implants in Latin America, valued at $8.8 million in 2003. Mexico is one of the few countries in Latin America where the thoracolumbar implants are over four times more expensive than cervical implants. Mexico has a small interbody fusion device market, as explained by the fact that the public health system does not pay for this type of implant.

Venezuela

The spinal implant market in Venezuela has suffered a reduction of about 30% due to economic problems and devaluation of the Bolivar, according to the 2003 data. Thoracolumbar implants represent 74.8% of the market due to the high incidence of degenerative diseases and fractures, and their cost is also higher than that of cervical implants. The market for interbody fusion is still in an incipient phase because of the elevated cost of the implants, the training required, and the acceptance of the use of this device.

CONCLUSIONS

The market of implants used in spinal surgery has been influenced by the economic, cultural, and educational factors of the different Latin American countries and, in general, has shown growth over the last few years. According to economic studies, the Latin American orthopedic device market will undergo strong growth over the next few years, and the most significant growth will be in Brazil and Mexico. The growth of the orthopedic device market will occur mainly regarding total hip and knee implants, thoracolumbar implants, and internal fixation devices. Reforms to improve the health care system in several countries and to increase training of surgeons in the use of orthopedic devices, and an aging population with the consequent likelihood of a high incidence of degenerative disease are the factors that will contribute to the growth of the implant market. The high level of poverty and unemployment are the main factors that still limit growth in several countries.

REFERENCE

1. Competitor insights for spinal implants 2003. Global spine series. Millennium Research Group. Latin American markets for orthopedic devices 2004. Global Orthopedics Series. Millennium Research Group.

34

Clinical Outcome Following Surgical Treatment of Spondylolysis

Brian J. C. Freeman

The pars interarticularis defect is unique to human beings, who by virtue of being bipedal transfer considerable weight through the pars interarticularis structure in the lumbar spine (1–3) (Fig. 34.1). Radiographic screenings have demonstrated an incidence of 4.4% in children between the ages of 5 and 7 years. The incidence of symptomatic pars defects in the young athletic population is much higher and is variously reported between 15% and 47% (4–7).

For those who fail conservative care, there are a number of surgical options. Direct repair of the pars defect has been shown to be effective for those with a *normal* disc, and it preserves intervertebral motion. Many different techniques have been described, including Buck's direct repair (8), Scott's wiring technique (9), Morscher's hook-screw (10), translaminar screws (11), pedicle screws with a V-shaped rod (12), and a cable screw construct (13).

Successful outcomes have been reported, ranging from 63% in one series (14) to 100% in another series (15). Predictors of successful surgical outcome include age less than 25 years, spondylolysis of less than 4 mm, absence of disc degeneration, positive response to local anaesthetic infiltration of the pars interarticularis defect, method of surgical repair, and motivation of the individual undergoing surgery (16).

For those patients with established disc degeneration identified on magnetic resonance imaging (MRI), many surgeons who have written on this topic would advocate investigation with lumbar discography to confirm the pain source. If discography confirmed the disc to be a pain source, most would advocate spinal fusion. Some authors have advocated surgical repair of the defect in combination with total disc replacement in such a case (Marnay T., personal communication). If spondylolysis is associated with a low-grade spondylolisthesis (Meyerding Grade 1 or 2), Dai et al. have suggested that direct repair of the defect and facet fusion produces acceptable results (17).

For those patients with a spondylolytic spondylolisthesis Grades 1 or 2 *without* objective neurologic deficit, most surgeons whose work is published would advocate fusion in situ; a minority would advocate *reduction* of the spondylolisthesis and fusion. One study compared anterior lumbar interbody fusion (ALIF) with instrumented posterolateral fusion (IPLF) for isthmic spondylolisthesis (Meyerding Grades 1 to 2) (18). No statistically significant difference was observed in clinical outcome between the two groups; satisfactory results were obtained in 85% of the ALIF group and 90% of the IPLF group. Another study of patients with isthmic spondylolisthesis reported *superior* long-term outcomes following noninstrumented posterolateral fusion compared to instrumented posterolateral fusion (19).

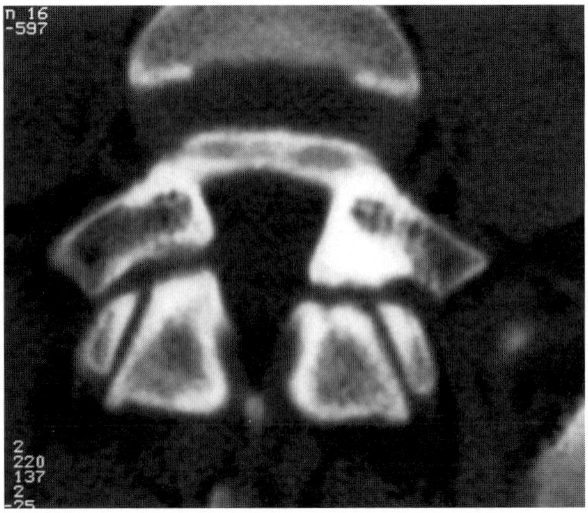

FIG. 34.1. Reverse-gantry computed tomograph showing bilateral spondylolysis at L5 in a 20-year-old.

THE BIOMECHANICAL EFFECTS OF SPONDYLOLYSIS AND ITS TREATMENT

Biomechanical studies performed on fresh frozen calf lumbar spines have shown that artificially induced bilateral interarticularis defects increase the intervertebral mobility not only at the involved level but also at the upper level adjacent to the lysis (20). The increased mobility of both the lytic segment and the adjacent level was significantly reduced by the Buck screw repair. However, if a pedicle screw system was applied across the involved segment, the mobility in the adjacent segment was *increased.* It would appear that fixation of the pars defect alone causes less adjacent-level mechanical stress than pedicle screw-rod fixation of the motion segment.

Deguchi et al. carried out a biomechanical comparison of various fixation techniques employed for the repair of spondylolytic defects (21). The procedures were carried out on calf cadaveric lumbar spines. The four techniques that were compared were Scott's wiring technique (wire loops passed around each transverse process and tightened under the spinous process); modified Scott's technique (wire loops around cortical screws placed in both pedicles and tightened under the spinous process); Buck's technique; and screw-rod-hook fixation. *All* fixation techniques significantly increased stiffness in the spondylolytic segment. The screw-rod-hook fixation and Buck's technique allowed the *least* motion across the spondylolytic defect when tested in flexion. The authors suggest that Buck's technique resists forces and movements in all directions, is low profile, and is less expensive than the screw-rod-hook system, but it remains technically demanding. Screw breakage or nerve root irritation requiring screw removal has occurred following Buck's technique (8,22).

Kip et al. carried out biomechanical testing of various pars defect repairs (23). He compared the Buck screw with the Morscher hook-screw and a modified Scott wiring technique. Overall, the Buck screw provided the stiffest and strongest repair (with a mean repair stiffness of 64% of the intact stiffness), followed closely by the Morscher hook-screw (with a mean repair stiffness of 52% of the intact stiffness). The figure 8 wiring repair (modified Scott repair) was the least stiff, with a mean repair stiffness of only 3% to 4% of the intact stiffness. The authors conclude that Scott wiring of pars defects is a tension band repair that is loaded *only* in flexion. It is used to repair a defect whose probable cause is repetitive hyperextension of the spine and should be questioned on biomechanical grounds. Nevertheless, it is interesting to note that similar *clinical* results have been obtained with both Buck's technique and Scott's wiring technique in some series (21).

CLINICAL OUTCOME FOLLOWING DIRECT REPAIR OF SPONDYLOLYTIC DEFECTS

The advantages of direct repair include a high rate of defect healing, preservation of intervertebral motion by avoidance of fusion across the disc, and restoration of anatomy.

BUCK'S TECHNIQUE

Buck (8) first reported the direct repair of a pars defect with a 4.5-mm stainless steel Arbeitsgemeinschaft für Osteosynthesefran or Association for the Study of Internal Fixation (AO) cortical lag screw in 1970 (Fig. 34.2). The defect was packed with cancellous bone graft and the patient was allowed to be mobile immediately following surgery. Kimura had described the insertion of bone-graft *without* internal fixation for spondylolysis and spondylolisthesis 2 years earlier (24). However, Kimura's technique required the patients to remain on bedrest for 2 months and was not universally popular. Buck initially reported on 16 patients with only 1 failure (8). In 1979, he updated his results to a 75-patient series, reporting satisfactory results in 88% (25). Several series of patients were then reported in the literature with success rates varying from 72% (22) to 95% (25) (Table 34.1).

Van der Werf et al. presented a series of 12 patients in 1985, with 8 good, 2 fair, and 2 poor results (26). There were two documented pseudarthroses in this series, one with a fair result and the other with a poor result. Pedersen and Hagen described 18 patients who underwent a direct repair using Buck's technique for a slip of Grade 1 or less (3). They reported 15 patients with a good or excellent result and 3 with a poor result (all with radiographic evidence of pseudarthrosis).

Roca et al. (27) reported on 15 patients with a slip of Grade 1 or less treated with the Buck method. There were 13 good results and 2 poor results (attributable to a

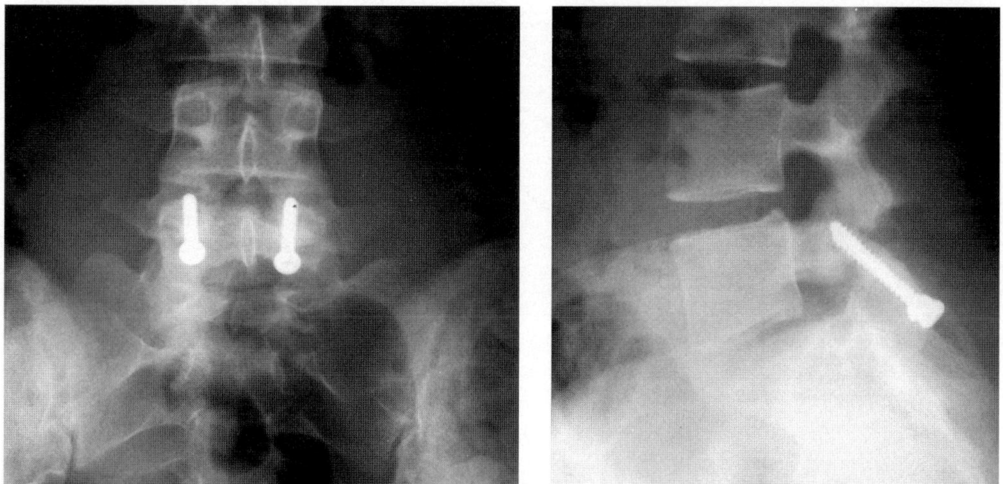

A B

FIG. 34.2. Anteroposterior (**A**) and lateral (**B**) radiographs showing a bilateral Buck repair 6 months after operation.

TABLE 34.1. *Published results of Buck's direct repair for spondylolysis*

Author	Year	Number of patients in series	Successful outcome (%)
Buck (8)	1970	16	94%
Buck (25)	1979	75	88%
Van der Werf et al. (26)	1985	12	83%
Pedersen and Hagen (3)	1988	18	83%
Roca et al. (27)	1989	15	87%
Bonnici et al. (28)	1991	24	88%
Suh et al. (32)	1991	10	90%
Hardcastle (33)	1993	10	90%
Dreyzin and Esses (22)	1994	11	72%
Tonino and Van der Werf (34)	1994	12	83%
Debnath et al. (16)	2003	19	95%

pseudarthrosis). In 1989, Bonnici et al. reported on 24 patients, 21 of whom obtained excellent results (28). Seventeen patients had adequate radiographic follow-up revealing 5 with screw loosening and 1 with a broken screw. Interestingly only 7 of 17 were noted to have healing of both defects radiographically, 5 patients had bridging of one defect, and 5 patients had no evidence of healing.

In 2003, Debnath et al. (16) reported on 22 young athletes who had undergone surgical treatment for lumbar spondylolysis; 19 of the patients underwent a Buck fusion, and 3 underwent a Scott fusion. Clinical outcome was assessed using the Oswestry Disability Index (ODI) (29), and the SF-36 (36-item Short-Form Health Survey) (30,31). The mean preoperative ODI was 39.5 (standard deviation 8.7), improving to 10.7 (standard deviation 12.9) at 2 years following surgery. The mean score for the *physical component* of the SF-36 improved from 27.1 (standard deviation 5.11) to 47.8 (standard deviation 7.7) with $p < 0.001$. The mean score for the *mental* component of health improved from 39.0 (standard deviation 3.97) to 55.4 (standard deviation 6.36) with $p < 0.001$ (Fig. 34.3). Of the 19 patients who underwent a Buck fusion followed by a strict rehabilitation

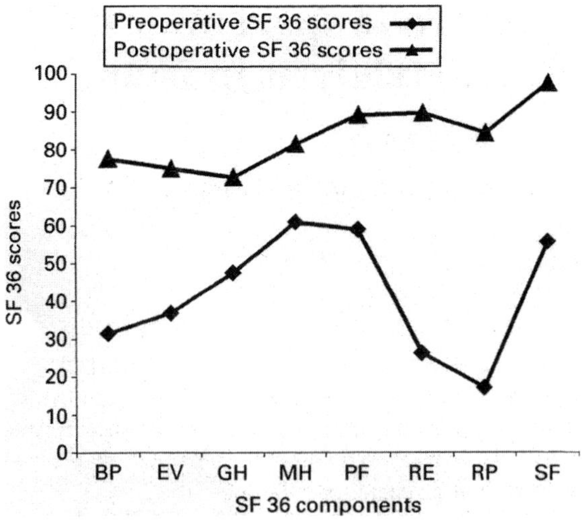

FIG. 34.3. Mean SF-36 scores in 22 young athletes before (*diamond line*) and 2 years following direct repair of lysis (*triangle line*) (16). Key: BP, bodily pain; EV, energy/vitality; GH, general health; MH, mental health; PF, physical function; RE, role limitation due to emotional problems; RP, role limitation due to physical problems; SF, social function.

program, 18 (95%) returned to sports activities after a mean of 7 months (range 4 to 10 months). For the one patient who did not return to sports, significant improvements in ODI and SF-36 were noted. Reverse-gantry computed tomography identified a solid fusion across the defect in this case. The outcome in the three patients treated by Scott fusion was *not* satisfactory; in two of the patients, the fusion did not result in union and they subsequently underwent revision to instrumented posterolateral fusion. The remaining patient showed no improvement in ODI and SF-36 scores despite a reverse-gantry CT scan confirming a sound union.

SCOTT'S WIRING TECHNIQUE

The Scott wiring technique (wire loops around each transverse process and tightened under the spinous process) was first documented by Bradford and Iza in 1985 (35) although they gave credit to James Scott for first suggesting the idea. Bradford and Iza reported on a series of 22 patients with 80% achieving good to excellent results and 90% obtaining a solid fusion of the pars defect. There were three cases of wire breakage. Subsequently Nicol and Scott (9) reported on 7 patients with 2- to 12-year follow-up. There was one case of wire breakage associated with nonunion requiring a revision to spinal fusion. In 1987, Scott (36) reported on his series of 31 patients; there were wire breakages in two of the patients (one of whom was symptomatic). In 1992, Johnson and Thompson reported on 22 patients treated by a modified Scott technique (wire loops around cortical screws placed in both pedicles and tightened under the spinous process) (37). In this series, there were two wire breakages, 19 patients under the age of 25 years had satisfactory results, and 2 of 3 patients over the 25 years had poor results.

Askar et al. in 2003 reported on a series of 15 patients under the age of 25 years with symptomatic spondylolisthesis with or without a Grade 1 slip treated by Scott wiring (Fig. 34.4) (38). Follow-up information was obtained in 14 of 15 patients at a mean of 10.9 years after surgery. Twelve of 14 had good or excellent results, but 2 of 14 had a poor result requiring further procedures for continued low back pain. The authors suggest Scott's wiring is technically easier than the Buck technique. The comparative results reported in the literature are shown in Table 34.2.

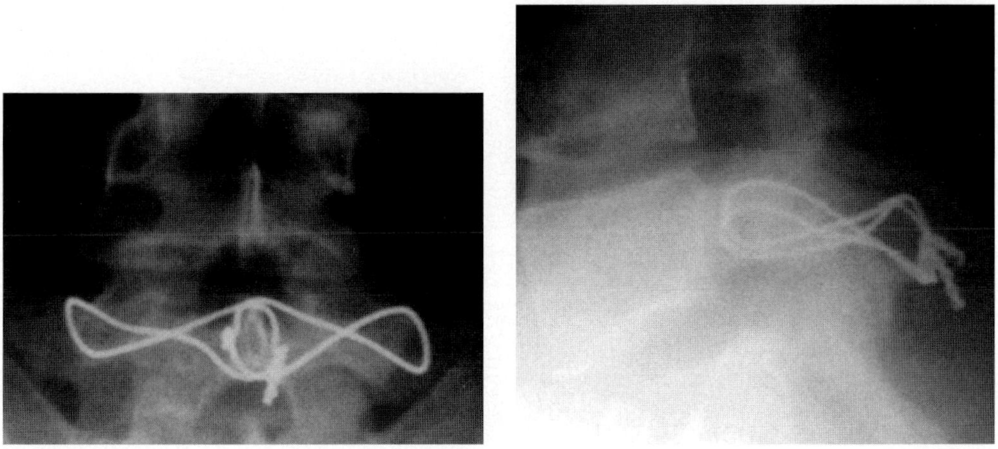

A B

FIG. 34.4. Anteroposterior (**A**) and lateral (**B**) radiographs showing Scott's wiring technique.

TABLE 34.2. *Published results of Scott's wiring technique*

Author	Year	Number of patients in series	Successful outcome (%)
Bradford and Iza (35)	1985	22	80%
Nicol and Scott (9)	1986	7	85%
Scott (36)	1987	31	93%
Johnson and Thompson (37)	1992	22	76%
Ascar (38)	2003	15	80%

MORSCHER'S HOOK-SCREW TECHNIQUE

In 1984, Morscher et al. (10) described a new method for treating a Meyerding Grade 1 lytic spondylolisthesis with a special hook-screw, whereby at least a partial reduction of a Grade 1 spondylolisthesis could be achieved (Fig. 34.5). The implant consisted of a specially developed screw with a cancellous thread at the tip and a machined thread at the base. A hook is laid over the lamina, and using a custom-made jig, the superior articular process is drilled. A screw is then passed through the hook into bone to obtain compression across the defect. Ten patients of 12 (83%) reported good or excellent results. The two patients with poor results had evidence of disc degeneration at the spondylolytic level before surgery. All cases were reported to heal with no screw breakage documented.

In 1990, Albassir et al. presented a series of 25 patients treated with the hook-screw technique (39). They reported 90% good or excellent results. Hefti et al. used the hook-screw technique to treat 33 patients (40). They describe the technique as simple and suggest that the method overcomes the difficulty of fixation in a dysplastic arch and avoids crossing the defect with a screw. Overall, they report 79% satisfactory results with a 73% fusion rate. A subgroup analysis revealed that for those patients under the age of 20 years old, 88% had satisfactory results, whereas in those patients over 20 years of age, only 71% achieved satisfactory results. There was one screw breakage noted in the series.

Sales de Gauzy et al. reported on 14 patients with symptomatic spondylolysis treated with the Morscher hook-screw (41). The mean age at surgery was 12 years of age (range 7 to 15 years) and the average follow-up was 33 months (range 16 to 66 months). Thirteen

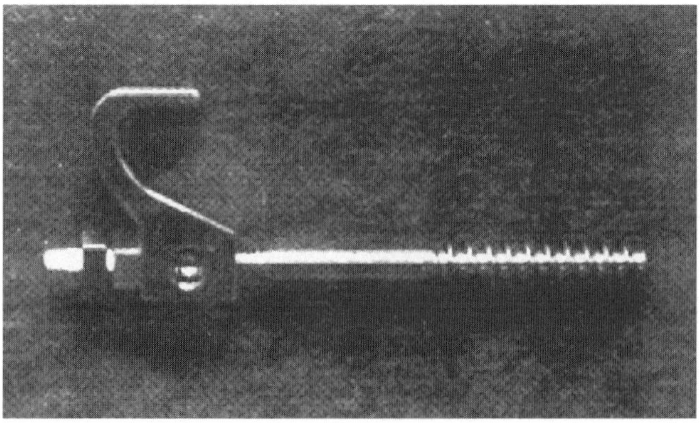

FIG. 34.5. Morsher hook-screw.

TABLE 34.3. *Published results for Morscher hook-screw technique*

Author	Year	Number of patients in series	Successful outcome (%)
Morscher et al. (10)	1984	12	83%
Albassir et al. (39)	1990	25	90%
Hefti et al. (40)	1992	33	79%
Sales de Gauzy et al. (41)	2000	14	93%
Ivanic et al. (42)	2000	113	78%

of 14 cases achieved excellent or good results, and 12 of 14 achieved a satisfactory fusion across the defect.

Ivanic et al. in 2003 reported on a retrospective study of 113 patients with spondylolysis undergoing direct repair with a hook-screw according to the Morscher technique (42). Before surgery, 46 patients underwent physical therapy without satisfactory or maintained improvement of their symptoms. The average follow-up period was 10.9 years (range 1 to 15.5 years), the pseudarthrosis rate overall was 13.3%. Further analysis revealed the pseudarthrosis rate for those patients under 20 years of age was 8.6%, and for those patients over the age of 20 years the pseudarthrosis rate was 35%. The average age at surgery was 16.9 years (range 7.5 to 39 years). Of the 15 pseudarthroses documented, 5 patients went on to have anterior arthrodesis. Among the group as a whole, 7 patients were noted to have loose implants, 2 requiring removal. There were 4 infections in the series. Taking these complications into account, the clinical success is estimated at 78% for this series. The published results for Morscher's hook-screw technique are shown in Table 34.3.

OTHER TECHNIQUES USED FOR DIRECT REPAIR

Gillet and Petit (12) reported on an original technique using a V-shaped rod and pedicle screws associated with direct bone grafting of the pars defect. Patients with established disc degeneration or *any* grade of spondylolisthesis were excluded from the series. Ten patients were considered eligible for pars repair over a 4-year period. The technique involves insertion of pedicle screws into the L5 pedicle followed by insertion of bone-graft into the decorticated defect. A 6-mm rod is then bent into a V-shape and placed *under* the L5 spinous process and fixed to the pedicle screws. The mean age for surgery was 26 years old (range 16 to 48 years). The clinical results suggested 7 of 10 patients had a good or excellent result, and 3 of 10 had a fair or poor result. The authors comment that nonunion could be overlooked because of difficulty in imaging the region postoperatively.

Songer and Rovin describe the repair of the pars interarticularis defect with a cable-screw construct (13). They emphasize the need to meticulously clean the pars defect with removal of soft tissue and exposure of bleeding bone. A pedicle cable screw is inserted into each L5 pedicle, a tricortical graft is inserted into the defect and a 1-mm double cable is then passed *underneath* the lamina and is split in two. The leader of each cable is then threaded through the hole in the pedicle screw and woven around the cranial end of the spinous process and through the loop at the other end of the cable. Each cable is then tensioned and crimped. Songer and Rovin operated on 7 patients (2 with acute fractures of the pars interarticularis) with a mean age of 20.5 years (range 12 to 32 years) and a mean follow-up of 25.5 months (range 19 to 37 months). They recorded 5 excellent and 2 good results using the modified Prolo score and documented fusion in all 7 cases. There was one cable failure.

PREDICTORS OF SUCCESSFUL SURGICAL OUTCOME FOLLOWING DIRECT REPAIR

Age

Scott initially used his wiring technique for spondylolysis at one or more levels in patients younger than 30 years (36). He subsequently reduced the upper age limit to 25 years. Few surgeons (at least those who have published on repairing this defect) would consider direct repair of a defect in the pars interarticularis in a patient over the age of 25 years old. Ivanic et al. (42) reported a pseudarthrosis rate of 8.6% in patients less than 20 years of age compared to 35% in patients over the age of 20 years. The authors advised caution in treating patients with a mature skeleton. Clearly, as the patient gets older, there is a much higher chance of disc degeneration in the spondylolytic segment, which may serve as a secondary pain source.

Size of Spondylolytic Defect or Degree of Spondylolisthesis

As the size of the defect increases, there is a gradual progression of the slip, with an increased risk of disc degeneration in some patients. Buck originally suggested that his technique was appropriate only in patients in whom there was a lysis of less than 3 or 4 mm (8). Debnath et al. (16) reported on 22 patients undergoing direct repair for lumbar spondylolysis: the mean size of the defect as determined by computer tomography was 3.5 mm (range 1 mm to 8 mm). Three patients had a spondylolytic defect that exceeded 4 mm and, despite this, achieved a successful outcome following surgery. Most surgeons would still contemplate a direct repair of the spondylolysis defect in patients who have a Meyerding Grade 1 spondylolisthesis. Fewer surgeons, however, would perform a direct repair of the pars defect in a Grade 2 spondylolisthesis (42).

Absence of Disc Degeneration on MR Image

Ideally, the disc at the spondylolytic level would appear entirely normal on the T2-weighted MR image. Loss of signal on this scan may indicate symptomatic disc degeneration; if doubt exists, lumbar discography should be carried out to ascertain the disc morphology and pain reproduction status. A positive discogram will significantly reduce the chance of a successful outcome following direct repair. Similarly, loss of signal in the *adjacent* disc should be appropriately investigated. Some authors regard Modic endplate changes at the spondylolytic level as a contraindication to direct repair.

Positive Response to Pars Infiltration

Suh et al. have suggested that pars infiltration gives an accurate prediction of successful outcome following pars repair (32). In their small series, pain relief, level of function, and likelihood of return to work were higher in patients preoperatively selected by Lidocaine infiltration of the pars defect. Wu et al. followed this protocol, identifying 93 cases with a positive response to pars infiltration (symptom reproduction and symptom relief) from a cohort of 275 patients with spondylolysis (43). The 93 patients identified underwent direct repair, with 91.3% obtaining good or excellent clinical results and 87% achieving a solid fusion.

Psychologic Profile of the Patient

Successful outcome depends in part on motivation. In one study reporting on surgery in professional athletes, the mental health SF-36 scores were high *before* surgery. These particular patients had much higher mental health SF-36 scores than did a group of patients with chronic discogenic low back pain. This factor may have contributed to the successful outcome reported in the series (16,30). It is well documented in the literature that patients with psychologic distress or those involved in personal litigation tend to do poorly after all types of spinal surgery.

Choice of Technique for Direct Repair

Biomechanical testing of pars repair has shown the Buck screw technique and the Morscher hook-screw technique to be the stiffest and strongest methods. Scott's wiring technique results in the least stiffness and strength (23). While one may question the wiring of pars defects on biomechanical grounds, the clinical results reported in the literature do not show an obvious difference between the screw and the wiring techniques. It is fair to say, however, that there are no published randomized controlled trials comparing the clinical outcomes of these various techniques.

THE ROLE OF SPINAL FUSION

Most adult patients with spondylolysis considered for surgical treatment have had the time for adjacent degenerative disc disease to develop or they may have established spondylolisthesis. Therefore, some form of lumbosacral fusion is the most common operation performed in these cases. Once disc degeneration is noted on an MR image either at the level of the spondylolisthesis or in an adjacent level, it is important to ascertain whether this disc or discs are contributing to the symptom of pain. Lumbar discography can be extremely useful in this situation if one takes note of the disc morphology and the pain reproduction.

In one study, 46 patients were diagnosed with spondylolysis and mild isthmic spondylolisthesis; 28 of the 46 patients had no spondylolisthesis, 11 patients had an associated Grade 1 spondylolisthesis, and 7 had an associated Grade 2 spondylolisthesis (17). Based on an MRI, 26 patients of the 46 were diagnosed with *adjacent*-level disc degeneration. In addition to the direct repair, these patients underwent a facet joint fusion across the degenerate disc level(s). The authors found no significant difference in outcome between those patients with a normal disc in whom the spondylolysis was treated with a direct repair and in those patients with a degenerate disc(s) who had a direct repair of the spondylolysis and additionally underwent a facet joint fusion at the adjacent level.

There are other surgeons who, given the presence of disc degeneration at the level of the spondylolysis, will carry out a direct repair of the spondylolysis in association with total disc replacement (Marnay T and Mayer M, personal communications). While this is an attractive concept to maintain motion in the intervertebral segment, the benefits of this combined procedure remain to be seen.

Regarding the various fusion techniques available, these include noninstrumented fusion, instrumented posterolateral fusion, anterior lumbar interbody fusion, posterolateral interbody fusion, and circumferential fusion. If spondylolysis is associated with spondylolisthesis, particularly in those *without* objective neurologic deficit, most surgeons who have published their work would suggest fusion in situ, whereas others may suggest reduction and fusion. One study compared anterior lumbar interbody fusion with instrumented posterolateral fusion for isthmic spondylolisthesis (Meyerding Grades 1 to 2) (18). No statistically significant difference was observed in clinical outcome between the two groups: satisfactory results were obtained in 85% of the anterior lumbar interbody fusion group and 90% of the instrumented posterolateral fusion group. In another study, patients with isthmic spondylolisthesis reported superior long-term outcomes following noninstrumented posterolateral fusion in comparison to instrumented posterolateral fusion (19).

REFERENCES

1. Wiltse LL, Widell EH, Jackson DW. Fatigue fracture: the basic lesion in isthmic spondylolisthesis. *J Bone Joint Surg Am* 1975;57:17–22.
2. Standaert CJ, Herring SA. Spondylolysis: a critical review. *Br J Sports Med* 2000;34: 415–422.
3. Pedersen AK, Hagen R. Spondylolysis and spondylolisthesis: treatment by internal fixation and bone-grafting of the defect. *J Bone Joint Surg Am* 1988;70:15–24.
4. Rossini F, Dragoni S. Lumbar spondylolysis: occurrence in competitive athletes: updated achievements in a series of 390 cases. *J Sports Med Phys Fitness* 1990;30:450–452.
5. Blanda J, Bethem D, Moats W, et al. Defects of pars interarticularis in athletes: a protocol for non-operative treatment. *J Spinal Disord* 1993;6:406–411.
6. Micheli LJ, Wood R. Back pain in young athletes: significant differences from adults in causes and patterns. *Arch Ped Adolesc Med* 1995;149:15–18.
7. Soler T, Calderon C. The prevalence of spondylolysis in the Spanish elite athlete. *Am J Sports Med* 2000;28: 57–62.
8. Buck JE. Direct repair of the defect in spondylolisthesis: preliminary report. *J Bone Joint Surg Br* 1970;52:432–437.
9. Nicol RO, Scott JHS. Lytic spondylolysis: repair by wiring. *Spine* 1986;11:1027–1030.
10. Morscher E, Gerber B, Fasel J. Surgical treatment of spondylolisthesis by bone grafting: direct stabilisation of spondylolysis by means of a hook screw. *Arch Orthop Trauma Surg* 1984;103:175–178.
11. Johnson JR, Kirwan EO. The long-term results of fusion-in-situ for severe spondylolisthesis. *J Bone Joint Surg Br* 1983;65:43–46.
12. Gillet P, Petit M. Direct repair of spondylolysis without spondylolisthesis, using a rod-screw construct and bone grafting of the pars defect. *Spine* 1999;24:1252–1256.
13. Songer MN, Rovin R. Repair of the pars interarticularis defect with a cable-screw construct: a preliminary report. *Spine* 1998;23:263–269.
14. Jeanneret B. Direct repair of spondylolysis. *Acta Orthop Scand* 1993;151:111–115.
15. Tokuhashi Y, Matsuzaki H. Repair of defects in spondylolysis by segmental pedicular screw hook fixation: a preliminary report. *Spine* 1996;21:2041–2045.
16. Debnath UK, Freeman BJC, Gregory P, et al. Clinical outcome and return to sport after surgical treatment of spondylolysis in young athletes. *J Bone Joint Surg Br* 2003:85: 244–249.
17. Dai LY, Jia LS, Yuan W, et al. Direct repair of defect in lumbar spondylolysis with mild isthmic spondylolisthesis by bone grafting with or without facet joint fusion. *Eur Spine J* 2001;10:78–83.
18. Kim NH, Lee JW. Anterior interbody fusion versus postero-lateral fusion with trans-pedicular fixation for isthmic spondylolisthesis in adults: a comparison of clinical results. *Spine* 1999;24:812–817.
19. Christensen FB, Hansen ES, Laursen N, et al. Long-term functional outcome of pedicle screw instrumentation as a support for postero-lateral spinal fusion. *Spine* 2002;27:1269–1277.
20. Mihara H, Onari K, Cheng BC. The biomechanical effects of spondylolysis and its treatment. *Spine* 2003;28:235–238.
21. Deguchi M, Rapoff AJ, Zdeblick TA. Biomechanical comparison of spondylolysis fixation techniques. *Spine* 1999;24:328–333.
22. Dreyzin V, Esses SI. A comparative analysis of spondylolysis repair. *Spine* 1994;19:1909–1914.
23. Kip PC, Esses SI, Doherty BI, et al. Biomechanical testing of pars defect repairs. *Spine* 1994;19:2692–2697.
24. Kimura M. My method of filling the lesion with spongy bone in spondylolysis and spondylolisthesis. *Orthop Surg* 1968;19:285–295.
25. Buck JE. Further thoughts on direct repair of the defect in spondylolysis. *J Bone Joint Surg Br* 1979;61:123.
26. Van der Werf GJ, Tonino AJ, Zeegers WS. Direct repair of lumbar spondylolysis. *Acta Orthop Scand* 1985;56:378–379.
27. Roca J, Moretta D, Fuster S, et al. Direct repair of spondylolysis. *Clin Orthop* 1989;246:86–91.
28. Bonnici AV, Koka SR, Richards DJ. Results of Buck screw fusion in Grade I spondylolisthesis. *J R Soc Med* 1991;84:270–273.
29. Fairbank JCT, Cooper J, Davies JB, et al. The Oswestry low back pain questionnaire. *Physiotherapy* 1980;66:271–273.
30. Grevitt M, Khazim R, Webb JK, et al. The short form 36 health survey questionnaire in spine surgery. *J Bone Joint Surg Br* 1997;79:48–52.
31. Jenkinson C, Coulter A, Wright L. Short form 36 (SF-36) health survey questionnaire: normative data of adults of working age. *BMJ* 1993;306:1437–1440.
32. Suh PB, Esses SI, Kostuik JP. Repair of pars interarticularis defect: the prognostic value of pars infiltration. *Spine* 1991;16(8 suppl):445–448.

33. Hardcastle PH. Repair of spondylolysis in young fast bowlers. *J Bone Joint Surg Br* 1993;75:398–402.
34. Tonino A, Van der Werf G. Direct repair of lumbar spondylolysis: 10-year follow-up of 12 previously reported cases. *Acta Orthop Scand* 1994;65:91–93.
35. Bradford DS, Iza J. Repair of the defect in spondylolysis or minimal degrees of spondylolisthesis by segmental wire fixation and bone grafting. *Spine* 1985;10:673–679.
36. Scott JHS. The Edinburgh repair of isthmic spondylolysis. *J Bone Joint Surg Br* 1987;69;491.
37. Johnson GV, Thompson AG. The Scott wiring technique for direct repair of lumbar spondylolysis. *J Bone Joint Surg Br* 1992;74:426–430.
38. Askar Z, Wardlaw D, Koti M. Scott wiring for direct repair of lumbar spondylolysis. *Spine* 2003;28:354–357.
39. Albassir A, Samson I, Hendrick L. Treatment of painful spondylolysis by the Morscher hook-screw. *Acta Orthop Belg* 1990;56:489–495.
40. Hefti F, Seelig W, Morscher E. Repair of lumbar spondylolysis with a hook-screw. *Int Orthop* 1992;16:81–85.
41. Sales de Gauzy J, Vadier F, Cahuzac JP. Repair of lumbar spondylolysis using Morscher material: 14 children followed for 1-5 years. *Acta Orthop Scand* 2000;292–296.
42. Ivanic GM, Pink TP, Achatz W, et al. Direct stabilisation of lumbar spondylolysis with a hook-screw. Mean 11-year follow-up period for 113 patients. *Spine* 2003;28:255–259.
43. Wu SS, Lee CH, Chen PQ. Operative repair of symptomatic spondylolysis following a positive response to diagnostic pars injection. *J Spinal Disord* 1999;12:10–16.

Subject Index

Note: Page references for figures are followed by an f and page references for tables are followed by a t.

R

S

T

V

W

Z